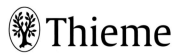

Interventional Breast Imaging

Ultrasound, Mammography, and MR Guidance Techniques

Uwe Fischer, MD
Professor
Women's Health Care Center
Göttingen, Germany

Friedemann Baum, MD
Women's Health Care Center
Göttingen, Germany

With contributions by
Friedemann Baum, Werner Boecker, Thomas Decker,
Uwe Fischer, Thorsten Kuehn, Susanne Luftner-Nagel

1295 illustrations

Thieme
Stuttgart New York

Library of Congress Cataloging-in-Publication Data is available from the publisher.

This book is an authorized and revised translation of the German edition published and copyrighted 2008 by Georg Thieme Verlag, Stuttgart, Germany. Title of the German edition: Diagnostische Interventionen der Mamma.

Portions of this work were translated by Ursula Vielkind, PhD, CTran, Dundas, Canada

Illustrator: Andrea Schnitzler, Innsbruck, Austria

© 2010 Georg Thieme Verlag,
Rüdigerstrasse 14, 70469 Stuttgart, Germany
http://www.thieme.de
Thieme New York, 333 Seventh Avenue,
New York, NY 10001, USA
http://www.thieme.com

Cover design: Thieme Publishing Group
Typesetting by Druckerei Sommer, Feuchtwangen
Printed in China by Everbest Printing Co. Ldt, Hong Kong

ISBN 978-3-13-146701-0   1 2 3 4 5 6

Contributors

Friedemann Baum, MD
Women's Health Care Center
Göttingen, Germany

Werner Boecker, MD
Professor
Gerhard-Domagk-Institute of Pathology
Münster, Germany

Thomas Decker, MD
Breast Screening Reference Pathology
Dpt. of Pathology
Dietrich-Bonhoeffer-Clinic
Neubrandenburg/Germany

Uwe Fischer, MD
Professor
Women's Health Care Center
Göttingen, Germany

Thorsten Kuehn, MD
Professor
Esslingen Hospital
Department of Gynecology and Obstetrics
Esslingen, Germany

Susanne Luftner-Nagel, MD
Women's Health Care Center
Göttingen, Germany

Preface

Imaging of the breast is primarily based on x-ray mammography, breast ultrasound, and MR mammography. Today, the full-field digital technique is well-established for the performance of x-ray mammography. Besides requiring less radiation exposure than conventional mammography, it offers additional advantages in the examination of young women and women with dense breast tissue by providing the opportunity to utilize a wide variety of postprocessing options. One of these options, the CAD System, has proven itself to be especially helpful in the detection of microcalcifications. Innovative aspects of modern breast ultrasound include the additional use of color duplex, 3D and 4D techniques. The third major examination method, MR mammography, has experienced a dramatic increase in its diagnostic significance. With the development of high-resolution MRI, MR mammography now possesses the highest sensitivity for the detection of both invasive and intraductal breast carcinomas.

Because of improved diagnostic imaging, the detection rate of small, nonpalpable carcinomas has increased. The current goal of early detection programs is the detection of breast cancer as an intraductal tumor, or as an invasive tumor under 1 cm in diameter. Patients with breast cancer detected at such an early stage generally have an excellent prognosis when treated appropriately.

With the increasing detection of early and/or small breast cancers, there is a growing necessity for image-guided diagnostic work-up of suspicious breast lesions. To obtain an accurate tissue diagnosis before definitive therapy is initiated, the primary tissue sampling of suspicious findings should be performed by percutaneous biopsy, and not by open surgery. Core needle biopsy of large palpable tumors may be performed under clinical guidance. However, tissue sampling of clinically occult findings should be performed using ultrasound, mammography, or MRI-guided core needle or vacuum-assisted needle biopsy. This procedural approach is in accordance with the course of action recommended for BI-RADS 4 and 5 findings in the recently revised European S3 guidelines for the early detection of breast cancer. By obtaining a definitive pathologic diagnosis before therapy, the number of unnecessary excisions for benign lesions has been substantially reduced. In addition, a pretherapeutic diagnostic work-up that confirms a breast carcinoma allows precise patient information and the appropriate planning of the surgical procedure, including the optimal strategy for lymphadenectomy.

Over the last several years, specialized and effective equipment has become available for the performance of percutaneous biopsies. Compatible biopsy equipment is available for use with all the different examination modalities. Large core biopsies (14 gauge to 19 gauge) and vacuum-assisted needle biopsies (8 gauge to 11 gauge) are currently the preferred biopsy methods. Fine-needle aspiration biopsies are presently reserved for a very few indications. In addition to biopsy equipment, there are a multitude of localization markers for the localization of lesions or target volumes before surgical excision. The spectrum of materials available includes localization wires in various configurations, clips and coils, and gel-markers visible on ultrasound.

Strategic approaches in breast diagnostics have also changed greatly in the last decades. In the 1970s, mammography and ultrasound were the predominant methods used in the diagnostic work-up of clinical findings. The fine-needle aspiration biopsy complemented these as part of what is referred to as the "triple test." With the development and improvement of technical and procedural options, it has become increasingly feasible to diagnose clinically occult carcinomas and reduce the development of late-stage disease (secondary prevention). It is conceivable that further diagnostic developments will increasingly allow the detection of breast cancer precursors. In this context, minimally invasive interventional methods would gain a greater importance (primary prevention).

This book deals solely with the presently established interventional methods used in breast diagnostics. Our goal is to give a complete compilation of the indications and procedural approaches for each particular method at the current, state-of-the-art level. The book is enriched by the addition of tips and tricks, as well as common sources of error.

The heart of this book is concerned with ultrasound-, x-ray-, and MRI-guided interventional techniques for the percutaneous acquisition of tissue samples and the pretherapeutic localization of lesions. The corresponding Chapters 4, 5, and 6 begin with a synopsis of the most important characteristic features of each diagnostic method (ultrasound, mammography, MR mammography). Relevant diagnostic evaluation criteria and lesion classification are particularly addressed. This creates the common basis of standardized terminology and assessment categories required for understanding the following discussions pertaining to the interventional techniques. The chapters continue with explicit information on the application of each intervention method and include typical practical examples. A pertinent statement from the European S3 guidelines and a description of the course of action in special casuistic examples supplement each section. The chapters include a checklist intended to facilitate the preparation and performance of breast interventions. These central chapters are supplemented by statements and information pertaining to practice guidelines (Chapter 1) and patient preparation before performing an intervention (Chapter 2).

Chapter 7 is a generously illustrated overview of the materials and equipment currently available for the performance of breast interventions. The special features of several exemplary systems are presented in detail. Chapters 8 and 9 describe the preparation of core biopsy specimens for histopathologic examination and specimen imaging to confirm correct sampling, respectively. Chapter 10 deals with the performance of galactography, a rarely indicated examination technique. It also includes a statement on up-to-date, direct visualization techniques of the ductal system, e.g., ductoscopy.

Recognizing patients with early breast cancer who do not need to undergo a full axillary lymph node dissection is one of the most important innovative advances in breast cancer therapy. For node-negative patients whose lymph node dissection has been limited to the sentinel node(s), therapy has been adjusted to the stage of disease and the risk of complications such as arm lymphedema has been avoided. Chapter 11 describes the indications, performance, and limitations of the sentinel node biopsy technique.

The second essential section of this book deals with the currently valid pathology reporting categories, i.e. the B-classification system for core and vacuum biopsy specimens. Chapter 13 describes the individual pathologic B-categories and the resulting consequences for an appropriate course of action. The reader of this chapter will quickly realize that patient management requires an interdisciplinary approach to correlate specific radiologic findings with pathology, and decide on further recommendations and/or treatment. This chapter is supplemented with informative images and clear, comprehensive tables and graphs. Chapter 12 deals with the essential aspects of fine-needle aspiration and cytologic assessment.

The last chapter is an assortment of instructive case studies. The reader is encouraged to analyze the ultrasonographic, mammographic, and MR-mammographic images of these histopathologically verified findings. This compilation of cases is a representative sample of predominantly small, occult lesions that would typically be assessed primarily by percutaneous intervention.

At this point, we would like to thank the many colleagues, friends, and family members for their contributions to the completion and success of this book. Special mention is due to Prof. Hans Werner Böcker and Prof. Thomas Decker, who spontane- ously agreed to co-author this book and write the chapters pertaining to the cytologic assessment of fine-needle aspiration biopsies and the pathologic assessment of percutaneously obtained specimens. Both men are indisputably two of the most experienced pathologists in the area of breast pathology. Prof. Thorsten Kühn is equally experienced in the area of axillary lymph node dissection and a pioneer of the sentinel node biopsy philosophy. His competent, informative chapter on this subject is a valuable asset to this book. We thank Dr. Susanne Luftner-Nagel for sharing her practical experience in the chapter on ultrasound-guided biopsies.

Support was also received from the medical industry by making interventional equipment and material available for testing and photo-documentation. Here we make special mention of Ms. Karin Samorra and Ms. Peggy Haas from GE Health Care, Mr. Heinz Gerhards from the Medicor Co., Mr. Hubert Noras from the Noras Co., Mr. Norbert F. Heske Sr. and Mr. Thomas Heske Jr. from the BIP Co., and Mr. Dominic Ansbergen from Ethicon.

Not to be forgotten, we thank Georg Thieme Verlag, Stuttgart, Germany for the competent and very pleasant support we received while preparing this book for print. Here we make special mention of Ms. Susanne Huiss, Ms. Martina Dörsam, and Ms. Gabriele Kuhn-Giovannini.

Finally, our deep-felt thanks go to all the members of our practice staff for their unfailing and constructive support of this project: our colleague Dr. Dorit von Heyden, and our staff members Anja El Hajab, Doris Hermes, Anke Küchemann, Ali Leicht, Gudrun Meyer, Jutta Rüschoff, and Christina Vujevic.

Uwe Fischer
Friedemann Baum

Table of Contents

Abbreviations

ACR	American College of Radiology
ADH	atypical ductal hyperplasia
AEPDT	atypical epithelial proliferation ductal type
ALH	atypical lobular hyperplasia
ALN	axillary lymph node
ALND	axillary lymph node dissection
ASCO	American Society of Clinical Oncology
B1–B5	breast needle biopsy classification system: 1 to 5
BCIRG	Breast Cancer International Research Group
BI-RADS	Breast Imaging Reporting and Data System (classification system according to ACR)
BW	body weight
C1–C5	cytology classification of malignancy system
CC	craniocaudal (view)
CGH	comparative genomic hybridization
CLIS	lobular carcinoma in situ
CNB	core needle biopsy
CT	computed tomography
CUP	cancer of unknown primary
DC	ductal carcinoma
DCIS	ductal carcinoma in situ
DEGUM	German Society for Ultrasound in Medicine
DGS	German Senology Association
DH	ductal hyperplasia
EBM	evidence-based medicine
EIC	extensive intraductal component
ER	estrogen receptor
FNA	fine needle aspiration
FNAB	fine needle aspiration biopsy
FNAC	fine needle aspiration cytology
FNR	False-negative rate
FOV	field of view
FPR	false-positive rate
G	good (PGMI)
G1–G4	pathologic grading categories 1 to 4
GE	gradient echo
HER2	human epidermal growth factor receptor 2
HF	high frequency
Hr	harmonic retrieval
HUT	ductal hyperplasia of usual type
I	inadequate (PGMI)
IBUS	International Breast Ultrasound School
ICDO	International Classification of Diseases for Oncology
IDC	invasive ductal carcinoma
ILC	invasive lobular carcinoma
INR	international normalized ratio
IR	inversion recovery
ITC	isolated tumor cells
IV	intravenous
LCIS	lobular carcinoma in situ
LM	lateromedial (view)
LN	lobular neoplasia
LOE	level of evidence
LOH	loss of heterozygosity
M	moderate (PGMI)
MIB	minimally invasive biopsy
MIP	maximum intensity projection
ML	mediolateral (view)
MLO	mediolateral oblique (view)
MR	magnetic resonance
MRI	magnetic resonance imaging
NCT	neoadjuvant chemotherapy
NSLN	nonsentinel lymph nodes
OCI	overall clinical image score
P	perfect (PGMI)
PET	positron emission tomography
PGMI	perfect, good, moderate, inadequate (quality assurance categorization for assessing mammograms)
pN	pathologic stage of lymph node
PPt	partial thromboplastin time
PPV	positive predictive value
pT	pathologic stage of primary tumor
pTis	histologically confirmed intraductal carcinoma in situ
SE	spin echo
SLN	sentinel lymph node
SLNB	sentinel lymph node biopsy
SLND	sentinel lymph node dissection
SM	smooth muscle
T	Tesla
TDLU	terminal ducal-lobular unit
TE	echo time
TE	tumorectomy
TGC	time gain compensation
TSE	turbo spin echo
UICC	International Union Against Cancer
US	ultrasound
VAB	vacuum-assisted biopsy
WHO	World Health Organisation

1 Patient Information, Guidelines, and Directives

U. Fischer

Patient Information

Patient information covering medical issues should put the patient in the position of being able to understand and evaluate the significance of an illness and its symptoms. It should encompass the benefits, risks, and side effects of medical procedures, but also warn against ineffective, unnecessary, and detrimental procedures. Like professional medical guidelines, comprehensive and objective patient medical information should be based upon the best available, up-to-date scientific research (evidence-based medicine [EBM]). The following is a small selection of the websites offering patient information:

www.cancer.net: American Society of Clinical Oncology
www.asbd.org: American Society of Breast Disease
www.lbbc.org: Living Beyond Breast Cancer
www.cancer.gov: National Cancer Institute
www.komen.org: Susan G. Komen for the Cure
www.nci.nih.gov: National Cancer Institute
www.cancer.org: American Cancer Society
www.nccn.org: National Comprehensive Cancer Network
http://breastcancer.about.com
www.healthcommunities.com

Guidelines

Medical guidelines, also called clinical practice guidelines or practice guidelines, are systematically developed decision-making aids for physicians, aimed to improve the quality of medical care by providing an up-to-date, scientific evidence-based statement on the knowledge and standards of the medical profession. As guidelines, they are designed to assist practitioners by providing an appropriate "decision and action corridor" for specific health problems, from which one can, and sometimes must, deviate when special circumstances justify an alternate approach. The implementation of guidelines lies within the responsible physician's margin of discretion for each specific medical case.

An evidence- and consensus-based guideline is a multidisciplinary expert group policy statement on the recommended approach to specific medical situations. Such a consensus is reached in a structured, defined, and transparent procedure, and is based on a thorough, systematic review and analysis of scientific research data, and on evidence derived from clinical experience and practice. As an example, S guidelines have been created by the German Association of Scientific Medical Societies (AWMF). The consensus process is undertaken in three developmental steps, S1 to S3.

- S1: Advisory statement created by an expert panel in an informal consensus.
- S2: Advisory statement created by an expert panel in a formal consensus process and/or on the basis of a formal systematic investigation and analysis of scientific evidence.
- S3: Advisory statement issued by an interdisciplinary expert panel after a structured process of consensus-building and explicitly including scientific evidence and all elements of systematic development: logic-, decision-, and outcome analysis.

Evidence-based medicine. EBM is the conscientious, explicit, and judicious use of the best scientific data currently available in making decisions concerning the medical care of individual patients. The practice of EBM requires integrating individual clinical expertise with the best available external clinical evidence and scientific data from systematic research. The categorization of research trials and publications according to EBM-criteria allows an evaluation of the strength of their scientific evidence. The levels of EBM are

- Level I: There is sufficient evidence of efficacy from the systematic meta-analysis of numerous properly designed randomized controlled trials.
- Level II: There is evidence of efficacy from at least one properly designed randomized controlled trial.
- Level III: There is evidence of efficacy from methodically well-designed trials without randomization.
- Level IVa: There is evidence of efficacy from clinical accounts.
- Level IVb: Represents the opinion of respected authorities, is based on clinical experience or on reports from expert committees.

Directives

A directive is an official instruction or guideline, which has a binding character, but is not of statutory nature. They are issued by institutions legitimized by the government, professional associations, or private sector organizations and are binding within the jurisdiction of the issuing institution. Nonobservance of a directive can have defined punitive consequences.

American College of Radiology (www.acr.org). The American College of Radiology (ACR) currently has approximately 30 000 members in the fields of diagnostic radiology, radiation oncology, medical physics, interventional radiology, and nuclear medicine. Besides providing a national accreditation program for mammography, the ACR publishes and updates the *Breast Imaging Reporting and Data System (BI-RADS) Atlas*, an innovative step in the standardization of terminology, categorization of findings, and reporting in mammography, breast ultrasound (US), and MR mammography.

European Guidelines for Quality Assurance of Mammography Screening. Leading politicians of the 12 countries belonging to the European Union resolved in 1985 to create a mutual project to reduce cancer mortality in Europe. Ultimately, the first edition of the *European Guidelines for Quality Assurance in Mammography Screening* resulted from this effort in 1993. This achievement, which is currently in the 4th edition (2006), was and is the essential basis for early detection programs in various European countries.

German National S3 guidelines for the Early Detection of Breast Cancer. In a concerted effort, 23 medical-technical societies, physicians associations, and nonmedical associations (e.g., self-help groups, womens' initiatives) have developed evidence-based guidelines for the early detection of breast cancer in Germany, called the S3 guidelines. These are primarily based on the statements in the European Guidelines. The aspired goal is a direct positive impact on the course of disease for women with breast cancer (early detection, diagnosis, therapy, and follow-up), as well as an optimization of the operational and organizational medical care structures. Especially noteworthy for their work in developing the S3 guidelines are the German Senology Association, the German Cancer Aid Society (Deutsche Krebshilfe e.V.), the German Cancer Society (Deutsche Krebsgesellschaft e.V.), and the World Society for Breast Health. The current version of the S3 guidelines was published in 2008.

German Radiology Association (www.drg.de). The German Radiology Association (Deutsche Röntgengesellschaft [DRG]) was established in Berlin in 1905 and is one of the oldest and most distinguished medical societies. It dedicates itself to promoting all branches of radiology, including basic science research, general diagnostic radiology, modern slice imaging techniques (computed tomography [CT], magnetic resonance imaging [MRI], US), and relevant special techniques such as duplex sonography. The German Radiology Association issues recommendations and guidelines pertaining to breast imaging diagnostics through its Breast Diagnostics Working Committee.

Throughout Europe, there are other specialized societies which deal with the diagnosis and treatment of breast cancer, hold conferences, provide advanced training, and develop quality assurance recommendations and guidelines. Here we make mention of the European Society of Mastology (EUSOMA) and the European Society of Breast Imaging (EUSOBI).

2 Patient Preparation

F. Baum

Medical history. Before performing a core needle or vacuum biopsy, it is important to exclude contraindications, most of which concern blood clotting. Most patients with a history of thromboembolisms (e.g., atrial fibrillation) are treated with coumarin derivatives. Patients with a history of arteriovenous occlusive disease, however, are usually taking acetylsalicylic acid (aspirin), but are occasionally treated with heparin. These patients are generally aware of their medications' effect on their coagulation status. This is also true for patients with an inherited coagulopathy such as clotting factor deficiencies (rare in women), platelet, and capillary disorders.

Patients who have taken an aspirin to alleviate pain or cold symptoms, however, are often not aware of the association with an increased bleeding risk. For this reason, patients must be asked if they have taken any of these medications or are aware of having a bleeding disorder before performing a minimally invasive biopsy. Occasionally, a patient undergoing anticoagulant therapy will require extensive preparation before a biopsy can be performed. It is not necessary, however, to do blood coagulation tests on patients with no known coagulation disorders or history of taking anticoagulant medication.

Anticoagulant medication. *Aspirin* intake should be stopped 10 days before performing an intervention to assure good thrombocyte aggregation. It is recommended that *heparin* treatment be discontinued at least 6 hours prior to biopsy. This, however, like the discontinuation of coumarin therapy, should be decided in collaboration with the patient's primary physician.

Temporary discontinuation of *coumarin* therapy (vitamin-K antagonist) should always be left in the hands of an experienced specialist. Heparin therapy should begin when the international normalized ratio (INR) falls below 2.5. The partial thromboplastin time (PTT) should then be raised to 60–80 seconds. A biopsy can be performed when the INR has fallen to 1.5.

Intravenous *heparin* therapy should be discontinued approx. 6 hours prior to biopsy. The PTT should then have fallen under 40 seconds by the time of biopsy. Heparin therapy can be reinitiated 6 hours after completion of the intervention. Continuation of vitamin-K antagonist medication should begin no earlier than 24 hours after completion of the intervention.

Endocarditis prophylaxis. Before performing any minimally invasive intervention, antibiotic prophylaxis is indicated in all patients with damaged heart valves or an artificial heart valve. In case of a penicillin allergy, ciprofloxacin is a good alternative.

Allergies. Before performing an intervention, a patient should be asked if there are any known allergies. In case of an *adhesive tape allergy*, the corresponding allergen should be avoided (**Fig. 2.1**). In special cases, the small stab incision may be sutured rather than using butterfly stitches (Steri-Strips; 3M, St. Paul, MN). Specific inquiry should be made about allergies against *local anesthetics*. In addition, *metal and collagen allergies* should be excluded before marker clips, coils, or localization wires are placed (**Fig. 2.2**). Before performing a magnetic resonance imaging (MRI) scan, *any contrast medium allergies* and *contraindications* (kidney function) should be taken into account.

Disinfection. As standard procedure, interventions should be performed under semisterile conditions. Due to the special circumstances of the intervention situation (ultrasound [US] gel, stereotactic holding system), it is not necessary to use sterile drapes. Care should be taken, however, to disinfect the skin with ethanol spray before local anesthesia is given and a stab incision is performed.

2

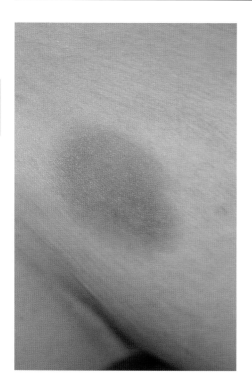

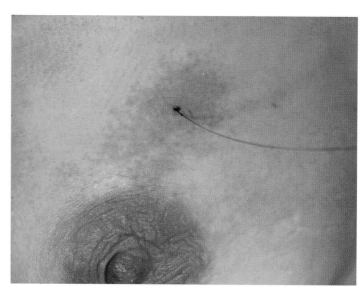

Fig. 2.1 Adhesive tape allergy.

Fig. 2.2 Nickel allergy after placement of localization wire.

3 Free-hand Localization Techniques

F. Baum

Open biopsy or excision of palpable lesions can be performed without the aid of preoperative localization as the surgeon can locate the lesion by palpation. In the absence of a palpable abnormality, however, preoperative localization is required to assure selective excision. This procedure is performed under ultrasound (US), mammographic (i.e., stereotactic), or magnetic resonance imaging (MRI) guidance.

Most mammographic findings requiring preoperative localization are clusters of microcalcifications. These can be localized by means of free-hand localization or stereotactic localization. The basic requirement for planning the localization of a mammographic finding is imaging of the breast in two orthogonal views (craniocaudal [CC] and lateromedial [LM]).

Wire Localization

Wire Localization (Berger Method)

Coordinate system. When applying the Berger method for freehand localization of a clinically occult lesion, the x- and z-axes of a coordinate system are drawn on the surface of the breast, the center of which (origin) is located at the nipple. By definition, the x-axis runs in the mediolateral (ML) direction, the z-axis in the CC direction of the body.

In a second step, one transfers the x- and z-axes and the lesion position from the mammographic images onto a coordinate system. To do this, the x- and z-axes are drawn onto a sketch of the breast. The ML image is placed with the thoracic wall edge parallel to the z-axis and the nipple on the x-axis. Now, a line parallel to the x-axis is drawn through the lesion to be localized

(**Fig. 3.1a**). The procedure is repeated using the CC image, placing the thoracic wall edge parallel to the x-axis and the nipple on the z-axis. Note that if placing the image above the coordinate system, the image must be reversed to have the medial and lateral film sides correspond to the correct side of the breast and coordinate system. Now a line parallel to the z-axis is drawn through the lesion onto the coordinate system (**Fig. 3.1a**). The intersection of the lines running through the lesion in both images reflects the position of the lesion in the breast. The distances from the nipple can be determined from coordinates on the x- and z-axes and the position of the lesion drawn onto the breast (**Fig. 3.1b**).

The breast must be held firmly to ensure accurate insertion of the localization needle. This can be done in either the CC or the ML position by having an assistant simulate mammographic compression with flat hands (**Fig. 3.2a, 3.2b**). Especially for the less-experienced physician, it is advisable to draw the calculated position of the lesion onto the breast because this can shift depending on the direction of compression. The depth of the lesion (y-axis = ventrodorsal direction) can be determined from the skin lesion distance in the CC and ML views.

Needle and wire placement. Before performing a preoperative localization, it is advisable to confer with the attending surgeon. If possible, the *approach* chosen for skin puncture should take the surgeon's preference into account. With experience, the free-hand technique allows a flexible approach (e.g., periareolar or axillary skin puncture, see below). The need for *local anesthesia* is dependent on the speed of skin puncture. If performed quickly, anesthesia is usually unnecessary because its administration is equally painful.

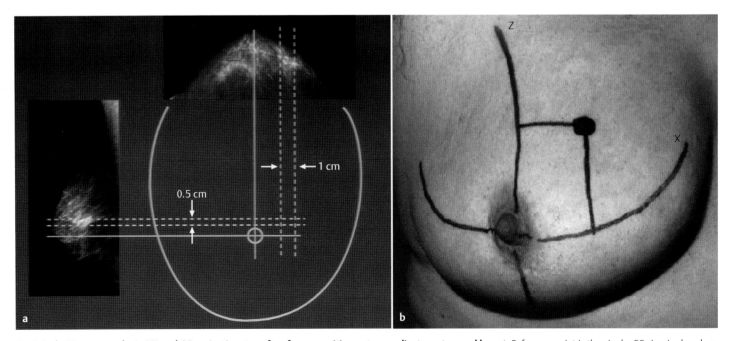

Fig. 3.1a, b Mammography in ML and CC projection, transfer of mass position onto coordinate system and breast. Reference point is the nipple. CC view is placed on reverse side to conform to coordinate drawing. Projection of mass position onto coordinate system (**a**). Transfer of coordinates onto the breast (**b**).

When choosing an approach other than directly over the lesion and perpendicular to the thoracic wall, the oblique distance between the skin puncture site and the lesion must be calculated because this is the depth to which the needle must be inserted (**Fig. 3.2c**).

Before advancing the hook wire, mammography should be performed in the CC and ML projections to document the correct position or reveal the need for correction (**Fig. 3.3e, 3.3f**). The objective is to puncture through the target lesion. The localization wire is advanced once the needle is in the correct position. The needle can be removed after mammographic reconfirmation (**Fig. 3.3g, 3.3h**). Small lesions may be encircled by the J-wire end. A preoperative localization may be considered successful if the localization wire lies within 1 cm of the lesion. In the follow-up and outcome monitoring, this should be attained in at least 90 % of cases. When using a repositionable J-wire, it is possible to bring the wire closer to the lesion by turning the needle/wire localizer so that the wire advances toward the lesion. Finally, postlocalization mammograms in two orthogonal views are performed (**Fig. 3.3i, 3.3j**). These mammograms are made available to the attending surgeon for his or her orientation.

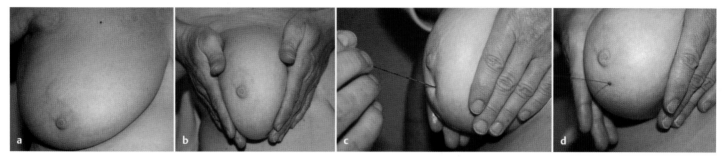

Fig. 3.2a–d Breast fixation during free-hand localization. Breast without fixation (**a**). Fixation of breast in mediolateral projection by laying hands flat onto both sides of the breast (**b**). Puncture of skin in periareolar position (**c**). Localization wire in place after removal of localization needle (**d**).

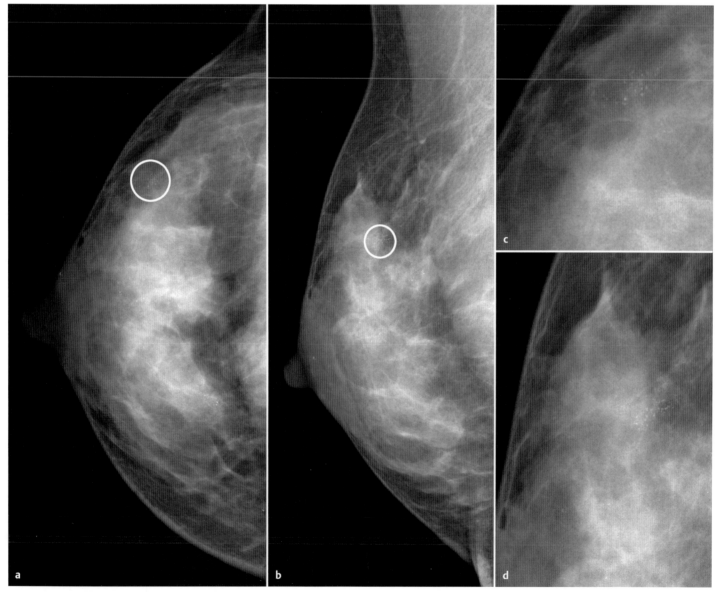

Fig. 3.3a–d Wire localization. Right mammogram in CC and ML projection (**a, b**). Close-up view of a pleomorphic cluster of microcalcifications in the upper outer quadrant (**c, d**). **e–h** See p. 7.

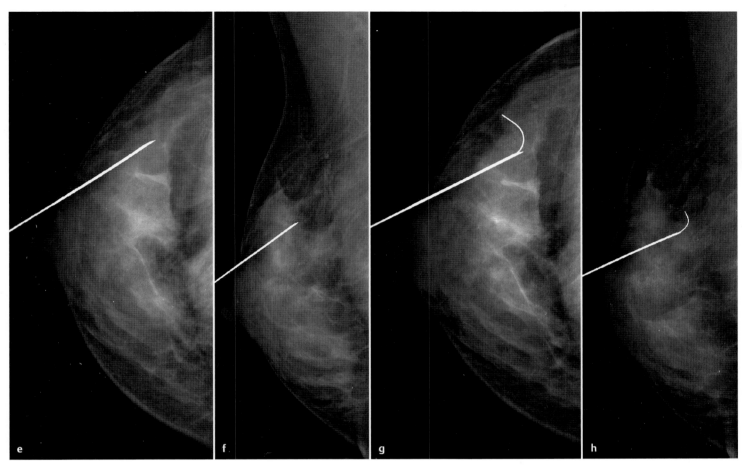

Fig. 3.3e–h Localization needle in place (CC and ML projection, **e, f**). Introduction of wire into breast tissue (**g, h**). **i–n** See p. 8.

3

3

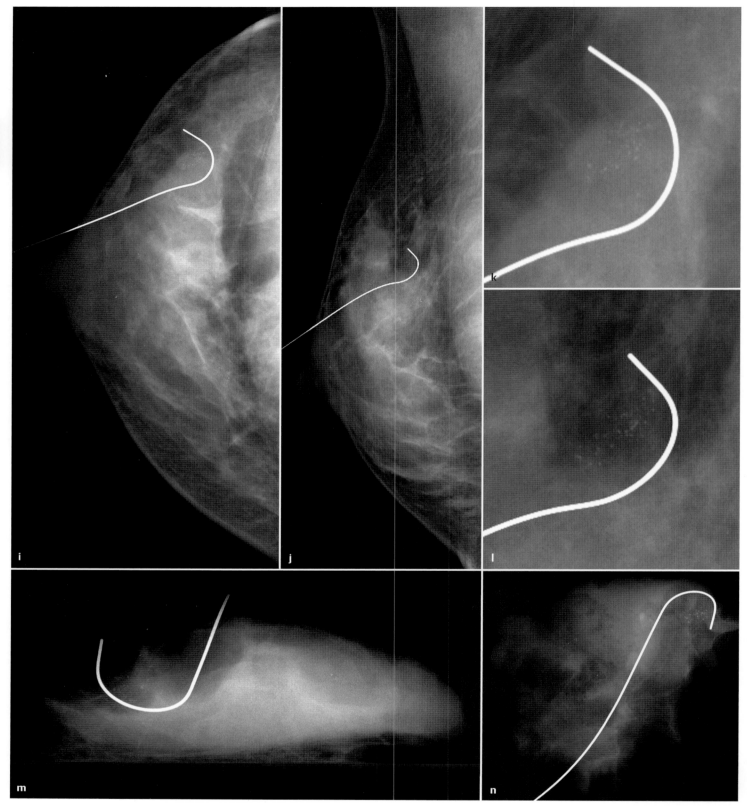

Fig. 3.3i–n Postlocalization mammogram after needle removal showing correct wire position (**i, j**). Close-up views: J-wire encircles microcalcification cluster (**k, l**). Specimen radiograph confirms complete excision (**m, n**). *Histology:* invasive lobular carcinoma (ILC).

Direct Free-hand Wire Localization

An experienced physician can perform a preoperative localization using the direct free-hand technique. In principle, it is very much like the localization of a lesion using the Berger method. Calculations are performed in a similar way based upon two orthogonal mammographic views (CC and LM). The lesion position is projected directly onto the breast, however, skipping the above-described step of projecting the lesion position onto a sketched breast with the coordinate system. Again, the distance between the skin puncture site and the lesion must be calculated because this is the depth to which the needle must be inserted (**Fig. 3.4**). Mammographic needle documentation, wire advancement, and final documentation of wire localization are as described above.

Tips and Tricks

- The performance of free-hand localization is simplest when choosing an approach that is as parallel and perpendicular to the coordinate axes as possible.
- In case of segmentally distributed or multifocal findings, it is advisable to localize the affected segment boundaries (**Fig. 3.5**).
- Large in situ carcinomas (>4 cm) are usually an indication for primary mastectomy. Preoperative needle biopsy of two or more sites can usually help determine whether this is the case.

3

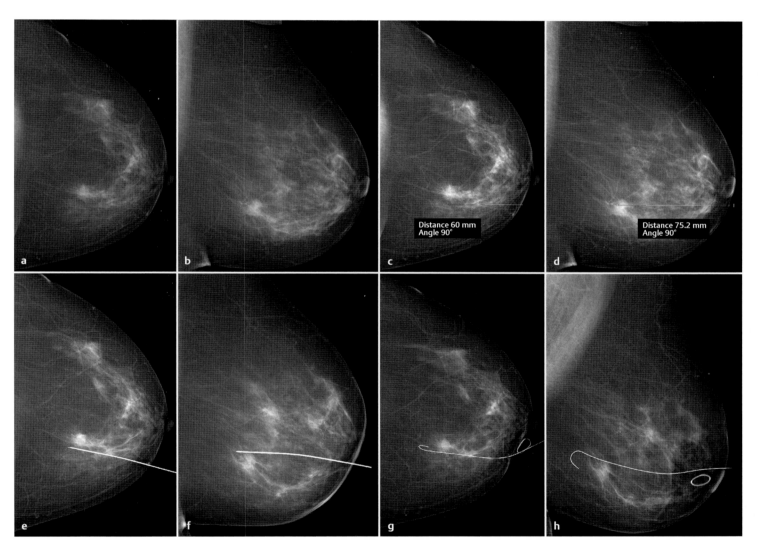

Fig. 3.4a–h Free-hand localization. Mammography in CC and LM projection showing suspicious mass in left lower inner quadrant (**a, b**). Measurement of lesion depth for periareolar needle insertion and perpendicular needle guidance (**c**). Note: The skin puncture site does not necessarily correspond to the mammographic skin borders (**d**). Correct needle position in CC and ML projection (**e, f**). Final documentation after removal of needle (**g, h**). The radiopaque gauze pad projects onto the skin puncture site (**h**).

3

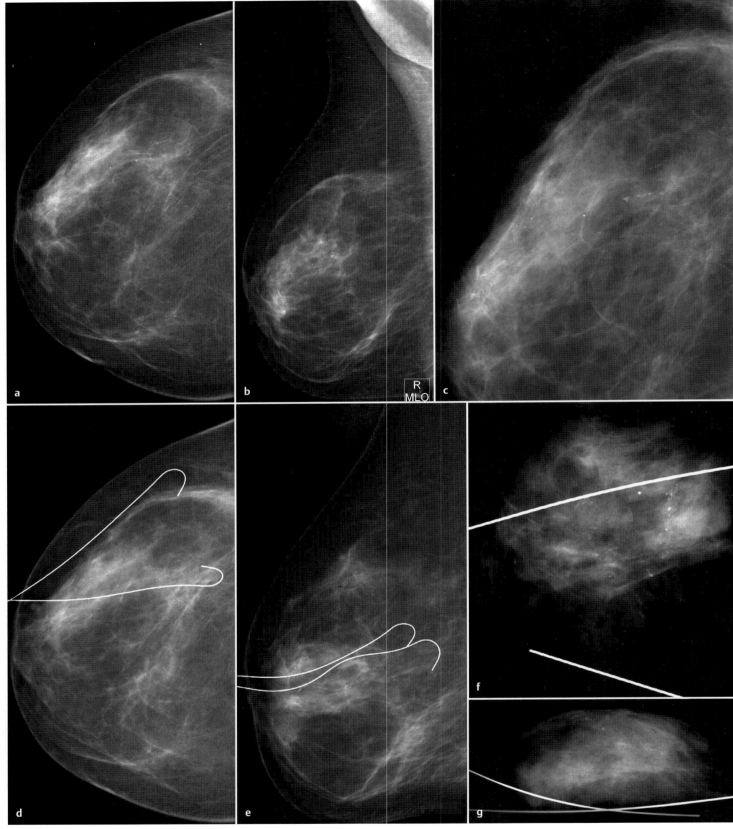

Fig. 3.5a–g Wire localization of segmental lesion. Mammography in CC and LM projection showing segmentally distributed, pleomorphic microcalcifications in the lateral aspect of the right breast (**a, b**). Magnification view in CC projection (**c**). Mammography in CC and LM projection showing localization wires along the medial and lateral borders of the segmental microcalcifications (**d, e**). Specimen radiograph in two orthogonal views. Microcalcifications are seen near excision borders (**f, g**).

Hook Wires

Various hook wires are available for preoperative localizations (**Fig. 3.6**). The wire tips have a single or double hook configuration. Which wire to choose depends on the breast consistency and the location of the lesion. In fatty tissue, the use of a double hook wire is usually favored because it provides better grip. If the lesion lies within an area of the breast with denser or more fibrous tissue, a single hook wire will have sufficient grip and will not dislocate.

Repositionable wires allow correction of the wire position even after having been advanced through the needle. Other wires cannot be pulled back into the needle once advanced.

Differences in wire properties affect the ease in handling. Some wires, for example, can easily be advanced through the needle. Others tend to bend or kink so that there is greater resistance during advancement, sometimes making it impossible to set the tip free. Wires with screw-type tips are no longer used for performing preoperative localizations.

3

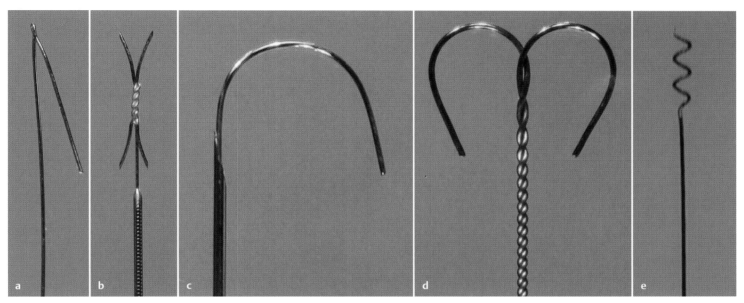

Fig. 3.6a–e Wire configurations. Nonrepositionable wires with a single hook (**a**) and a double hook (**b**). Repositionable wires with a single hook (**c**) and a double hook (**d**). Obsolete screw-type tip (**e**).

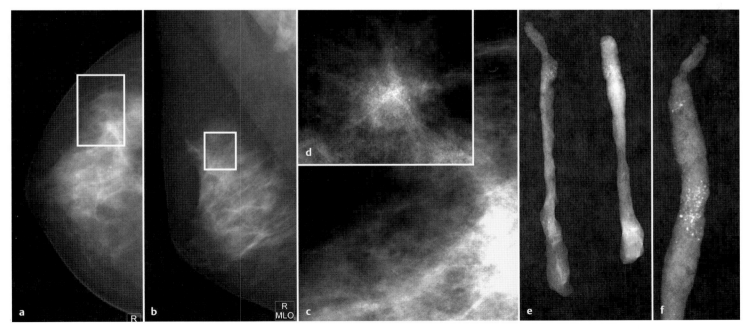

Fig. 3.7a–f Wire localization requiring position corrections. Mammography in CC and mediolateral oblique (MLO) projection showing clustered, amorphous microcalcifications in the upper outer quadrant of the right breast (**a, b**). Close-up views (**c, d**). Specimen radiograph after vacuum biopsy (**e, f**). **g–m** See p. 12.

3

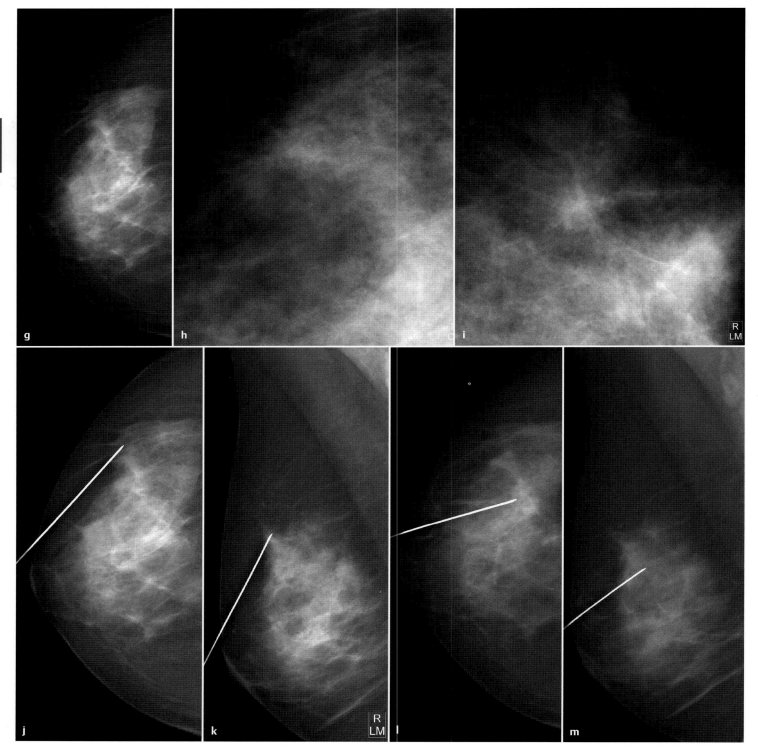

Fig. 3.7g–m Histology: atypical ductal hyperplasia (ADH). Mammography in CC projection (**g**) and magnification views in CC and LM projections show remaining microcalcifications (**h, i**). Incorrect needle position after free-hand preoperative localization (**j, k**). Correct needle position after repositioning (**l, m**). **n–u** See p. 13.

Tips and Tricks

Free-hand localization does not always result in optimal needle positioning. Correction requires calculation and spatial envisioning of which changes must be made to attain an optimal position. In most cases, the needle must be retracted to just under the skin before pushing it forward again in the new direction (**Fig. 3.7j–m**).

When using a repositionable wire, it is still possible to retract the wire back into the needle and perform a correction after the wire has been advanced. This can only be done, however, as long as the needle has not been removed from the breast. When using a J-wire, it is possible to bring the wire closer to the lesion by turning the needle with the retracted wire so that the wire advances toward the lesion when set free (**Fig. 3.7o, p**).

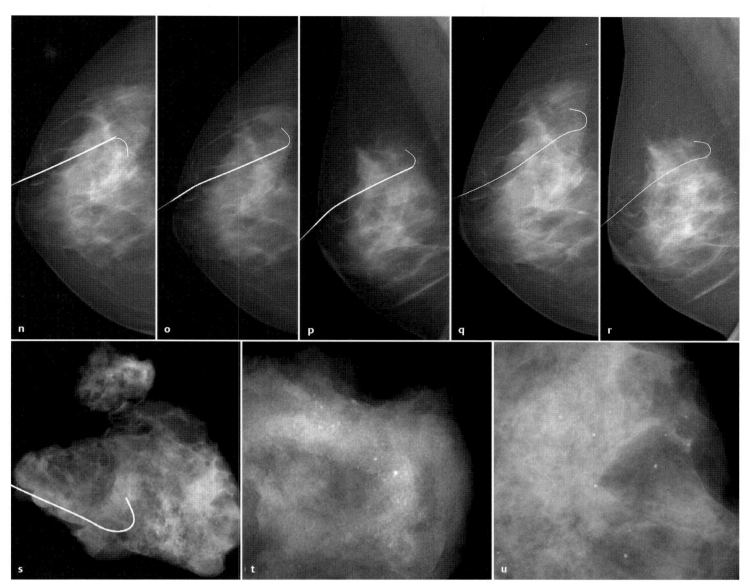

Fig. 3.7n–u Hook released in direction opposite from microcalcifications after wire advancement (**n**). Mammography in CC and LM projection after repositioning of wire (**o, p**). Final documentation after removal of needle (**q, r**). Specimen radiograph shows further microcalcifications (**s–u**). *Histology:* ADH.

3

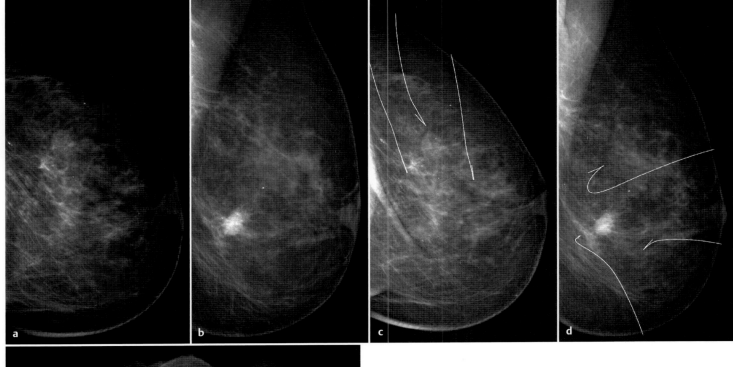

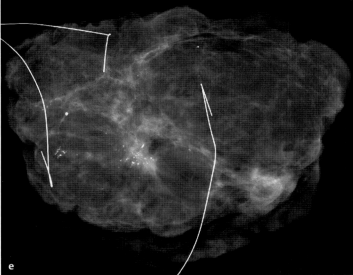

Fig. 3.8a–e Wire localization of target volume. Lesion with associated microcalcifications. Mammography in CC and LM projection showing mass with regionally distributed, pleomorphic microcalcifications in the lateral aspect of the left breast (**a, b**). Mammography in CC and LM projection after localization of target volume borders (**c, d**). Specimen radiograph (**e**). *Histology:* invasive ductal carcinoma (IDC) with extensive intraductal component.

Problems and Solutions

Free-hand localization of a lesion in a soft, deformable breast is often very difficult. In such cases it is advisable to calculate the lesion position, then transfer and draw the coordinates onto the breast using the Berger method or directly. To draw the x- and z-coordinates onto the breast, the breast should be compressed in each respective projection (**Fig. 3.2b**). In this way, lesion displacement due to compression is accounted for and it is possible to retain a good orientation.

Localization of regionally distributed findings sometimes requires placement of several localization wires at the borders of the target volume (**Fig. 3.8**). It is advisable to confer with the attending surgeon when planning the procedure.

Occasionally, large hematomas may develop after performance of a percutaneous biopsy. This can lead to a substantial displacement of breast findings. If the attending surgeon wishes, the dorsal border of such a hematoma can be localized with a second wire after localizing the suspicious lesion (**Fig. 3.9**).

3

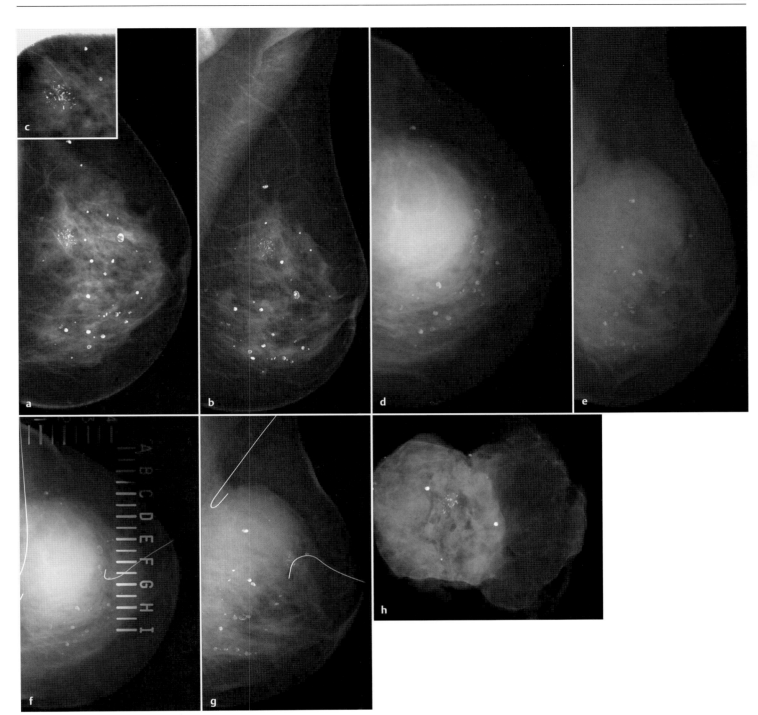

Fig. 3.9a–h Wire localization with hematoma. Mammography in CC and MLO projection showing clustered, amorphous microcalcifications in the central aspect of the left breast (**a, b**). Magnification view in CC projection (**c**). Mammography in CC and LM projection showing large hematoma after US-guided large core needle biopsy (CNB) (histology: IDC) (**d, e**). Wire localization of the microcalcification cluster at the ventral aspect of the hematoma and of the dorsal border of the hematoma (**f, g**). Specimen radiograph (**h**). *Histology:* IDC.

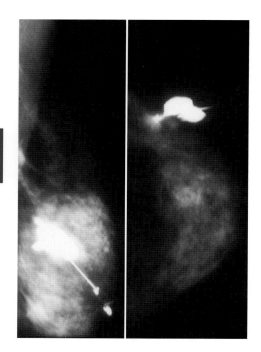

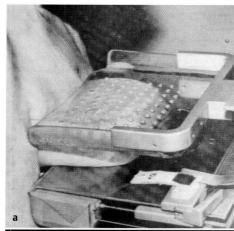

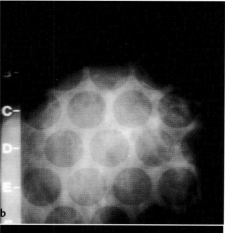

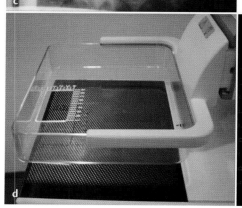

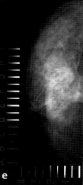

Fig. 3.10 Dye localization. Mammography in CC and LM projection: dye injection (coal and radiocontrast medium suspension) after needle localization. Low-quality older mammograms document this obsolete localization method.

Fig. 3.11a–e Localization using fenestrated compression device or coordinate system. Fenestrated compression device (**a**). Scout film showing lesion (**b**). Insertion of needle through hole nearest lesion (**c**). Images **a–c** from 1978. Localization using coordinate system (**d, e**). Localization compression device with large window and coordinate markings (**d**). Mammography in CC projection and coordinate markings (**e**).

Dye Localization

In the past, localizations were performed using dyes instead of localization wires, clips, and coils. After mammographic needle localization, a dye such as methylene blue or a coal suspension was injected into or near the lesion to mark it (**Fig. 3.10**). The surgeon then had to dissect his or her way to the nonpalpable finding until the visible dye marking confirmed locating the correct position. Because lesions can be more easily located intraoperatively after wire localization, this method has completely eliminated the use of dyes for this purpose.

Fenestrated Compression Devices

Before the development of stereotactic localization equipment, preoperative localization was performed either free-hand or using a fenestrated compression device. The fenestrated compression paddle has regularly spaced openings through which a localization needle can be inserted (**Fig. 3.11**). After taking the scout film, usually in CC projection, the appropriate opening can be determined and the needle inserted perpendicularly to the skin. A check film should be taken before removing compression. The needle should pass through the lesion, as it may retract slightly when compression is removed. After recording the correct needle position, compression is lifted and the breast compressed at a right angle to the original film (LM projection). The second check film shows whether the needle must be withdrawn or inserted further to the correct depth, again well into or slightly past the lesion. The wire can then be introduced after verification of the correct position. Final mammographic documentation in two orthogonal views is performed for verification of the final wire position.

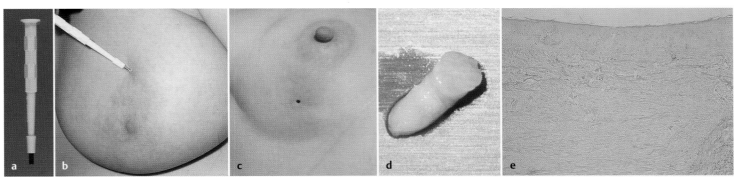

Fig. 3.12a–e Skin punch biopsy. Equipment: round-shaped cutting knife attached to handle (**a**). Knife edge is pushed completely through skin layers after local anesthesia (**b**). Skin defect (**c**). Tissue cylinder (**d**). *Histology* of **c:** erythema migrans (Lyme disease) (**e**).

Skin Punch Biopsy

A skin biopsy is sometimes necessary in the diagnostic work-up of breast skin abnormalities. A punch biopsy can be easily performed using a round-shaped cutting knife attached to a plastic handle. After local anesthesia of the skin, the metal cutting cylinder is pushed perpendicularly, using a turning/twisting motion, deep into the skin and subcutaneous tissues. The acquired tissue cylinder is approx. 3 mm in diameter and 6 mm in length (**Fig. 3.12**).

Tips and Tricks

To retrieve the tissue cylinder easily, it is helpful to angle the cutting cylinder before removal. If the tissue cylinder remains attached in the breast, it can be grasped with sterile tweezers and cut at the base with a scalpel.

4 Ultrasound-guided Interventions

S. Luftner-Nagel

Breast Ultrasound

Significance of Breast Ultrasound

After mammography, ultrasound (US) is the second most important diagnostic breast imaging tool. Aside from its use in distinguishing between cystic and solid lesions, the device-related technical advances of the last years have afforded breast US an excellent capacity for differentiating between benign and malignant solid findings. Modern equipment technology and standardized examination technique make breast US an excellent diagnostic tool. In the hands of an experienced examiner, it has a sensitivity of 57–90% and a specificity of 60–90%.

Indications

Dense parenchyma. Breast US is an important adjunct to mammography in the early detection of breast cancer. This is especially true when breast tissue composition is dense (American College of Radiology [ACR] density types III–IV) where the mammographic detection of noncalcifying breast cancer is limited. Many workgroups also favor the employment of breast US for women with scattered fibroglandular densities (ACR density type II). Studies have shown that an additional 3–4 per 1000 clinically and mammographically occult breast cancers can be detected through the adjunctive use of breast US in women with dense breast tissue. Importantly, these additionally detected tumors do not differ in size or stage from the mammographically detected, clinically occult breast cancers. Hence, experienced ultrasonographers can detect most focal masses with a diameter greater than 5–10 mm.

Ambiguous palpable findings. Breast US is obligatory in the diagnostic work-up of ambiguous areas of palpable thickenings or lumps, with or without correlating findings on mammography or magnetic resonance (MR) mammography. In addition, it is a helpful adjunctive tool in the evaluation of clinically occult, mammographic, or MR mammographic findings.

In women under 35 years of age, breast US is the diagnostic examination of first choice for working up ambiguous clinical findings. With this approach it is often possible to clearly assess a clinically conspicuous finding as harmless (e.g., bland cyst) and avoid unnecessary diagnostic imaging. If US reveals an ambiguous correlating finding, further work-up including mammography is mandatory.

Core needle biopsy. US-guided minimally invasive biopsy of ambiguous findings is an accurate, rapid, safe, and cost-efficient method for harvesting representative tissue. For these reasons, US-guidance is preferred over other biopsy guidance techniques in the diagnostic and preoperative setting. A retrospective US examination should always be performed when an ambiguous focal mass is detected on mammography or MR mammography, and is also recommended even when the primary examination has shown no conspicuous findings ("second-look" US). Detection of a correlating lesion is often facilitated in awareness of lesion size, configuration, and position, and can then be subjected to a US-guided large core needle biopsy (CNB).

Technique and Methodology

Breast examination. Breast US is a real-time examination of breast sections. The patient is examined in the supine position with her arms raised and hands placed under her head or neck. The examination of a patient with large breasts can be facilitated by elevating the side to be examined (e.g., by placing pillows under the ipsilateral shoulder/back) to achieve a more even distribution of breast tissue on the chest wall. The transducer is best held at its base and moved primarily by wrist motions. A gel-like solution is applied to the skin to promote US wave transmission through the skin. Care should be taken that contact between the transducer and the breast is uniform and perpendicular to the surface. The weight of the transducer and hand is usually sufficient pressure to ensure good US wave transmission. As a rule, exerted pressure should be as light as possible, but as heavy as necessary to obtain good images. A systematic examination of the breast can be achieved by moving the transducer in the mediolateral direction with overlapping sagittal scan planes. Especially in the examination of large breasts, it is often helpful to image the lateral aspects in transversal planes. Radial imaging is particularly good for the assessment of ductal structures. Because US is a dynamic examination, it is possible to assess and document the spatial dimensions of a finding by rotating the scan plane. This is important to differentiate a true, 3D lesion from a pseudolesion seen in only one plane. By varying/increasing compression exerted with the transducer, US wave transmission through breast tissue is improved and the elasticity of a lesion can be assessed.

Axillary examination. The US examination of the axilla should be performed routinely in follow-up patients after breast cancer and in patients with a suspicious breast finding. The detection of suspicious axillary lymph nodes is usually a contraindication for the performance of a sentinel lymph node biopsy in patients with breast cancer. In such cases, a conventional axillary dissection is indicated.

Quality Assurance Guidelines

Requirements. The ACR has defined technical standards for the diagnostic and performance monitoring of imaging equipment in its ACR Practice Guidelines and Technical Standards (http://www.acr.org/SecondaryMainMenuCategories/quality_safety/guidelines/toc.aspx).

The following are the minimal technical device specifications for the performance of breast US as published by the German Association of Statutory Health Insurance Physicians, last revised on April 1, 2009.

Quality Assurance Guidelines: Minimal Technical Device Specifications

- **Operating mode requirement:** B-mode
- **Scan format:** linear array
- **Transducer frequency:** ≥7.0 MHz
- **Transmit focal setting:** electronically variable focal zone for optimal lateral resolution
- **Transceiver aperture:** variable with chosen focal zone
- **Reception amplification:** variable time gain compensation (TGC)
- **Dynamic range:** at least 60 dB
- **Field of view:** width ≥3–8 cm, penetration depth ≥6 cm
- **Echo acquisition:** ≥15 images/second
- **Image documentation:** image documentation on a digital or analogous medium in accordance with archiving requirements. The following data must be included: B-mode image with distance scale, measured values, measuring marks, transducer frequency or frequency range, focal zone position, patient identification, date of examination, transducer designation, and study center. The inclusion of a pictograph showing transducer position and orientation is recommended.
- **Bit depth:** ≥8 bit
- **Technical image quality (organ/body area):** imaging of the breast
- **Technical image quality (characteristic image features):** differentiation between
  - internal structures of the breast, including vascular and ductal structures
  - solid and cystic structures

The enormous technical advances made in the last years have recently been factored in the required device specifications described above. Transducers are available with higher frequencies and good penetration depths. Besides the frequency, signal processing is also an important factor in determining image quality. A special focusing technique employed by modern US equipment, for example, makes images with exceptionally high quality possible.

The German Society for Ultrasound in Medicine (DEGUM) has taken great effort in developing a state-of-the-art statement on technical device specifications and in improving US training guidelines. One of its workgroups has compiled the following list of criteria to promote better technical quality assurance, taking the advances of modern US equipment into account (**Table 4.1**).

International guidelines. The 4th edition of the *European Guidelines for Quality Assurance in Breast Cancer Screening and Diagnosis* includes for the first time a chapter pertaining to multidisciplinary aspects of quality assurance in breast diagnostics. Relating to ultrasonography of the breast, it requires that the examiner be highly experienced and especially trained in breast US, and that the transducer frequency be at least 7.5 MHz, but optimally at 10 MHz or higher.

The International Breast Ultrasound School (IBUS: http://www.ibus.org) and the American College of Radiology (ACR: http://www.acr.org) have also issued up-to-date international guidelines.

Table 4.1 Minimal and recommended (in parentheses) device specifications for the performance of breast US*

Image quality in the clinical situation
128 gray levels per pixel
Good differentiation of breast tissue components
Depiction of structural irregularities in breast tissue
Depiction of tumor border irregularities
Distinct depiction of cysts ≥4 mm (elevated standard ≥2 mm)
Distinct depiction of tumors ≥10 mm (elevated standard ≥5 mm)
Penetration depth of at least 4 cm with good spatial resolution
Depiction of a 20-gauge needle in breast parenchyma along the image plane

Technical requirements
Documentation: digital or hardcopy (multiformat film, video printer, Polaroid)
Transducer frequency >5 MHz or multifrequency transducer (must fulfill quality assurance standards on phantom tests)
Scan rate >12 images/second
Field of view >3.8 cm
Incorporated acoustic stand-off if near field resolution is not sufficient
Monitor display: patient I.D., date, transducer, caliper, body marker (or indication of localization, e.g., as text), capacity, time gain compensation (TGC), preset, depth scale
Safety standards meeting US safety regulations
Free-hand biopsy or using a biopsy guide with virtual monitor visualization of needle pathway (5-mm lesion must be accessible at every depth)

* As per the German Society for Ultrasound in Medicine (DEGUM)

Terminology and Diagnostic Criteria in Breast Ultrasound

In analogy to the well-established ACR Breast Imaging Reporting and Data System (BI-RADS) categorization of mammographic findings, an ACR International Expert Working Group has developed a categorization system for US criteria of breast findings (BI-RADS-US). The resulting US lexicon has provided a consistent and universally understood terminology that serves as the basis for a standardized characterization of sonographic breast lesions, and thereby minimizes intra- and interobserver variability. The DEGUM's Breast Ultrasonography Working Group has modified and expanded the ACR BI-RADS-US lexicon to reflect the group's own experience (see **Table 4.4**).

DEGUM Ultrasound BI-RADS features. The following features are included in the BI-RADS-analogous DEGUM criteria for ultrasonographic findings in the breast:
- **Parenchymal density** (parenchyma volume/total breast volume): classified into four density types (**Table 4.2**)
- **Structural composition of breast tissue:** homogeneous, inhomogeneous (**Table 4.3**)
- **Lesion description:** shape, orientation, margin, lesion boundary, echo pattern, posterior acoustic features, calcifications, compressibility, mobility, surrounding tissue alterations (**Table 4.4**)

Table 4.2 Breast density*

Type I	Fibroglandular tissue <25%	Fatty breast
Type II	Fibroglandular tissue 25–50%	Partial involution
Type III	Fibroglandular tissue 50–75%	Dense breast tissue
Type IV	Fibroglandular tissue >75%	Extremely dense breast tissue

* A statement regarding breast tissue density should include a description of the tissue structure, i. e., architecture (e. g., inhomogeneous breast tissue with reduced sensitivity for the detection of small breast cancers).

Table 4.3 Göttingen ultrasound-sensitivity model: four-category system for evaluating the sensitivity of breast US*

Category	Background echotexture	Sensitivity
1	Homogeneous, equivalent to parenchyma	Very good
2	Homogeneous, mixed fat/parenchyma equivalent	Good
3	Homogeneous, fat equivalent	Limited
4	Inhomogeneous	Very limited

* Modified categorization of breast US sensitivity according to echogenicity patterns.

Table 4.4 Evaluation criteria for breast lesions*

Criteria	Low level of suspicion	Higher level of suspicion
Shape	Round, macrolobulated	Irregular
Orientation	Parallel to the skin	Perpendicular to the skin
Margin	Circumscribed	Indistinct, angular, microlobulated, spiculated
Lesion boundary	Abrupt interface	Echogenic halo without sharp demarcation
Echogenicity, echo pattern	Anechoic, hyperechoic	Hypoechoic (relative to fat)
Internal structure	Homogeneous	Inhomogeneous
Posterior acoustic features	Enhancement	Shadowing
Posterior shadowing at borders	Bilateral	
Calcifications	Macrocalcifications	
Surrounding tissue alterations	Compression due to displacement	Architectural distortion, retraction
Compressibility	Good	Little or none
Mobility	Good	Little or none
3D pattern	Compression pattern	Retraction pattern
Vascularity	None	Present in or immediately adjacent to lesion
Lymph nodes	Possessing high central echogenicity (hilus)	Hypoechoic, sometimes indistinct or angulated margins
Ductal pattern	Regular	Solid internal structures, abrupt caliber changes or stoppage

Note: * The dynamic criteria compressibility and mobility cannot be evaluated in the static image. These must be assessed during the performance of the US examination. 3D data can only be acquired using special equipment and are, like vascularization data, not mandatory.

Tips and Tricks

Similar to the succinct description of the overall breast composition in the mammography report, the breast US report should also include a statement indicating the relative possibility that a lesion could be missed due to breast composition. It is important to communicate this information to the primary clinician, alerting him or her to the fact that the sensitivity of the examination in detecting small cancers is limited in certain women. With this goal in mind, it seems of little value to use the categories described in **Table 4.2**, which classify a breast according to the relative volume of parenchyma. Instead, the degree of homogeneity or heterogeneity of breast tissue has a greater influence on the sensitivity and specificity of the breast US examination. This information should be included in the examination report (**Table 4.3**).

The standard feature descriptors used to characterize US findings are listed in **Table 4.4** and illustrated in **Fig. 4.1**.

In addition to the ACR BI-RADS-US features, the DEGUM has introduced the criteria compressibility, mobility, and 3D pattern, as well as a description of ductal structures and lymph nodes. The vascular criteria were expanded to include a quantification of vascular structures and a description of the vascular pattern.

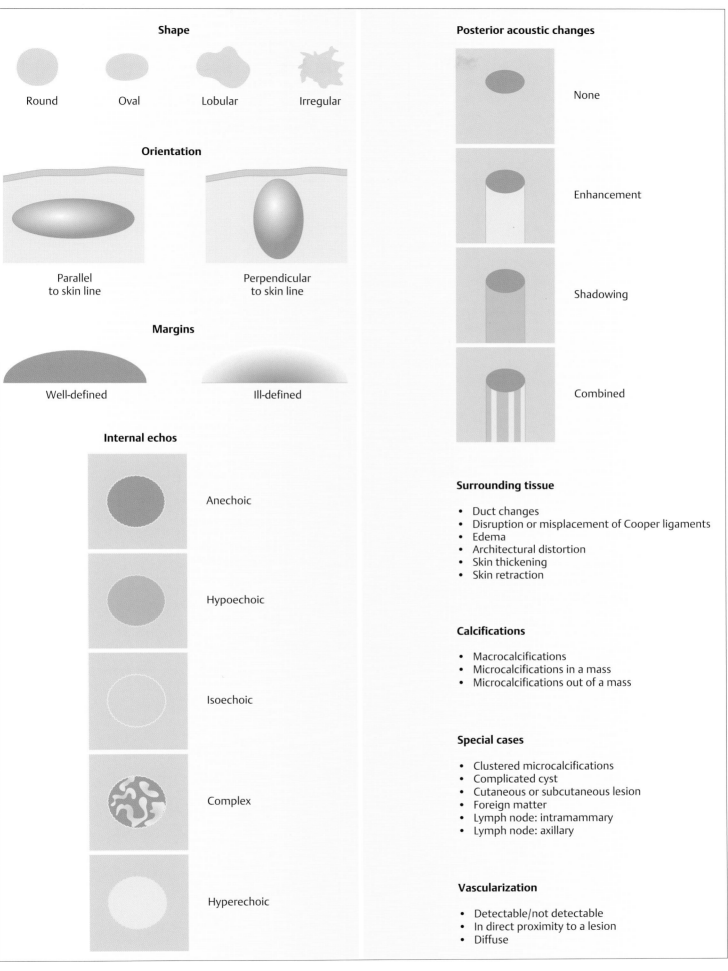

Shape

Round   Oval   Lobular   Irregular

Orientation

Parallel
to skin line

Perpendicular
to skin line

Margins

Well-defined   Ill-defined

Internal echos

Anechoic

Hypoechoic

Isoechoic

Complex

Hyperechoic

Posterior acoustic changes

None

Enhancement

Shadowing

Combined

4

Surrounding tissue

- Duct changes
- Disruption or misplacement of Cooper ligaments
- Edema
- Architectural distortion
- Skin thickening
- Skin retraction

Calcifications

- Macrocalcifications
- Microcalcifications in a mass
- Microcalcifications out of a mass

Special cases

- Clustered microcalcifications
- Complicated cyst
- Cutaneous or subcutaneous lesion
- Foreign matter
- Lymph node: intramammary
- Lymph node: axillary

Vascularization

- Detectable/not detectable
- In direct proximity to a lesion
- Diffuse

Fig. 4.1 Schematic illustration of sonographic lesion criteria.

DEGUM-US-BI-RADS categories. The DEGUM-US-BI-RADS categories encompass categories 0 to 5 in contrast to the ACR BI-RADS-US categories 0 to 6. The significance of category 0 has also been modified. Category 0 stipulates that an additional imaging evaluation is necessary before a final assessment can be made. It is not used, however, to indicate that a lesion has been identified that needs further work-up, but rather that the sensitivity of the examination is limited due to breast composition (e.g., inhomogeneous or fat-equivalent echotexture = Göttingen US-sensitivity category 3–4) or macromastia. Category 6, which is used in the ACR BI-RADS-US lexicon to signify a biopsy-proven malignancy, was not adopted for use by the DEGUM Breast Ultrasonography Working Group. Instead, because of the importance of categorizing breast US findings according to their sonographic features and keeping this information available for statistical analysis, category 6 is reported separately in the overall final assessment and does not replace the DEGUM-US-BI-RADS category. By retaining the DEGUM-US-BI-RADS categories 1–5, it is possible to correlate each categorized lesion with the final diagnosis (confirmed by stability over time or histopathology). This analysis is a prerequisite for the evaluation of the appropriateness and usefulness of the individual assessment criteria, as well as for the determination of the carcinoma prevalence in each assessment category, and is thus a quality assurance tool. The necessity and potential for improvements and adjustments of a BI-RADS evaluation and categorization system can only be realized based on such an analysis. In addition, outcome monitoring is necessary for the assessment of a physician's individual performance and the success of the early breast cancer diagnosis program.

When assigning a US-BI-RADS category to an US lesion, previous US examinations should be taken into account and, if relevant, indicated in the report (**Table 4.5**).

Ultrasound-guided Percutaneous Core Needle Biopsy

Indications

Percutaneous biopsy of the breast is performed to provide a definitive diagnosis of ambiguous imaging findings, and to verify a breast cancer diagnosis before treatment (e.g., surgery, neoadjuvant chemotherapy). If a suspicious breast lesion is found in the primary US examination, or if a correlating lesion is identified in the "second-look" US examination after having been primarily detected on mammography or MR mammography, then the percutaneous biopsy should be performed under US-guidance. As this method requires no additional complex equipment or patient preparation, it is the most simple, rapid, and cost-efficient method for harvesting representative tissue, and is preferred over the other alternative techniques. As a real-time examination, an US-guided biopsy can be directed exactly and followed on the monitor. Targeted tissue sampling is thus possible in the majority of cases, independent of lesion location. The high rate of representative tissue acquisition from US-guided biopsies has been proven in many studies.

Axilla. Performing a CNB in the axillary region is associated with a higher complication rate due to the topographic proximity to large vascular and neural structures. For this reason, it is often preferable to perform a fine-needle aspiration biopsy (FNAB) of suspicious axillary lymph nodes. Larger lesions, however, may be core biopsied without great risk. In some cases, it is advisable to adjust the throw to the shorter setting.

Table 4.5 Ultrasound Breast Imaging Reporting and Data System according to the German Society for Ultrasound in Medicine (DEGUM) adapted from US BI-RADS

Category	Assessment	Examples	Carcinoma-risk	Consequence
0	Final assessment not possible	Macromastia, extreme fibrocystic changes with inhomogeneous attenuation	Not known	Additional evaluation
1	Negative	No lesion, architectural distortion, or skin thickening found	0%	Routine follow-up
2	Benign finding	Cyst, lymph node, breast implant, unchanged scar or fibroadenoma	0%	Routine follow-up
3	Probably benign finding	Solid, oval, parallel to skin, circumscribed, fibroadenoma-like mass, complicated cyst, grape-like conglomerate of microcysts	<2%	Short term follow-up*, optional CNB
4	Suspicious abnormality	Solid mass without typically benign features, or with one or more malignant features	4A: 2–30% 4B: 30–60% 4C: 60–90%	Pathologic evaluation (CNB)
5	Highly suggestive of malignancy	Solid mass with several features of malignancy	90–100%	Pathologic evaluation (CNB)
Overall BI-RADS 6	Pathologically verified breast cancer by CNB or VAB	Not applicable	100%	Initiation of appropriate definitive therapy

* Size increase or development of suspicious features at follow-up examination results in an upgrading of the BI-RADS category. Stability of solid lesion features and size results in downgrading the BI-RADS category.

Note: At the end of the diagnostic chain (clinical exam, mammography, US, MR mammography, percutaneous biopsy), the final diagnosis is stated in the medical report and given a BI-RADS category 1–6.

Objective

A clearly benign result after percutaneous core needle biopsy of ambiguous breast findings can obviate surgery, avoiding unnecessary breast scar formation and costs. The preoperative verification of a breast cancer diagnosis, on the other hand, allows appropriate patient information and detailed planning of the surgical intervention, including the possibility of performing a sentinel node biopsy. When neoadjuvant chemotherapy is planned, all relevant immunohistochemical analyses (e. g., receptor status, c-erbB2 gene status, etc.) can be performed on the obtained CNB specimens.

Materials

There are several devices available that are specialized for the performance of large core breast biopsies. These consist of a hand piece with a spring mechanism and a biopsy needle. The biopsy needle consists of an inner needle with a sampling chamber and an outer cannula with a cutting edge. Most systems provide a choice between two penetration depths. There are two major types of biopsy guns: semiautomatic and fully automatic.

After loading the spring mechanism of a *semi-automatic* gun (see **Figs. 7.10, 7.11, 7.12, 7.13, 7.14, 7.15, 7.16**), the inner stylet is manually advanced into the lesion or region of interest. The outer cutting cannula is rapidly advanced by pushing a trigger button, capturing the specimen tissue. The sample can then be retrieved from the notch.

In contrast, after loading a *fully automatic* biopsy gun (see **Figs. 7.17, 7.18, 7.19, 7.20, 7.21, 7.22**), the biopsy needle is positioned before the lesion. During fire, the stylet rapidly penetrates target tissue and is followed by split-second automatic fire of the outer cannula, cutting and capturing the specimen in a one-step operation. Fully automatic biopsy guns are available as complete sterile disposable systems and as reusable systems (handgun) fitted with sterile needles.

Normally, multiple core specimens are obtained to retrieve sufficient tissue material for pathologic assessment and definitive diagnosis. To avoid having to puncture the skin and cause additional breast trauma for every tissue sample, a *coaxial introduction needle* (see **Figs. 7.30, 7.31, 7.32, 7.33, 7.34, 7.35**) is placed to establish a tract through which the biopsy needle is guided to the breast lesion. After US-guided insertion and positioning in the breast, the stylet is removed and the biopsy needle is inserted into the coaxial needle cannula until it abuts. After confirmation of correct needle positioning, it can then be fired into the lesion to take a tissue sample. Fine adjustments of the needle position are made before each additional firing, permitting tissue sampling from different areas within the lesion.

Procedure

The reflective and refractive properties of US must be taken into account when performing an US-guided biopsy. Structures that are perpendicular to the angle of ultrasonic pulse incidence are optimally visualized. US-guided CNB should encompass the following steps:

- Verification of biopsy indication and receipt of informed consent.
- Preinterventional mammography (depending on patient age: bilateral two views / unilateral one view).
- Patient positioning:
  - lesion in *medial* aspect of breast: patient supine with raised ipsilateral arm.
  - lesion in *lateral* aspect of breast: patient supine or supine-oblique with raised ipsilateral arm. Elevating the ipsilateral side by placing towels or cushions under the shoulder/back is recommended. Further cushioning to support the raised arm provides for a comfortable, relaxed patient (**Fig. 4.2**).
- Examiner positioning:
  - lesion in *lateral* aspect of breast: Examiner should sit on the ipsilateral side of the patient. The US monitor can be viewed best if located on the contralateral side of the patient (**Fig. 4.3**).
  - lesion in *medial* aspect of breast: It is usually best if the examiner sits on the contralateral side of the patient to access the lesion more easily. The US monitor should stand on the opposite (ipsilateral) side so that the examiner can follow the intervention from a comfortable position (**Fig. 4.4**).
- Preinterventional *documentation* of the suspicious lesion in two orthogonal planes:
  - statement of lesion size: three dimensions.
  - statement of lesion localization: side, clock face, distance from the nipple.
- Determination of *biopsy direction*, taking the following factors into consideration:
  - transducer is held in the nondominant hand.
  - lesion is optimally visualized.

4

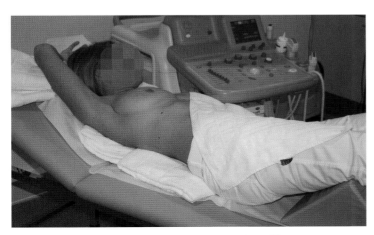

Fig. 4.2 Patient's position for US-guided biopsy of a lateral lesion.

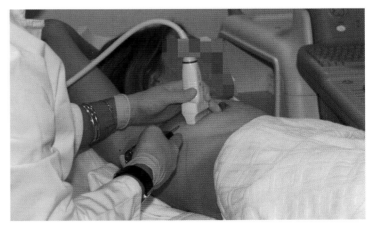

Fig. 4.3 Examiner's position for US-guided biopsy of a lateral lesion.

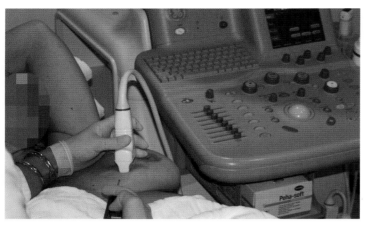

Fig. 4.4 Examiner's position for US-guided biopsy of a medial lesion.

- biopsy needle is guided as horizontally as possible, parallel to the chest wall and transducer (**Fig. 4.5a**), exactly under the middle of the transducer and in the image plane (**Fig. 4.5b**).
- because the breast is soft, it is usually possible to press the distal end of the transducer into the breast to achieve horizontal skin contact (**Fig. 4.5c**).

- Determination of *skin puncture localization*:
  - initially image the lesion 1–2 cm from the proximal end of the transducer.
  - puncture skin at least 1 cm from transducer end (**Fig. 4.6a**).
  - if lesion is deep, distance should be greater, especially if breast is firm and its surface curved (**Fig. 4.6b**). Occasionally, it is necessary to select a longer needle.
  - after skin puncture, the transducer is slid parallel to the needle and toward the puncture site (**Fig. 4.6c, d**) to visualize the needle in maximum length (**Fig. 4.6e, f**).

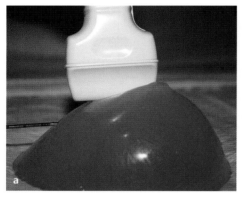
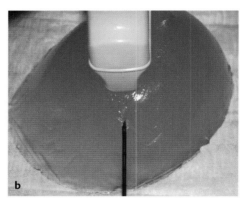
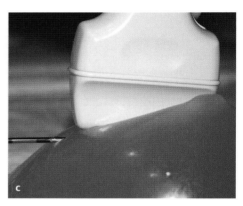

Fig. 4.5a–c Needle guidance for biopsy on US phantom. After the skin puncture, the lesion is visualized near the center of the monitor image. The biopsy needle is guided horizontally and parallel to the chest wall and the transducer (**a**). Be sure to keep the needle in the image plane (**b**). Horizontal transducer/skin coupling is achieved by lightly pressing the distal end of the transducer into the breast (**c**).

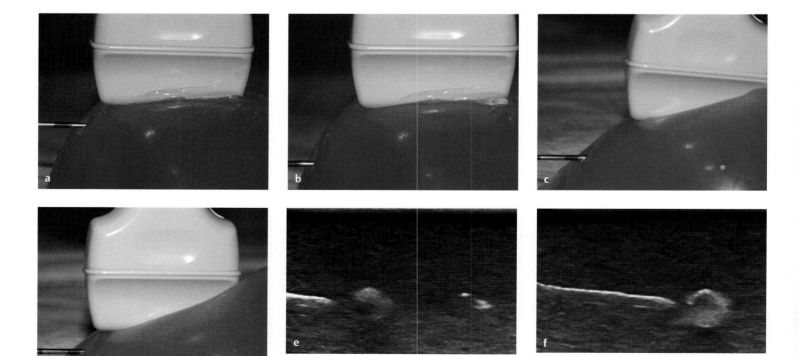

Fig. 4.6a–f Skin puncture positions for lesions at different depths. For a lesion near the breast surface, skin puncture is chosen approx. 1 cm from the proximal transducer end (**a**). For a deep lesion, skin puncture should be chosen further from the transducer (**b**) and is dependent upon breast firmness and surface curvature (**b, c**). To visualize the needle in full length, the transducer is slid toward the skin puncture site after inserting the needle (**c, d**). Corresponding monitor image before and after sliding the transducer toward the puncture site (**e, f**).

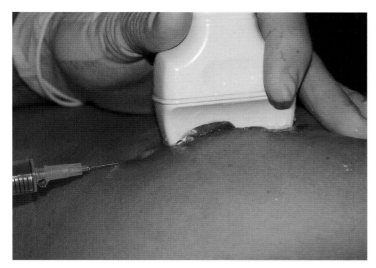

Fig. 4.7 Application of local anesthesia.

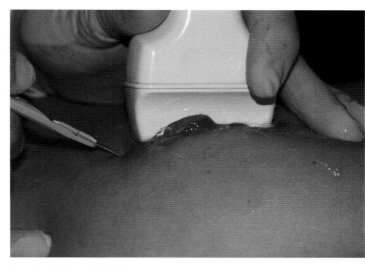

Fig. 4.8 A skin stab incision.

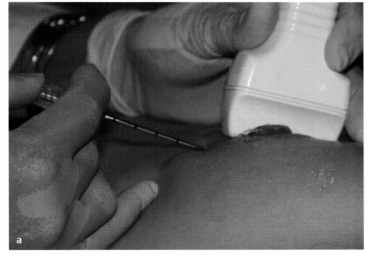

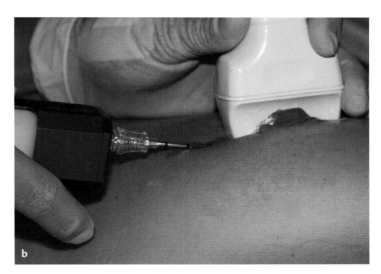

Fig. 4.9 Insertion of a coaxial introduction needle (a) and a biopsy needle (b).

- Skin and transducer disinfection before application of sterile gel and putting on gloves.
- Local anesthesia of the skin (wheal) (**Fig. 4.7**) and soft tissues under US-guidance toward lesion:
  - 1% local anesthetic.
  - *Note*: care must be taken not to obscure the visualization of small lesions when injecting local anesthesia in surrounding tissue.
- Skin incision (**Fig. 4.8**).
- Demonstrate the firing sound of the biopsy gun to the patient before beginning procedure (best outside patient's field of view).
- Introduce and position coaxial introduction needle before lesion under US-guidance (**Fig. 4.9a**):
  - lesion should be visualized near middle of monitor image.
  - needle direction must be kept parallel to the long axis of the transducer and visualized in full length.
- Remove stylet from coaxial needle and insert biopsy needle (**Fig. 4.9b**). Perform fine adjustment of needle position and prefire documentation (**Fig. 4.10a**).
- Warn patient before firing.
- Trigger biopsy (≥4 samples are recommended, long throw adjustment).

- Postfire documentation in two projections (one documentation per lesion, **Fig. 4.10b–d**).
- Remove needle and process sample (4% neutral buffered formaldehyde).
- Dress puncture site:
  - clean breast and puncture site with alcohol.
  - apply adhesive skin closure strips and sterile bandage.
  - cool and compress for approx. 15 minutes.
- Written documentation:
  - include technical data, biopsy access, complications.
  - state whether biopsy was representative, questionably representative, or not representative.
- Correlate imaging with histology: plausible and acceptable? Rebiopsy?

Tips and Tricks

Practice on phantom. Optimal visualization of the needle during an US-guided biopsy requires the ability to envision in three dimensions while coordinating the needle and transducer movements effectively. It is especially important to keep the lesion in the image plane, and the needle and transducer axes parallel to each other. Achieving the prefire situation may require multiple adjustments of both needle and transducer posi-

4

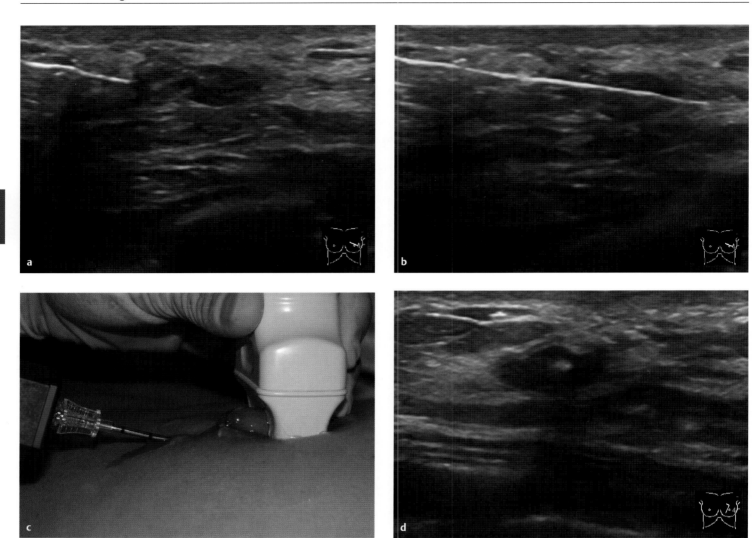

Fig. 4.10a–d   Obtaining a core specimen under US guidance. Prefire (**a**). Postfire (**b–d**).

tions. Practice is the best way to improve technique and assuredness. A commercial (**Fig. 4.11**) or self-made phantom is suitable for this purpose. A self-made phantom can easily be created, for example, by taking a turkey breast and inserting targets (e. g., olives, small grapes with seeds, etc.) into incisions of varied depth on one side, then wrapping it into a plastic freezer bag.

Mobile lesions. Mobile lesions are sometimes difficult to keep under the transducer. It often helps to wedge the lesion with the transducer into a position in the breast where it is less mobile. It is sometimes sufficient to exert more compression and/or to press the distal end of the transducer into the breast.

Incomplete needle firing. With time, the spring of older biopsy guns can lose strength and elasticity. After firing an automated core biopsy gun, the outer cutting sheath may not complete the cutting process after the inner needle has been thrust forward. This occurs most often when the lesion is fibrotic and very firm. In such cases the cutting process can be completed manually by removing the needle from the gun and pushing the outer sheath to its end position before removing the needle from the breast.

Dorsal lesions near the chest wall. When biopsying dorsal lesions, it is especially important that needle guidance is parallel to the chest wall. To achieve this, the skin puncture site must usually be more than 1 cm away from the proximal transducer end. For lateral lesions, it helps to elevate the ipsilateral side of the body. Occasionally, it might be necessary to choose a longer biopsy needle. Injection of local anesthesia between the chest wall and the lesion can increase the distance between them and facilitate biopsy. It is also possible to lift the lesion away from the thoracic wall with the needle tip before firing, thereby improving the

angle at which biopsy is performed. If there is increased risk of complications (pneumothorax), a short throw setting can be selected.

Fragmented, hemorrhagic samples. After the first few samples have been harvested, the following samples tend to become increasingly fragmented and hemorrhagic. Sampling from different regions of a large lesion can alleviate this problem. When sampling a small lesion, however, special care must be taken with the first biopsies to insure that adequate material is harvested before the quality of the samples becomes insufficient.

Impairment of lesion visualization. In the course of performing a percutaneous biopsy of a lesion, air is introduced into the biopsy region. There is usually also a small amount of bleeding. Both of these factors can impair visualization, especially of small or primarily less conspicuous lesions (**Fig. 4.12**). This is another important reason to be especially accurate when performing the first biopsies of small lesions. Also, injecting local anesthesia into the tissues near a lesion can decrease the ability to identify a small or inconspicuous lesion and make biopsy futile.

Small lesion. After percutaneous biopsy of a small lesion less than 5 mm in diameter, it is possible that the lesion has been completely excised and/or later detectability significantly reduced. This can cause difficulties if preoperative localization is required. If this is anticipated, a coil marker can be released into the biopsy cavity for later US or stereotactic localization. Alternatively, 16- or 18-gauge needles (normally less preferred than 14-gauge) can be used for biopsy. An experienced examiner can also reduce the number of samples taken. In some cases, the postbiopsy hematoma can be identified and localized using magnetic resonance imaging (MRI) 2–4 weeks after biopsy (**Fig. 4.13**).

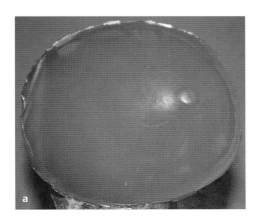

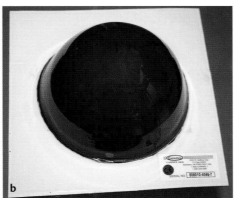

Fig. 4.11a, b US phantoms. Breast biopsy phantom BB-1 (PTW Co., Freiberg, Germany.) (**a**), US-biopsy phantom RMI 429 (Gammex-RMI Co., Middleton, WI) (**b**).

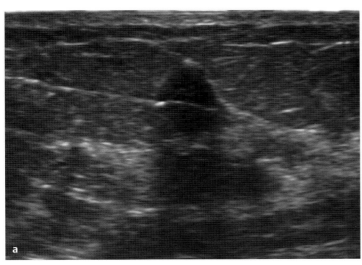

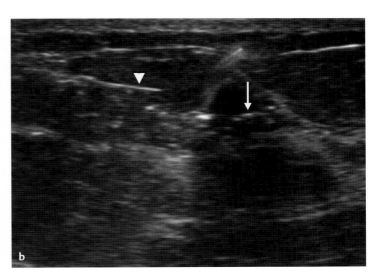

Fig. 4.12a, b Impairment of lesion visualization. Postfire image after first sampling (**a**). Prefire image before second sampling (**b**) showing artifacts due to air in biopsy channel (↓) after first biopsy (▼ = biopsy needle).

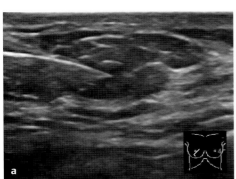

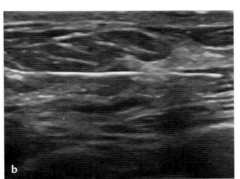

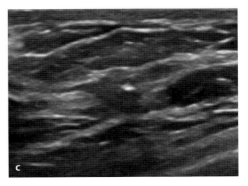

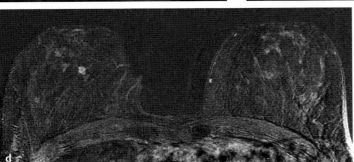

Fig. 4.13a–d Small tubular breast cancer in the right breast. US-guided CNB: prefire (**a**), postfire (**b**), postfire in cross section (**c**). MRI subtraction image (**d**). After retrieval of three tissue samples, the lesion could no longer be reliably reproduced on US. Preoperative localization was then performed under MRI guidance.

Static 3D-Volumetric Ultrasound / Real-Time 4D Ultrasound

Today, routine breast US, as well as the performance and documentation of US-guided biopsies and preoperative localizations are usually accomplished using a 2D technique. Recently, 3D and 4D US have been increasingly employed. During US-guided interventions, 4D US provides real-time visualization of the needle in all three planes. In the case of percutaneous biopsy, it permits the differentiation between a central or peripheral hit, and a missed biopsy (**Fig. 4.14**). In the case of a preoperative localization, the localization wire can be exactly placed. *3D targeting* entails correlating the biopsy needle or localization wire position to the targeted lesion in all three sonographic planes. A 3D-volumetric US

printed image can also provide the basis for high-quality double reading.

Sources of Error and Specific Complications

The correct and reliable performance of an US-guided CNB requires good visualization of both the target lesion and the biopsy needle in one image plane. To achieve this, the examiner must be able to think in three dimensions and have experience and practice in the coordinated handling of the biopsy device and transducer. **Figures 4.15, 4.16, 4.17, and 4.18** demonstrate some of the most common sources of error.

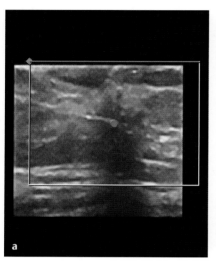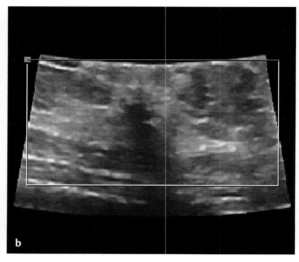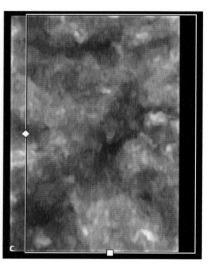

Fig. 4.14a–c US-guided biopsy using 3D volume US. Marking the needle tip in the first plane (**a**) (red spot) allows easy identification of the needle tip in the other planes and confirmation that the needle has been placed correctly within the lesion (**b, c**).

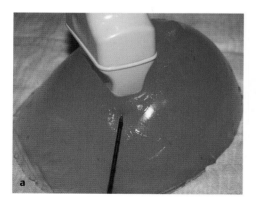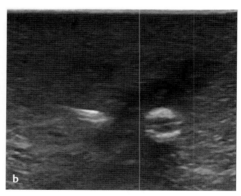

Fig. 4.15a, b Suboptimal needle visualization. The needle is not parallel to the long axis of the transducer. The needle is not visualized in full length if the transducer is rotated during the examination (**a**). Because the needle is only partially visualized in the image plane, it is not possible to identify the needle tip reliably (**b**).

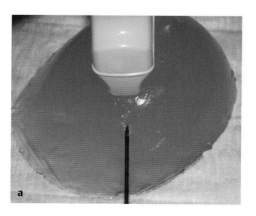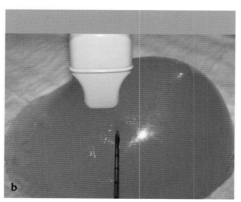

Fig. 4.16a, b Suboptimal needle visualization. The needle is not in the image plane. During the examination, the transducer can become misaligned with the needle axis (**a, b**). The needle is therefore no longer under the transducer and cannot be visualized.

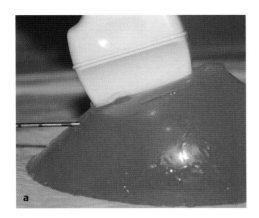

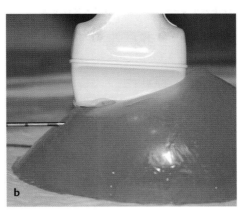

Fig. 4.17a, b Suboptimal needle visualization. The needle axis is at an angle to the transducer axis. If the transducer is lightly placed on the breast surface, the breast curvature causes the transducer axis to be at an angle to the chest wall (**a**), impairing visualization of the horizontal needle. To position the transducer parallel to the chest wall and needle, the distal end of the transducer is gently pressed into the breast (**b**).

4

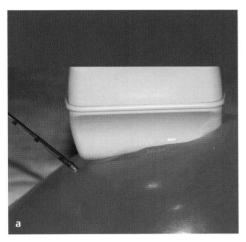

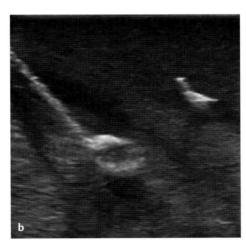

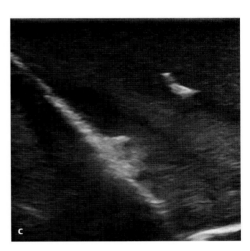

Fig. 4.18a–c Unfavorable skin puncture site. If the skin puncture site is chosen too close to the proximal transducer end (**a**), reaching a deep lesion while keeping a horizontal needle axis will be impossible. The needle axis must then be directed toward the chest wall resulting in a higher complication risk and impaired needle visualization: prefire (**b**), postfire (**c**).

Thorax puncture. US-guided biopsy is performed under visual monitoring and always as parallel to the thoracic wall as possible. Theoretically, it is possible to puncture the thorax, pleura, or pericardial cavity if the needle is directed toward the chest wall during biopsy. Life-threatening complications could result in such cases.

Fistula. In rare cases, performing a percutaneous biopsy on a lactating breast can result in the development of a fistula.

Missed biopsy. US-guided percutaneous biopsy performed by an experienced examiner has a high accuracy rate of over 95%, including tumors ≤5 mm diameter. In rare cases, however, the biopsy misses the target and no representative material is harvested (false-negative). Benign results should always be critically evaluated to confirm that histopathology correlates with the imaging findings.

Checklist: Ultrasound-guided Core Needle Biopsy

1. Verify indication, informed consent.
2. Mammography, usually in two views.
3. Preintervention-US documentation.
4. Positioning of patient and examiner.
5. Positioning of US unit.
6. Determination of biopsy direction and skin puncture site.
7. Disinfection and local anesthesia.
8. Sterile gel and gloves.
9. Demonstration of firing sound to patient.
10. Stab incision and insertion of coaxial needle under visual monitoring.
11. Removal of stylet and insertion of biopsy needle.
12. Prefire documentation.
13. Trigger biopsy after fine adjustment and warning patient.
14. Postfire documentation.
15. Retrieve sample.
16. Repeat biopsy procedure as often as required.
17. Postinterventional dressing of puncture site.

Ultrasound-guided Vacuum-assisted Biopsy

Indications

The larger lumen, vacuum-assisted biopsy (VAB) is an alternative to CNB for definitive pathologic diagnosis of suspicious breast lesions. It is the most costly and elaborate of the described biopsy techniques. The consensus of the Minimal Invasive Breast Interventions Working Group (AG MiMi) of the German Senology Association (DGS) has defined four recommended indications for performing US-guided VABs (**Table 4.6**).

Which findings to include in the spectrum of indications for the performance of VAB is still controversial. The inclusion of small suspicious lesions as a diagnostic indication for VAB seems especially questionable: later lesion imaging will be significantly impaired and difficulties will arise if further evaluation or localization is necessary. Using a smaller biopsy caliber might be advantageous in such a case; however, if VAB is performed for the diagnostic evaluation of a small lesion, then it is highly recommended to place a marker coil in the biopsy cavity to facilitate localization at a future date.

Whether a clearly benign finding should be removed from the breast is predominantly dependent upon patient wishes. Good patient management makes this therapeutic indication for VAB dispensable.

Specific Complications

Bleeding. Excessive bleeding can occasionally occur during US-guided VAB, making the further identification and demarcation of a lesion difficult. Thus, it is often problematic to assess whether a lesion has been successfully removed after completion of the intervention. In case of doubt, it is recommended to perform a short-term follow-up examination 6 months after biopsy. Before biopsy, the patient should be informed about the possibility that residual lesion may remain in the breast.

Impaired visualization of small lesions after vacuum-assisted biopsy. The diagnostic VAB of small lesions often results in the complete excision. In the case of proven malignancy, it is prudent to place a marker in the biopsy cavity to facilitate preoperative localization. The decision of whether or not to place a marker, however, is made on an individual basis. This should be discussed with the patient at the outset, especially because if histopathology is benign, the marker coil/clip will remain in the breast permanently. As an alternative, it is sometimes possible to localize

the biopsy cavity under US-guidance for 1–2 weeks after biopsy. Also, contrast-enhanced MRI can usually identify the biopsy region over several weeks after VAB, providing another, albeit expensive, alternative method for preoperative wire localization.

Materials

Various hand-held VAB devices are currently available for use in US-guided breast interventions (see **Figs. 7.23, 7.24, 7.25, 7.26**). In contrast to VAB systems used for stereotactic interventions, devices designed for use under US-guidance have no jet-mechanism (except the Vacora System; Bard Biopsy Systems, Tempe, AZ). Before beginning with the intervention, therefore, the biopsy needle is placed between the thorax and the dorsal edge of the lesion and not before the lesion.

Procedure

The procedure for performing aVAB is, in principle, the same as that for performing a CNB. Before beginning with the intervention, the needle should be placed so that the lesion is between the needle and the transducer. In this position, the dorsal attenuation caused by the needle will not interfere with visualization of the lesion during biopsy. The tissue samples are harvested by incremental needle rotation unilaterally toward the lesion. When performing a diagnostic VAB, the acquisition of at least 12 tissue samples with an 11-gauge needle is recommended. If other needle sizes are used, harvesting of the volume equivalent is recommended. When performing a therapeutic VAB, the tissue is harvested until the lesion is removed.

Ultrasound-guided Fine-needle Aspiration

The significant disadvantages of performing a fine-needle aspiration for cytology (FNAC) on solid lesions are the high inadequate sample rate, and the expertise required of the cytopathologic specialist. Because automated CNB provides better sensitivity, specificity, and positive predictive value for both benign and malignant lesions, FNAC is no longer recommended for the routine biopsy of breast lesions.

Indications

Simple cysts. The main indication for the performance of fine-needle aspiration (FNA) is to drain a simple, symptomatic cyst, thus relieving pain promptly and/or eliminating a lump causing apprehension. Occasionally, a cyst will refill within a few days or weeks.

Another indication is to differentiate between a cystic and solid lesion when US is ambiguous. If no fluid is aspirated, an US-guided CNB should be performed for histopathologic assessment.

Suspicious lymph nodes. The pathologic evaluation of suspicious lymph nodes or lesions in the axillary and other lymphatic drainage regions is usually performed as a FNAB because of the higher complication rate associated with core needle biopsy. The specificity of cytology for the differentiation between inflammatory and metastatic lymph nodes is high, making the FNAB a suitable alternative to CNB for this indication.

Table 4.6 Employment of US-guided VABs according to the recommendations of the Minimal Invasive Breast Interventions Working Group (AG MiMi) of the German Senology Association (DGS) 2004

Diagnostic use
Mismatch between histopathology and diagnostic imaging after CNB and remaining suspicion of malignancy (BI-RADS 4/5)
Suspicious lesion of approx. 5 mm diameter (BI-RADS 4/5)

Therapeutic use
Intraductal/intracystic lesions (e. g., singular papilloma)
Clearly benign, symptomatic lesion (e. g., fibroadenoma)

Materials

To be able to perform an US-guided FNA with one hand while holding the transducer with the other, a syringe with a fine needle is fitted into a special handle (syringe pistol, **Fig. 7.1**). This handle is constructed so that it is possible to guide the needle under visual monitoring and create a vacuum in the syringe by drawing back the plunger with one hand.

Procedure

In preparation for the performance of a FNA, a 10- or 20-mL syringe with a fine needle (e.g., 20-gauge) is fitted into the special handle described above. Local anesthesia is not usually required, but is recommended to avoid patient discomfort and distress. Visualization of the needle during FNA is achieved in the same way as when performing a core needle biopsy. It is important not to draw back the plunger before skin puncture and needle advancement into the lesion. Only when visual confirmation of the needle inside the lesion is made should a vacuum be created inside the syringe by drawing back the plunger as far as possible. To attain material for cytology of solid lesions, the needle is passed through the lesion rapidly with an "in and out" motion several times, varying direction within the lesion (**Fig. 4.19**). The vacuum is then neutralized by slowly releasing the plunger before the needle is removed from the breast. Samples are usually prepared on cytology slides as shown in **Figs. 8.1, 8.2, 8.3, and 8.4**. Slides are then labeled and usually air-dried.

Ultrasound-guided Localization

Indications

US-guided preoperative wire localization is indicated for lesions that are not easily distinguished on palpation, can be identified on US, and have been proven malignant or yielded a risk lesion (e.g., atypical ductal hyperplasia [ADH], radial scar, lobular carcinoma in situ [LCIS]) on CNB. An exact localization facilitates the complete excision of the targeted lesion while minimizing the amount of healthy surrounding tissue removed.

On rare occasion, a lesion may be preoperatively localized without prior histopathologic assessment. This is the case if percutaneous biopsy is not possible or contraindications exist.

Materials

Localization wires. There are several preoperative localization wires available with good sonographic imaging properties. As a rule, they consist of a localization wire inside a cannula. They differ primarily in the configuration of the wire tip, which determines whether the wire can be withdrawn into cannula for repositioning, and the security with which it is fastened in fatty or fibrous breast tissue (see **Figs. 7.41, 7.42, 7.43, 7.44, 7.45, 7.46, 7.47, 7.48, 7.49**).

Coils/Clips

Marker clips and coils are used less often in the preoperative situation than are wires. There are several different markers available, including gel pellets that provide good US visibility for several weeks (see **Figs. 7.50, 7.51, 7.52, 7.53, 7.54, 7.55, 7.56, 7.57, 7.58, 7.59, 7.60**). Thus, an inconspicuous US lesion diagnosed in one medical facility can be marked by releasing a marker into the biopsy cavity for later preoperative localization in another medical facility. When initial biopsy has been preformed under stereo-

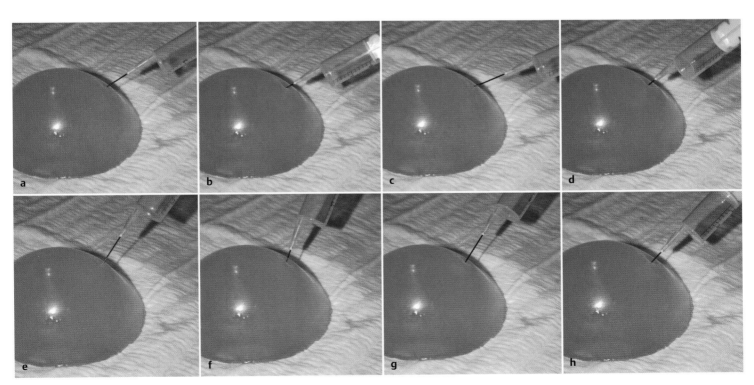

Fig. 4.19a–h FNAB

tactic or MRI guidance, a gel marker released into the biopsy cavity can provide a surrogate target for US-guided localization. The insertion of a metal coil or clip marker also provides a simple means to landmark the original borders of a malignant lesion before administration of neoadjuvant chemotherapy, making a preoperative US-guided or stereotactic localization possible when the breast lump becomes impalpable and radiologically undetectable.

Procedure

Visualization of the needle during an US-guided localization is achieved in the same way as when performing a CNB. Once the localization needle is positioned in the target lesion, the thin wire can be advanced into the breast and the cannula removed, leaving the wire in place.

Needle path. It is no longer necessary to take the surgical approach into account when deciding on the skin puncture site and needle pathway for preoperative wire localization. Many studies have substantiated the fact that tumor cell displacement or track seeding is not a relevant factor in the rate of local recurrence and overall survival after breast surgery and postoperative radiotherapy. The wishes of the attending surgeon should be taken into consideration, however.

Optimally, the localization wire should penetrate the target lesion through to the distal edge. The minimum requirement is that the wire lie less than 1 cm away from the lesion. When localizing large lesions, it is sometimes advantageous to place several wires at the surgically relevant borders instead of in the lesion center. After US-guided localization, a mammographic documentation in two planes should be performed for lesions also visible on mammography. Lesions that are not primarily seen on mammography can, however, sometimes be allocated to mammographic structures in the post-localization mammogram.

Good Practice Recommendations*

A preoperative localization wire should be placed ≤1 cm from the target lesion in ≥90% of cases. If possible, the lesion should be penetrated and the wire should not project more that 2 cm past the distal lesion border. When localizing a nonmass lesion, two or more markers/wires can be placed at the surgically relevant borders without adhering to the 1-cm limit.

* European S3 guidelines: Early Breast Cancer Detection

Clinical Cases

Clinical Case 1: Failed Reproduction of Lesion Visualization after Ultrasound-guided Core Needle Biopsy (Fig. 4.20)

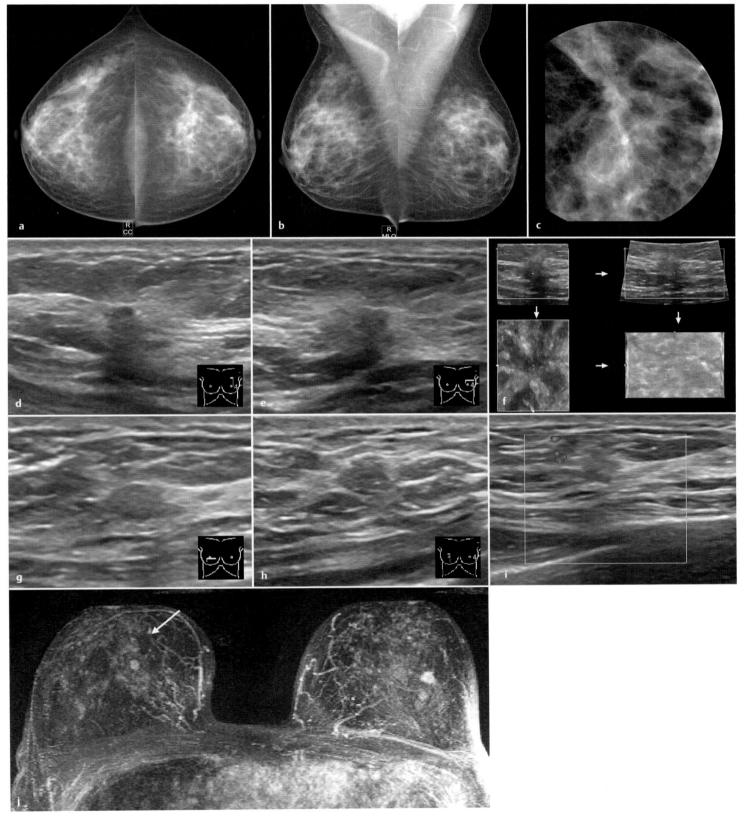

Fig. 4.20a–j Failed reproduction of lesion visualization after US-guided CNB:
Routine examination of a 58-year-old woman who presented without clinical symptoms.

a–c Bilateral digital mammography in two planes and spot compression from left CC view.

d–e Correlating US lesion in upper outer quadrant of left breast.

f 3D image.

g–i Incidental ultrasonographic finding in lower aspect of right breast with power Doppler image (**i**).

j MR mammography: Maximum intensity projection (MIP) shows hypervascularized lesions correlating with US findings in both breasts. **k–v** See p. 34.

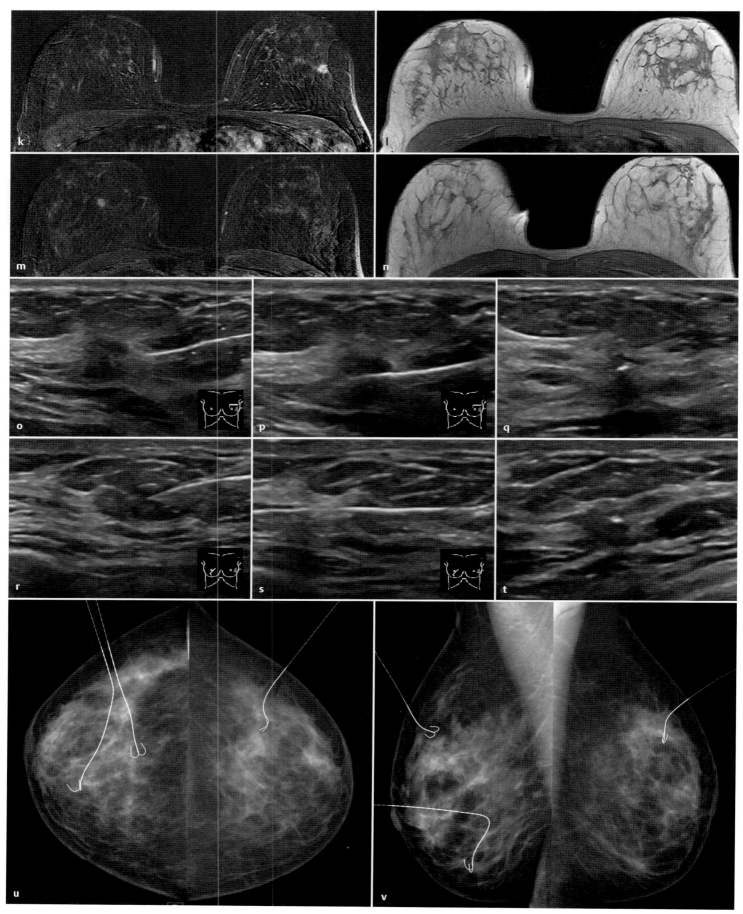

Fig. 4.20k–v

k–n MR mammography: subtraction slice images with corresponding precontrast T1-weighted images (**l, n**).

o–q Left US-guided CNB: prefire, postfire, cross-section image. *Histology*: well-differentiated invasive ductal carcinoma (IDC), B5b, G1.

r–t Right US-guided CNB: prefire, postfire, cross-section image. *Histology*: well-differentiated IDC, B5b, G1.

u, v Bilateral digital mammography in two planes: The left lesion was preopera-

tively localized under US guidance. The right lesion could not be reproduced on US after biopsy and required MR-guided localization. In view of the verified malignancy in the right breast, a further focal hypervascularization was preoperatively localized (arrow in **j**). *Final histology, left*: invasive partially solid, partially tubuloductal breast cancer, pT1c, $_{sN}$N0(1), G2. *Final histology, right caudal lesion*: invasive tubular breast cancer, pT1a, $_{sN}$N0(2), G1. *Final histology, right craniomedial lesion*: intraductal epithelial proliferations without cellular atypia.

Clinical Case 2: US-guided Vacuum-assisted Biopsy due to Mismatch (Fig. 4.21)

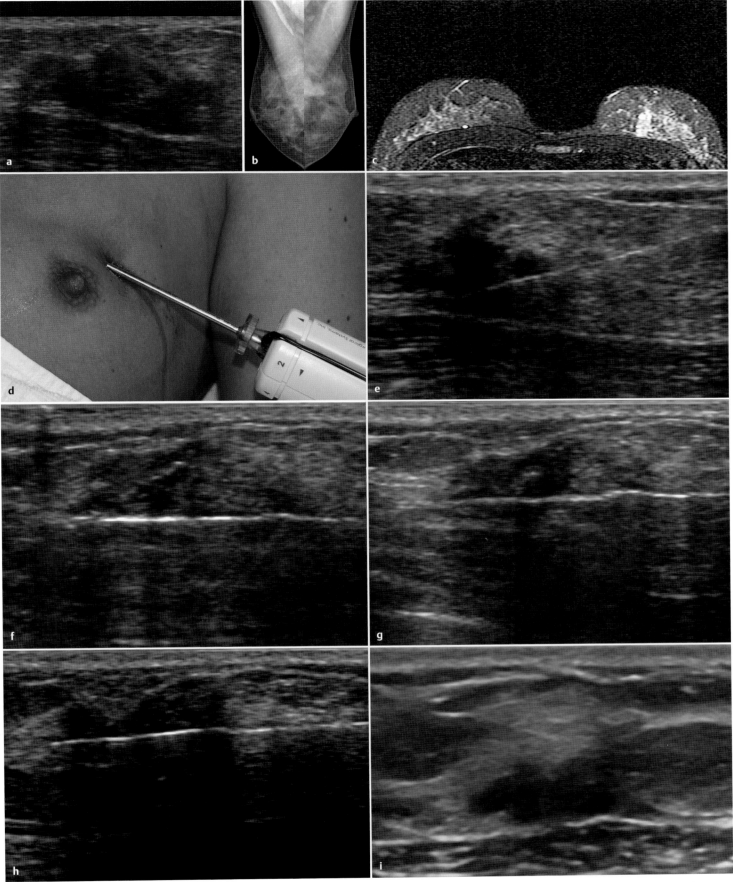

4

Fig. 4.21a–i US-guided VAB due to questionable correlation between image findings and CNB histology (mismatch): A 36-year-old woman with a palpable abnormality in the upper aspect of the left breast located medially from a surgery scar. CNB revealed atypical ductal hyperplasia.
a Correlating US finding.
b Bilateral digital mammography in mediolateral oblique projection showing correlating lesion.

c MR mammography: subtraction image with corresponding asymmetric hypervascularization (MR BI-RADS 4).
d US-guided VAB of the left breast.
e US documentation before beginning procedure.
f–h US documentation during VAB.
i Follow-up US examination after 6 months. *Histology*: Adenosis.

4

Clinical Case 3: Fine-needle Aspiration Biopsy of Axillary Lymph Node (Fig. 4.22)

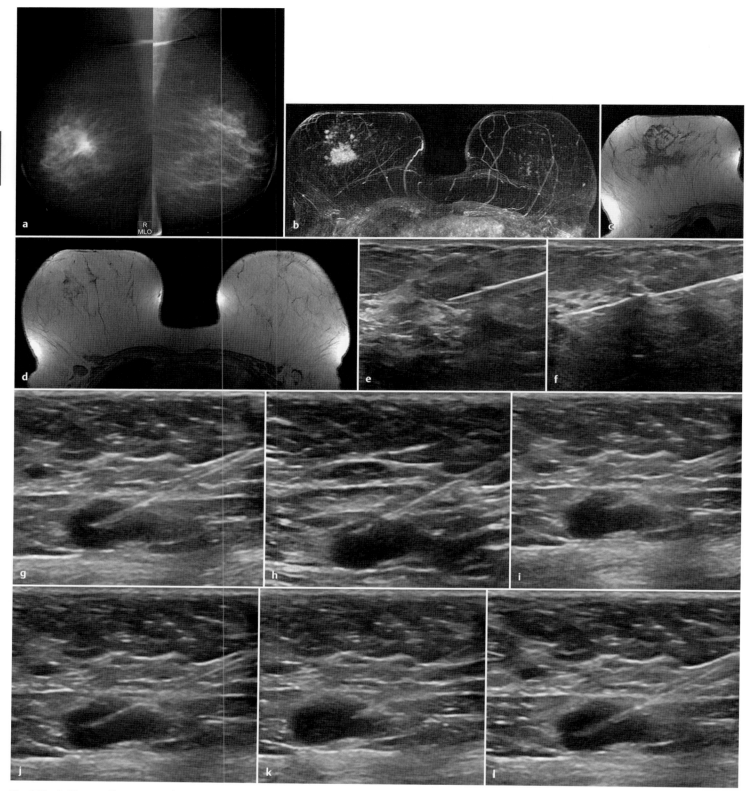

Fig. 4.22a–l   Fine-needle aspiration for cytology (FNAC) of suspicious lymph node in the right axilla: A 75-year-old woman with a BI-RADS 5 finding in the right breast.

a Bilateral digital mammography in MLO projection.
b MR mammography: MIP image.
c MR mammography: precontrast T1-weighted image of tumor.

d MR mammography: precontrast T1-weighted image shows suspicious right axillary lymph node.
e, f Right US-guided CNB: prefire, postfire.
g–l US-guided FNAC of suspicious lymph node. *Cytology:* lymph node metastasis of carcinoma compatible with a metastasis of a ductal carcinoma (IDC) of the breast.

Clinical Case 4: Ultrasound-guided Core Needle Biopsy of Microcalcifications (Fig. 4.23)

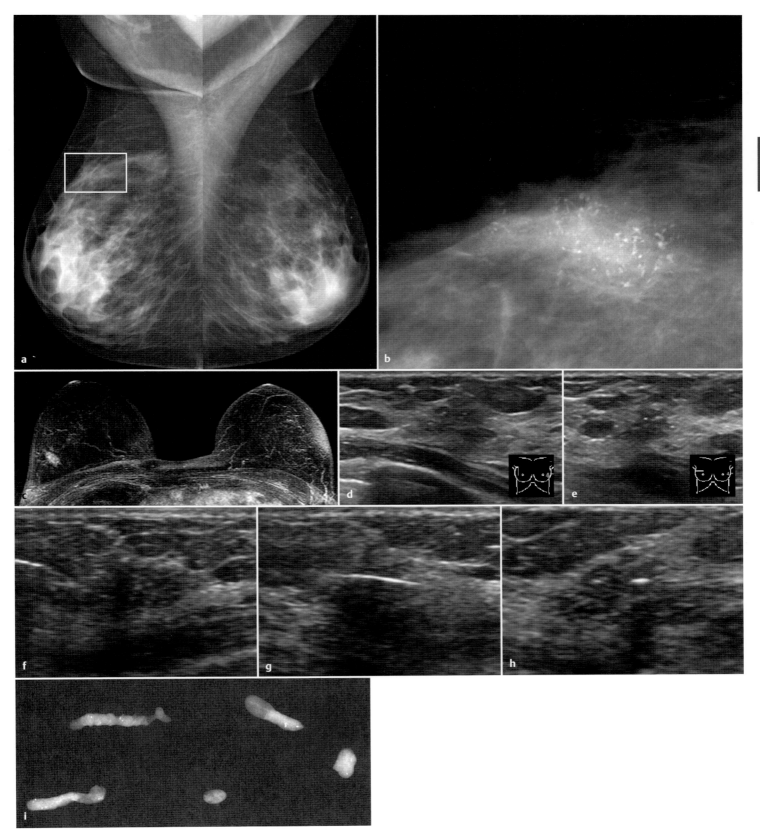

4

Fig. 4.23a–i US-guided CNB of microcalcifications primarily detected on mammography: Routine examination of a 67-year-old woman who presented without clinical symptoms.
a Bilateral digital mammography in MLO projection.
b Digital magnification mammography of lateral right breast in cc view.

c MR mammography: MIP image.
d, e US image of right upper outer quadrant.
f–h Right US-guided CNB: prefire, postfire, cross-section image.
i Specimen radiography. *Histology:* DCIS, B5a.

Clinical Case 5: Fine-needle Aspiration Biopsy to Differentiate between Cystic and Solid Lesion (Fig. 4.24)

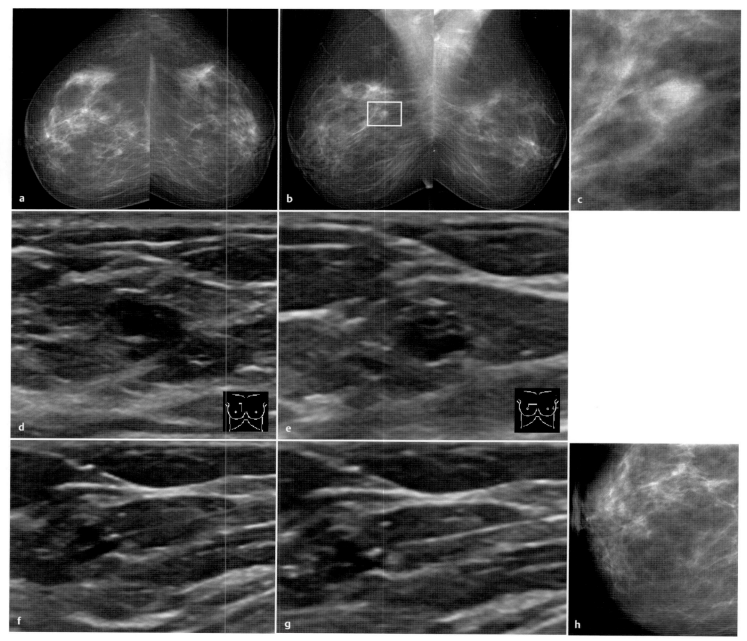

Fig. 4.24a–h FNAC to differentiate between cystic and solid lesion: An early detection examination of 44-year-old woman who presented without clinical symptoms.
a, b Bilateral digital mammography in two planes.
c Close-up view of central area in MLO view showing new mass.

d, e US images of right upper inner quadrant.
f, g Fine-needle aspiration for FNAC.
h Spot compression of medial right breast in cc view after FNAC. No reproduction of the small mass seen in **a**.

Clinical Case 6: Clip- and Coil-marking (Fig. 4.25)

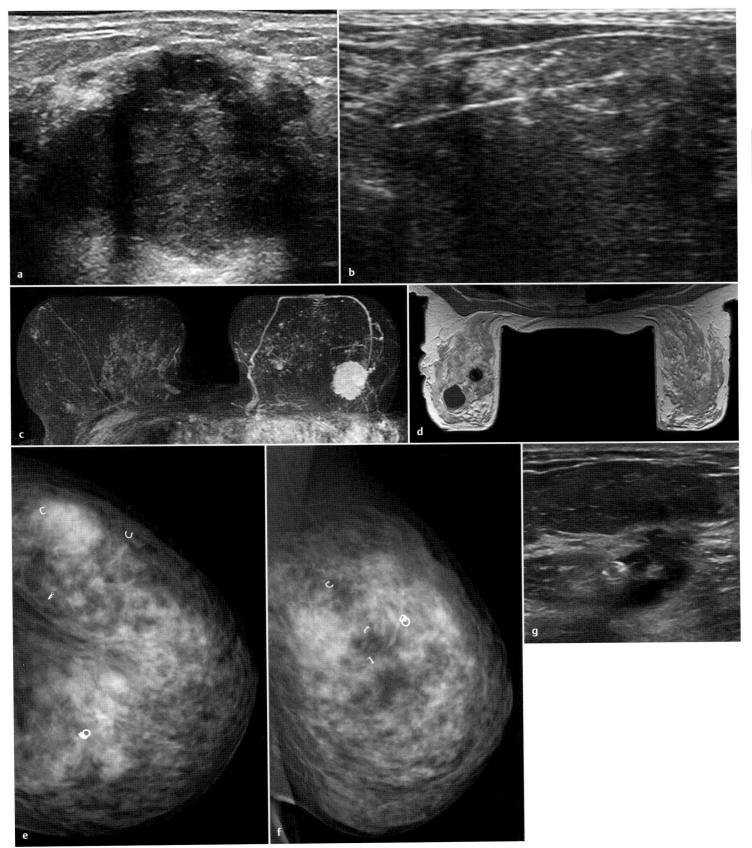

Fig. 4.25a–g US-guided clip-marking of tumor borders (BI-RADS 6) and MRI-guided coil-marking of second suspicious lesion in the left breast before neo-adjuvant chemotherapy: A 51-year-old woman presented with a palpable mass in the left breast. She was diagnosed with a hematoma after a US-guided CNB.
a US of left palpable mass.
b US-guided puncture before releasing one of three marker clips at cranial, caudal, and medial tumor borders. Lateral border is subcutaneous. Dorsal border is the thoracic wall.

c Pretherapeutic MR mammography: MIP image.
d MR mammography: precontrast T1-weighted image with coil marker in second suspicious lesion in right upper inner quadrant (BI-RADS 5).
e, f Mammographic documentation of the right breast in two planes. Good differentiation of coil (US) and clip (MRI) markers.
g US image of coil marker.

Clinical Case 7: Silicone Granuloma after Bilateral Augmentation with Silicone Implants (Fig. 4.26)

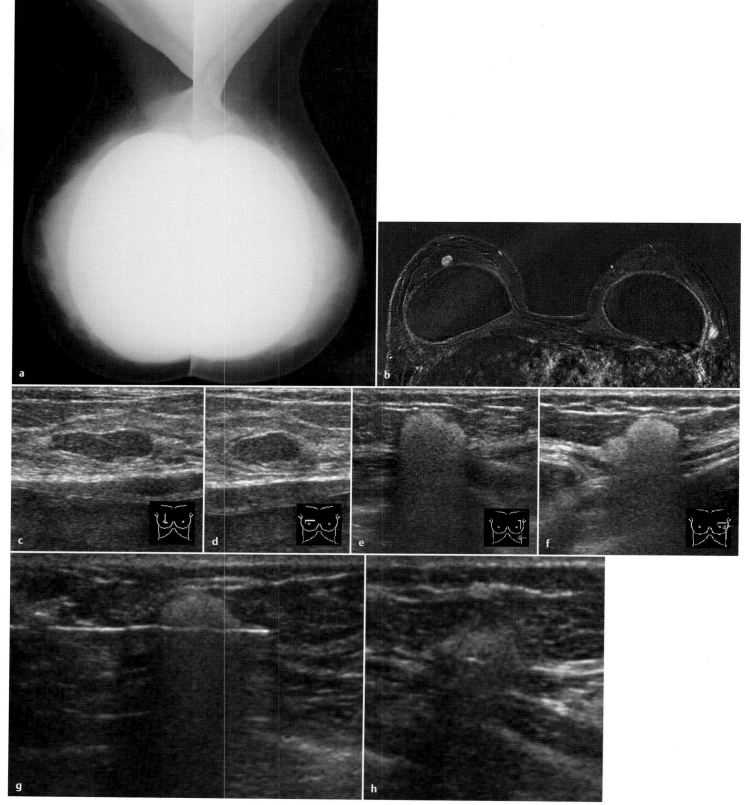

Fig. 4.26a–g Silicone granuloma after bilateral augmentation with silicone implants: Routine examination of a 41-year-old woman who presented without clinical symptoms.
a Bilateral digital mammography in MLO projection.
b MR mammography: subtraction image.

c, d US image of cranial aspect of the right breast.
e, f US image of left upper outer quadrant.
g, h Left US-guided CNB: prefire, postfire. *Histology*: Fragments of a lymph node with pronounced foreign body granulomatous lymphadenitis, compatible with a silicone granuloma. No malignancy.

Clinical Case 8: Collagen Clip-marking (Fig. 4.27)

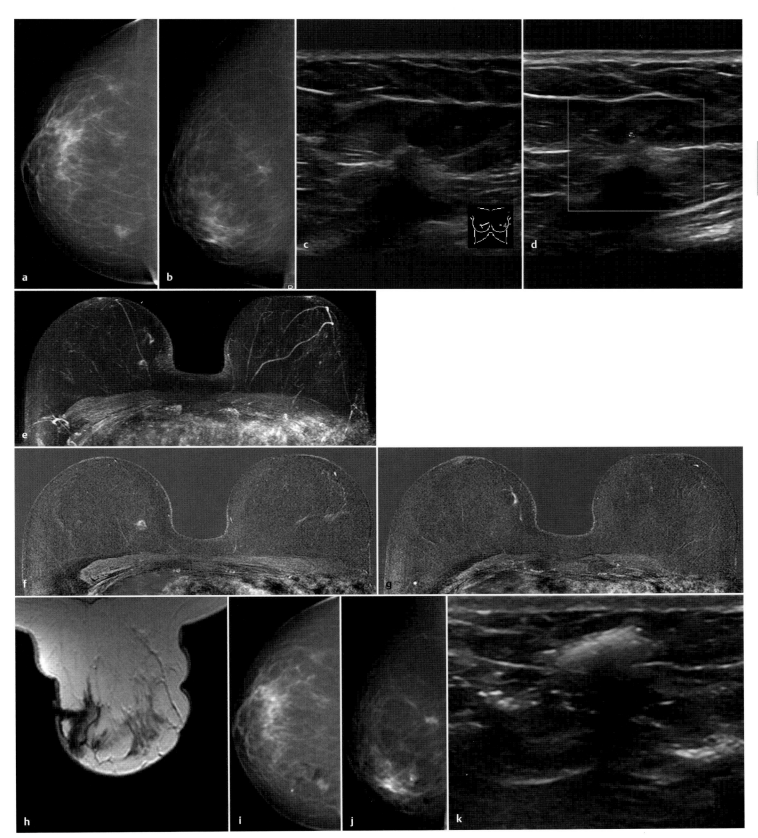

Fig. 4.27a–k US visualization of collagen-clip marker after MRI-guided clip-localization of suspicious MR mammography lesion: A 51-year-old woman was diagnosed with a BI-RADS 6 finding in the right upper inner breast quadrant after CNB.
a, b Bilateral digital mammography in two planes.
c, d Correlating US lesion in upper inner quadrant of the right breast.
e MR mammography: MIP image showing linear hypervascularization caudomedially from index tumor.

f, g MR mammography: corresponding subtraction images slices.
h MR mammography: postcontrast T1-weighted image with clip localization of suspicious linear hypervascularization for later US-guided localization at a different institute.
i, j Mammographic documentation in two planes.
k US image of collagen clip. *Histology, right index tumor:* IDC, G2. *Histology, right linear hypervascularization:* DCIS, G1.

4

Further Reading

American College of Radiology (ACR). ACR-BI-RADS®-Ultrasound. In: ACR Breast Imaging Reporting and Data System. Breast Imaging Atlas. Reston, VA: American College of Radiology; 2003

Berg WA, Gutierrez L, NessAiver MS, et al. Diagnostic accuracy of mammography, clinical examination, US, and MR imaging in preoperative assessment of breast cancer. Radiology 2004;233(3):830–849

Burbank F. Mammographic findings after 14-gauge automated needle and 14-gauge directional, vacuum-assisted stereotactic breast biopsies. Radiology 1997;204(1):153–156

Kaplan SS. Clinical utility of bilateral whole-breast US in the evaluation of women with dense breast tissue. Radiology 2001;221(3):641–649

Kolb TM, Lichy J, Newhouse JH. Comparison of the performance of screening mammography, physical examination, and breast US and evaluation of factors that influence them: an analysis of 27,825 patient evaluations. Radiology 2002;225(1):165–175

Kolb TM, Lichy J, Newhouse JH. Occult cancer in women with dense breasts: detection with screening US—diagnostic yield and tumor characteristics. Radiology 1998;207(1):191–199

Konsensusempfehlung zur Anwendung und Indikationen der Vakuumbiopsie der Brust unter Ultraschallsicht. Arbeitsgemeinschaft Minimalinvasive Mammainterventionen (AG MiMi) der Deutschen Gesellschaft für Senologie (DGS). 2004

Krainick U, Meyberg-Solomayer G, Majer I, et al. Minimal invasive Mammabiopsien: die Vakuumbiopsie (VB) mit dem Handheld (HH) Mammotome™ unter Ultraschallsicht – Erfahrungen und Indikationsspektrum des Brustzentrums Tübingen. Geburtshilfe Frauenheilkd 2002;62 : 346–350

Liberman L, Dershaw DD, Rosen PP, Abramson AF, Deutch BM, Hann LE. Stereotaxic 14-gauge breast biopsy: how many core biopsy specimens are needed? Radiology 1994;192(3):793–795

Liberman L, Feng TL, Dershaw DD, Morris EA, Abramson AF. US-guided core breast biopsy: use and cost-effectiveness. Radiology 1998;208(3):717–723

Liberman L. Percutaneous imaging-guided core breast biopsy: state of the art at the millennium. AJR Am J Roentgenol 2000;174(5):1191–1199

Madjar H, Ohlinger R, Mundinger A, et al. [BI-RADS-analogue DEGUM criteria for findings in breast ultrasound—consensus of the DEGUM Committee on Breast Ultrasound]. Ultraschall Med 2006;27(4):374–379

Madjar H. Kursbuch Mammsonographie. Ein Lehratlas nach den Richtlinien der DEGUM und der KBV. 2nd ed. Stuttgart: Thieme; 2005

Parker SH, Burbank F, Jackman RJ, et al. Percutaneous large-core breast biopsy: a multi-institutional study. Radiology 1994;193(2):359–364

Parker SH, Jobe WE, Dennis MA, et al. US-guided automated large-core breast biopsy. Radiology 1993;187(2):507–511

Perry N, Broeders M, de Wolf C, et al. European Guidelines for Quality Assurance in Breast Cancer Screening and Diagnosis. 4th ed. Luxembourg: Office for Official Publications of the European Communities; 2006

Pisano ED, Fajardo LL, Tsimikas J, et al. Rate of insufficient samples for fine-needle aspiration for nonpalpable breast lesions in a multicenter clinical trial: The Radiologic Diagnostic Oncology Group 5 Study. The RDOG5 investigators. Cancer 1998;82(4):679–688

Schulz KD, Albert US, eds. Stufe-3-Leitlinie Brustkrebs-Früherkennung in Deutschland. Munich: Zuckschwerdt; 2008

Schulz-Wendtland R, Krämer S, Lang N, Bautz W. Ultrasonic guided micro-biopsy in mammary diagnosis: indications, technique and results. Anticancer Res 1998; 18(3C, 3C)2145–2146

Weismann C, Hergan K. [Current status of 3D/4D volume ultrasound of the breast]. Ultraschall Med 2007;28(3):273–282

5 Stereotactic Interventions

F. Baum

X-Ray Mammography

Significance of X-ray Mammography in Breast Diagnostics

X-ray mammography is currently the standard diagnostic imaging modality for the early detection of breast cancer. It is the most effective method for the detection of calcifying early-stage breast cancer and has a high sensitivity for the detection of suspicious masses in fatty and fibroglandular breast tissue. Nevertheless, the diagnostic sensitivity of x-ray mammography in dense breast parenchyma (American College of Radiology [ACR] density types III and IV) is significantly limited, and noncalcifying tumors (70% of all breast cancers) are often obscured in such mammograms. Studies indicate that the mammographic sensitivity for the detection of breast cancer is reduced to approximately 40% in extremely dense breast tissue (ACR density type IV), and to approximately 60% in heterogeneously dense breast tissue (ACR density type III). The specificity of mammography is approximately 80–90%.

Indications

Screening mammography is the term used for x-ray mammography incorporated in early breast cancer detection programs aimed at women without clinical symptoms with the goal of detecting cancer in its early stages, thus reducing breast cancer mortality. International professional associations vary in their recommendations with regard to screening, but most agree on examination intervals between 1 and 2 years beginning at 40 to 50 years of age. Women presenting with clinical symptoms indicative of breast cancer undergo *diagnostic mammography. Follow-up mammography* after breast cancer treatment is recommended biannually for the affected breast for the first 3 years after diagnosis, and annually for the contralateral breast. High-risk women may initiate a mammogram screening program at the age of 30 years, or at an age 5 years younger than the youngest affected family member.

Technique and Methodology

The low energy x-rays used in mammography produce high-contrast images that differentiate between normal breast tissue and possible abnormalities. Special film-screen combinations and digital detectors promote high spatial resolution. Breast compression while undergoing a mammography is necessary for optimal image quality. Compression spreads tissue out so that small abnormalities are less likely to be obscured, allows a lower x-ray dose to be used to image the breast, and minimizes motion artifacts and x-ray scatter.

Standard mammographic projections are the craniocaudal view (CC) and the mediolateral-oblique view (MLO). A strict mediolateral (ML) or lateromedial (LM) view may be additionally performed for optimal spatial orientation. Magnification views and focal/spot compression views are the most common special mammography views used to facilitate evaluation.

At present, two techniques are available for the performance of mammography: a conventional film-screen technique and a digital technique. The digital technique offers several advantages. Postprocessing, including window leveling for optimal contrast and brightness, image inversion, and zooming, as well as the application of a computer-aided detection system (CAD), can be used to help interpret digital mammograms. Digital radiographic images can be stored and sent electronically, and the required radiation dose is reduced by 25 to 30% in comparison to conventional film-screen mammography. Digital tomosynthesis mammography and dual-energy contrast-agent–enhanced digital subtraction mammography are digital applications currently under investigation.

Quality assurance. All components of mammographic imaging are regularly subjected to quality assurance checks. This is true for factors involved in the performance of an examination, as well as those pertaining to image processing and digital imaging.

The quality of mammographic images is evaluated and categorized according to the PGMI (perfect, good, moderate, inadequate) rating system (**Table 5.1**). The criteria used for evaluation relate to image labeling, film processing, and breast positioning, as well as to standard views. Mammograms performed after breast conservation therapy, reduction mammoplasty, or breast augmentation are not included in the quality evaluation.

Table 5.1 PGMI classification system

PGMI classification
P = perfect
G = good
M = moderate
I = inadequate
Quality assurance standards*
>75% of image pairs should be classified as P or G
>97% of image pairs should be classified as P, G, or M
<3% of image pairs should be classified as I

* One evaluation is given to an image pair (right and left MLO view, right and left CC view).

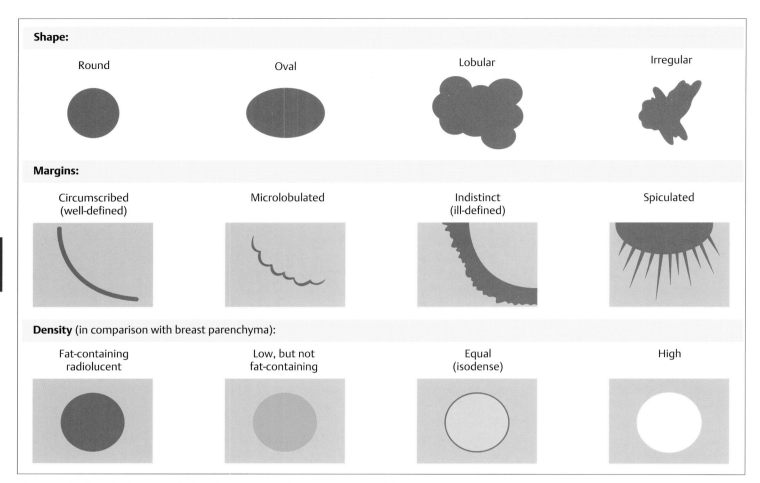

Shape:

Round   Oval   Lobular   Irregular

Margins:

Circumscribed   Microlobulated   Indistinct   Spiculated
(well-defined)   (ill-defined)

Density (in comparison with breast parenchyma):

Fat-containing   Low, but not   Equal   High
radiolucent   fat-containing   (isodense)

Fig. 5.1 Evaluation criteria for mass lesions. Definitions used for shape, margins, and density.

Terminology and Diagnostic Criteria in X-ray Mammography

The ACR BI-RADS Mammography Lexicon is the basis for mammographic image analysis. Findings are described using a standardized language, and categorized according to the probability of malignancy.

Masses and densities. A *mass* is a space-occupying lesion seen in two different projections. A *density* is a potential mass seen in only one projection. The assessment of these lesions takes the features shape, margins, and density into account (**Fig. 5.1**). If the shape of a lesion is oval or round, it is more likely to be benign than an irregularly shaped or spiculated lesion. Circumscribed margins are usually a sign of benignity; indistinct margins could indicate malignancy. The probability of malignancy is lower for low-density lesions than for high-density lesions.

Calcifications. Calcifications can be divided into two groups according to their size. *Macrocalcifications* are usually benign. *Microcalcifications* (<0.5 mm) are sometimes associated with malignancy. A description of calcifications should include their morphology and their distribution (**Fig. 5.2**). Morphologically they are divided into *typically benign* calcifications, e.g., round or punctate, *intermediate concern* calcifications, i.e., amorphous or coarse heterogeneous, and *higher probability of malignancy* calcifications, i.e., fine-pleomorphic and fine-linear branching.

Distribution modifiers describe the arrangement of the calcifications as grouped or clustered (<2 cm³), linear, segmental, regional, or diffuse. A cluster of microcalcifications might indicate malignancy. A segmental or linear arrangement, however, is considered more suspicious of malignancy.

To facilitate assessment of microcalcifications, a matrix is currently being employed in clinical studies (**Fig. 5.3**).

Architectural distortion. An architectural distortion is an alteration of the normal breast without an associated visible mass, and is another criterion used in mammographic assessment. If not associated with prior surgery or trauma, further diagnostic workup is required.

ACR BI-RADS mammography assessment categories. The purpose of a structured analysis and consistently using standardized language in the description of breast lesions is to help categorize these according to their probability of malignancy, and thus aid in decision making as to what consequences to take. The ACR BI-RADS for mammography has defined seven categories for lesion assessment (**Table 5.2**).

Microcalcifications:

Distribution:

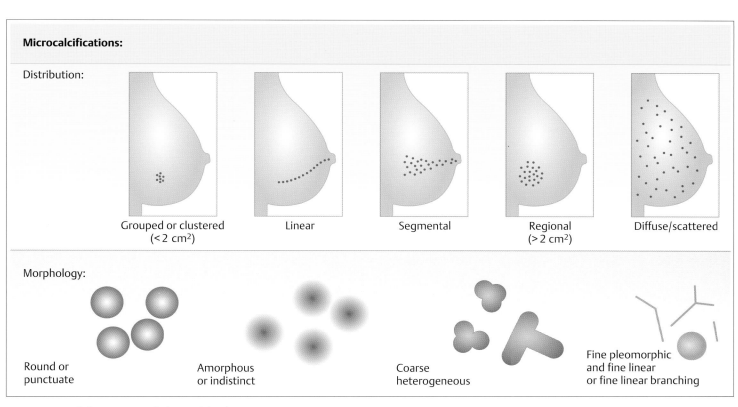

| Grouped or clustered (< 2 cm²) | Linear | Segmental | Regional (> 2 cm²) | Diffuse/scattered |

Morphology:

| Round or punctuate | Amorphous or indistinct | Coarse heterogeneous | Fine pleomorphic and fine linear or fine linear branching |

Fig. 5.2 Microcalcifications. Morphology and distribution patterns.

Table 5.2 American College of Radiology BI-RADS mammography categories from Fischer, U., Baum, F.: Diagnostische Interventionen der Mamma, Georg Thieme Verlag, 2008

Category	Assessment	Examples	Carcinoma risk	Consequence
0	Incomplete	Focal asymmetry, partially obscured, iso-dense mass	Not known	Additional imaging evaluation, retrieval of prior mammograms
1	Negative	No lesion, architectural distortion, or skin thickening found	0%	Routine follow-up
2	Benign finding(s)	Fat-containing lesions, lymph node, implant, secretory or popcorn calcifications, unchanged fibroadenoma or architectural distortion due to surgery scar	0%	Routine follow-up
3	Probably benign finding	Noncalcified circumscribed fibroadenoma-like mass, focal asymmetry, cluster of round (punctate) microcalcifications	<2%	Short-term follow-up*, optional CNB or VAB
4	Suspicious abnormality	• Partially ill-defined mass • Grouped, pleomorphic microcalcifications • New cluster of fine-pleomorphic microcalcifications	• 4A: 2–30% • 4B: 30–60% • 4C: 60–90%	Pathologic evaluation (CNB)
5	Highly suggestive of malignancy	• Solid mass with several typical features of malignancy • Mass with suspicious microcalcifications • Linear-branching microcalcifications	90–100%	Pathologic evaluation (CNB or VAB)
Overall BI-RADS† 6	Pathologically verified breast cancer by CNB or VAB	Not applicable	100%	Initiation of appropriate definitive therapy

* Size increase or development of suspicious features at follow-up examination results in an upgrading of the BI-RADS category. Stability of solid lesion features and size results in downgrading the BI-RADS category.

† At the end of the diagnostic chain (clinical exam, mammography, US, MR mammography, percutaneous biopsy), the final diagnosis is stated in the medical report and given an overall BI-RADS category 1–6.

5

5

	Morphology		
Distribution	Typically benign	Intermediate concern	Higher probability of malignancy
Diffuse/ scattered	2	3	4B
Grouped or clustered (<2 cm²)	3	4A	4C
Regional	4A	4B	4C
Segmental	4A	4C	4C
Linear/ branching	4B	4C	5

Fig. 5.3 Matrix to assess suspiciousness of microcalcifications according to Müller-Schimpfle. The x-axis shows increasing suspiciousness of morphology to the right. The y-axis shows increasing suspiciousness of distribution toward the bottom. The corresponding BI-RADS classification is indicated at the crossing.

Basic Principles of Stereology

The design of all stereotactic breast intervention systems is the same. They must provide for breast positioning and compression, acquisition of scout and stereo x-ray-images, determining and transferring target coordinates, and guiding the needle/biopsy instrument to the exact target position.

Lesion depth. The principle for determining the depth of a target lesion is the same for all stereotactic systems. First, a scout image demonstrating the abnormality in the biopsy window is acquired. Then, two images are acquired at +15° and –15° angles to form the stereo pair (**Fig. 5.4**).

The resulting shift of a target reference point on these images is proportional to the lesion depth (position in the z-axis): the further away an abnormality is from the image detector, the greater the distance of the abnormality shift is in the stereo pair. Knowing the angle at which the x-ray tube is pivoted for acquiring the stereo pair (+15° and –15°), modern digital systems automatically calculate the depth of an abnormality based on the tangent function of the right triangle shown in **Fig. 5.5**.

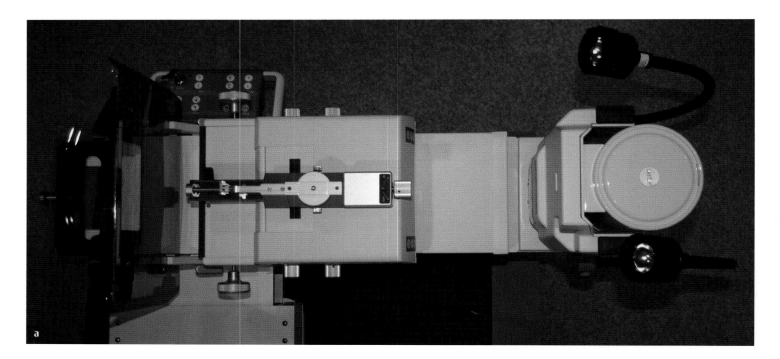

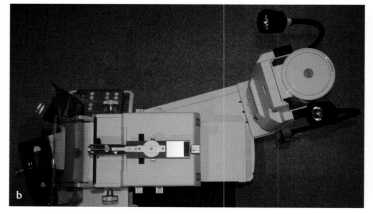

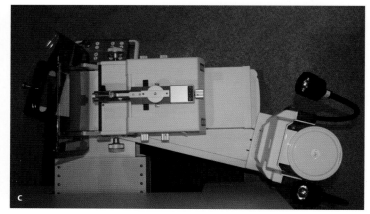

Fig. 5.4a–c Stereotactic table viewed from above (without patient padding). X-ray tube in neutral, 0° position (**a**), and after pivoting 15° to the right (**b**) and left (**c**).

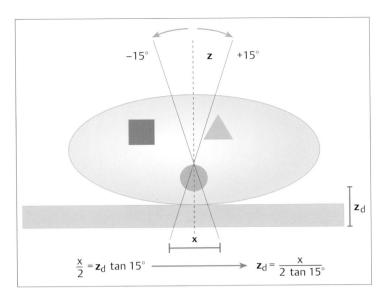

$$\frac{x}{2} = z_d \tan 15° \longrightarrow z_d = \frac{x}{2 \tan 15°}$$

Fig. 5.5 Lesion depth. The displacement of a lesion in the image plane (x) by pivoting the x-ray tube ± 15° correlates to the distance of the lesion from the detector (z_d).

Stroke margin. Modern stereotactic biopsy systems also monitor the stroke margin. The stroke margin is the distance between the needle tip and the detector/breast support after firing the biopsy gun. When the stroke margin falls below the tolerance value, firing the biopsy gun runs the risk of injuring breast tissue and skin on the distal breast surface, as well as damaging the unit detector. This can be a painful and expensive undertaking.

Calculation of the stroke margin requires knowledge of the needle tip's end position after firing. Because this is dependent upon the needle length and stroke—and the stroke of different biopsy needles varies—the unit must be programmed accordingly to ensure accuracy. This can be accomplished in different ways. Most equipment manufacturers provide a computer file containing all available needle lengths for selection at the beginning of an intervention. Alternatively, the needle tip position can be calibrated using a notch and bead sight. Using this method, the target cannot be marked before calibration has been completed.

Calibration. Verification of the accuracy of the stereotactic system's calibration is performed daily or prior to use by comparing the correct or standard measurements assigned to a point in space with the measurements made by the stereotactic system. Each stereotactic system has its own specific add-on calibration target. A consistency check must be performed once a month.

To test the Lorad table (**Fig. 5.6a**), a calibration needle is first set to the zero position in the notch and bead sight. Then the x-, y-, and z-coordinates are manually set at 10, 20, and 30 mm. The needle tip is marked in the stereo pair images and the coordinates shown by the stereotactic unit must match these values.

The Fischer table (**Fig. 5.6b**) uses a phantom with needle tips that are localized stereotactically. Correct calibration is indicated by the exact agreement of the phantom and biopsy needle tip positions.

Specific Patient Information

Before beginning the procedure, the patient must be informed in detail about what she may expect. Most are especially surprised to hear that the greatest problem they will probably encounter is having to lay still in the prone position for 30–45 minutes. Explaining the procedure steps gives the patient a feeling of security and helps the patient to maintain the patience required for the procedure. The need for repeated x-ray imaging to check the needle position as well as the necessity of harvesting multiple samples should be discussed. It is also important to reaffirm that no anticoagulant medication such as aspirin or coumarin derivatives have been taken, and to ascertain whether the patient has had prior allergic reactions to local anesthetics, adhesive bandages, and nickel (localization wire, clip). The patient should be informed about possible complications such as bleeding, infection, and allergic reactions. Note that after the intervention, the biopsy area will be cooled and compressed for approx. 30 minutes. If microcalcifications are to be biopsied, the patient should know that the tissue cores will be radiographed to ensure that they contain the calcifications sampled, and that this signifies correct sampling.

It is advisable to demonstrate the noises associated with firing the biopsy gun and harvesting the biopsy cores before beginning the procedure.

Possible problems. Certain situations can create problems for performing stereotactic interventions and should be discussed with the patient when appropriate. These include (1) the *thin breast*, which is not of sufficient compressed width to accept the length of the needle throw; (2) *very fine microcalcifications*, which are sometimes difficult to detect on stereo images, and (3) the *mass lesion*, which is sometimes difficult to target appropriately for correct coordinate calculation. In particular, lesions near the chest wall or skin can make a stereotactic intervention difficult to perform.

Stereotactic Vacuum-assisted Biopsy

Vacuum-assisted biopsy (VAB) is the standard method for performing a stereotactic biopsy. Instead of acquiring tissue samples by a spring-loaded movement of the biopsy needle (large core biopsy), vacuum biopsy instruments suction tissue into a side notch (sampling chamber), and depending on the biopsy system, shear the specimen by slowly advancing the rotating inner or outer cutting cannula (**Fig. 5.7**). The biopsy specimen is then either transported by vacuum through the cannula to the specimen collection chamber, or removed from the breast with the needle through a coaxial introduction needle. The main advantages of VAB are that a larger tissue volume is removed, and that the sampling notch can be rotated 360° so that multiple contiguous cores can be obtained around the centrally located needle. Professional associations recommend obtaining ≥ 12 samples when using an 11-gauge needle.

VAB has a higher sensitivity than core biopsy in the stereotactic diagnostic work-up of suspicious microcalcifications. This is due to sampling error encountered when performing a core biopsy of microcalcifications (**Fig. 5.8**). Because conventional core biopsy obtains noncontiguous cores of tissue, it is possible for the separate cores to miss passing through the tissue containing the target calcifications.

5

5

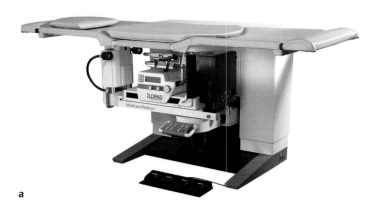

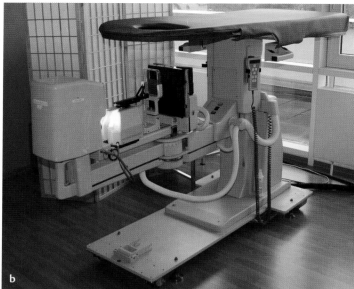

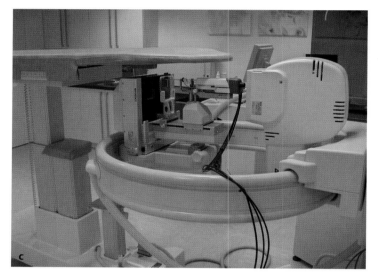

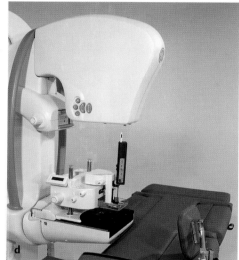

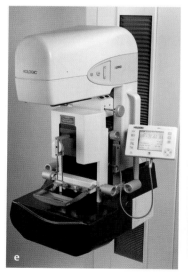

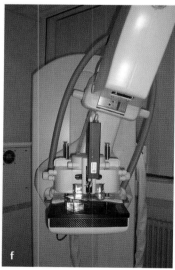

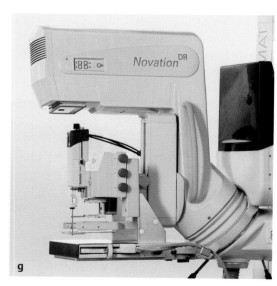

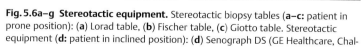

Fig. 5.6a–g Stereotactic equipment. Stereotactic biopsy tables (**a–c:** patient in prone position): (**a**) Lorad table, (**b**) Fischer table, (**c**) Giotto table. Stereotactic equipment (**d:** patient in inclined position): (**d**) Senograph DS (GE Healthcare, Chalfont St., Giles, UK). Stereotactic equipment (**e–g:** patient in sitting position): (**e**) Selenia Digital Mammography (Hologic, Bedford, MA), (**f**) Senograph DS, (**g**) Siemens Novation (Siemens Medical Solutions, Erlangen, Germany).

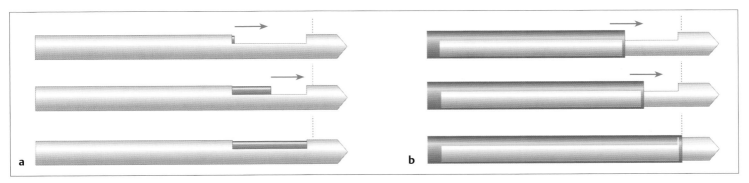

Fig. 5.7a, b Sampling method for two different vacuum-assisted devices. After vacuum suction pulls the breast tissue into the sample notch of the biopsy needle, the rotating cutter shears the specimen from the adjacent tissue. The Mammotome (Ethicon Endo-Surgery, Cincinnati, OH) and ATEC systems (Suros Surgical Systems, Inc., Indianapolis, IN) have an inner rotating cutting stylet (**a**). The Vacora system (Bard Biopsy Systems, Tempe, AZ) has an outer cutting cannula (**b**).

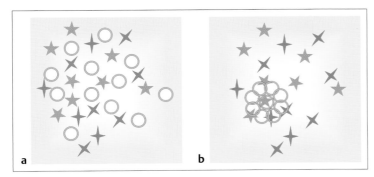

Fig. 5.8a, b Sampling error. Large CNB of microcalcifications with sampling error (**a**). Vacuum biopsy obtains representative samples containing microcalcifications by acquiring contiguous specimens around central needle position (**b**). (Circles = biopsy cores, stars = microcalcifications).

Indications and Goals

The most common indications for the performance of VAB are mammographic findings in the BI-RADS categories 4 and 5 that do not have a correlating ultrasound (US) finding. With the carcinoma risk of these lesions ranging from 2 to 100%, one cannot forgo histologic assessment. Occasionally, findings in the BI-RADS category 3 are also subjected to biopsy (e.g., patient wishes).

The main indication for performing a stereotactic VAB is the histologic assessment of suspicious microcalcifications. The goal of performing stereotactic VAB is to avoid unnecessary surgery when ambiguous imaging findings are found to be benign on histology, and to verify a breast cancer diagnosis for optimal preparation before definitive treatment. In rare cases, VAB can be used to completely excise small borderline lesions, avoiding the need for surgical excision.

European S3 Guidelines for the Performance of Percutaneous Breast Biopsies

Percutaneous breast biopsy is indicated for histologic assessment of imaging findings in the BI-RADS categories 4 and 5. The goal is to verify breast cancer for better planning before definitive therapy is initiated, as well as to rule out cancer and avoid unnecessary open surgery for lesions of benign histology.

ACR Practice Guidelines for the Performance of Percutaneous Breast Biopsies

Indications for percutaneous breast biopsies include, but are not limited to, the following: lesions assessed as highly suggestive of malignancy (BI-RADS Category 5) to confirm the diagnosis so that definitive treatment options can be selected; lesions assessed as suspicious abnormalities (BI-RADS Category 4); multiple suspicious masses, particularly in a multicentric distribution to facilitate treatment planning; and lesions assessed as probably benign (BI-RADS Category 3) when there are valid clinical indications, rebiopsy when initial biopsy results are discordant with the imaging assessment.

Suspicious microcalcifications. Microcalcifications constitute the most common indication for the performance of stereotactic VAB. Usually, there is no correlating finding on US. Taking into account that the average positive predictive value (PPV) is 40% for microcalcifications in the BI-RADS categories 4 and 5, it is indispensable that the indication for performing open surgery be verified by prior percutaneous biopsy. Specimen radiography allows the peri-interventional verification of successful sampling. Confirmation of target calcifications in the biopsy cores substantiates that the sample is representative.

Mass lesions. Aside from microcalcifications, mass lesions detected on mammography are another indication for stereotactic biopsy, provided they are not seen on US. It is recommended that biopsy be performed as a VAB. In justified cases, however, it may be performed as an automated core needle biopsy (CNB). When there is the possibility that the whole mass lesion may be removed by the needle biopsy procedure, a clip marker should be placed at the biopsy site.

The stereotactic determination of a mass lesion's depth is sometimes very difficult. In contrast to the situation when biopsying microcalcifications, where a calcification can be singled out to serve as a target, choosing a reference point in the +15° and −15° stereo images of a mass lesion is not possible if no distinguishing mark can be identified.

Architectural distortion. Architectural distortions can also be percutaneously biopsied by means of a stereotactic VAB. If histology reveals a radial scar, open biopsy is warranted because there is a possible association with carcinoma development, usually of the tubular type, in the periphery of such lesions.

Density. A density, which is seen in only one mammographic projection, is a special case. After it is imaged in the scout view, it is usually also discernible in the +15° and –15° stereo images, making it subject to percutaneous biopsy.

Materials

Mammotome biopsy system. The Mammotome biopsy system (Ethicon Endo-Surgery, Cincinnati, OH) was introduced in the late 1990s and was the first vacuum biopsy system on the market. In contrast to the devices used for US-guided and MRI-guided interventions, the needle holder of the stereotactic VAB device is equipped with a spring-loading mechanism (**Fig. 5.9a**). Once the needle has been placed in the holder and advanced to the target position, a vacuum is created by an external vacuum pump connected to the probe by tubing. After the biopsy specimens are sheared from the breast, they are transported inside the needle to the specimen collection chamber and retrieved (**Fig. 5.9b**). After rotating the needle, the cutting procedure is repeated and the next specimen harvested without having to remove the biopsy needle from the breast.

Vacora system. The Vacora system (Bard Biopsy Systems, Tempe, AZ) is a very compact system that can be used for all image-guided VABs without requiring modification (**Fig. 5.10**). This system has an internal spring-loading mechanism and vac-

uum pump. Because the specimens must be retrieved after each sampling by removing the biopsy needle from the breast, a coaxial introduction needle is used. For stereotactic interventions, the system uses a needle guide onto which the coaxial introduction needle is mounted to facilitate the repeated removal and replacement of the biopsy device.

ATEC system. When used for performing a stereotactic biopsy, the ATEC (automated tissue excision and collection) system (Suros Surgical Systems, Inc., Indianapolis, IN) is mounted onto a special spring-loading fixture, which allows the needle to be fired into the breast (**Fig. 5.11a, b**). Once the needle is placed in the desired position, the biopsy can be performed rapidly by manually rotating the biopsy device after each specimen cutting and retrieving all specimens at the end of the procedure from the specimen collection chamber (**Fig. 5.11c**). As for the Mammotome device, the vacuum is created by an external vacuum pump.

All VAB units have special fixtures with which they can be mounted onto the different stereotactic biopsy systems.

Procedure

Access path and patient positioning. Before beginning a stereotactic VAB, it is necessary to have a mammography examination of the affected breast in two orthogonal views available (**Fig. 5.12a–d**). Knowing the exact location of the target abnor-

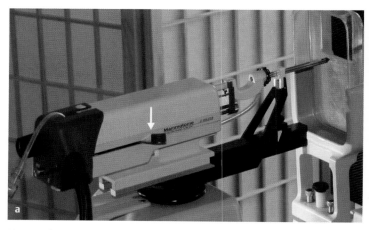
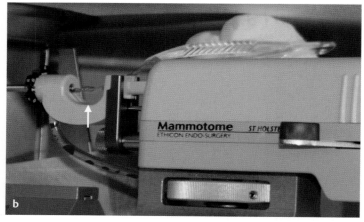

Fig. 5.9a, b Mammotome system (Ethicon Endo-Surgery, Cincinnati, OH). VAB needle holder for stereotactic biopsy. Cocking lever for the jet mechanism is seen on the side of the system (arrow) (**a**). Specimen collection window for specimen retrieval (arrow) (**b**).

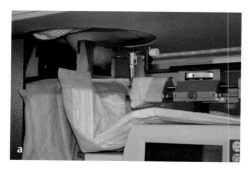
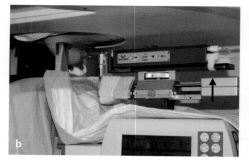
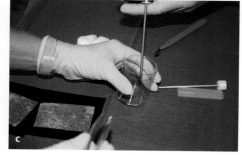

Fig. 5.10a–c Vacora stereotactic vacuum biopsy device (Bard Biopsy Systems, Tempe, AZ).
a Special fixture with needle guide for fastening coaxial introduction needle, and gun-carrier for the introduction and removal of the biopsy unit during the procedure.

b Vacora biopsy unit mounted on carrier. Tilt lever at back end of biopsy unit fastens the system in place (arrow).
c Specimen retrieval after each cutting process. Release of the specimen into a plastic receptacle protects against blood splattering.

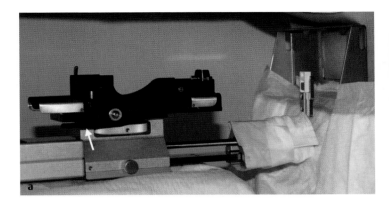

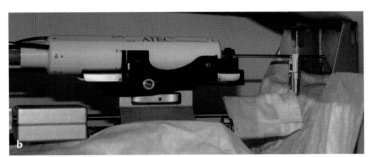

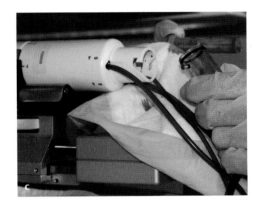

Fig. 5.11 a–c ATEC stereotactic vacuum biopsy device (Suros Surgical Systems, Inc., Indianapolis, IN).
a Special fixture with spring mechanism for jet advancement of needle. Cocking lever is seen on the side of the system (arrow).
b ATEC system mounted on carrier. Tubing attachments to external vacuum pump.
c Removal of specimen retrieval chamber at the end of completed biopsy procedure.

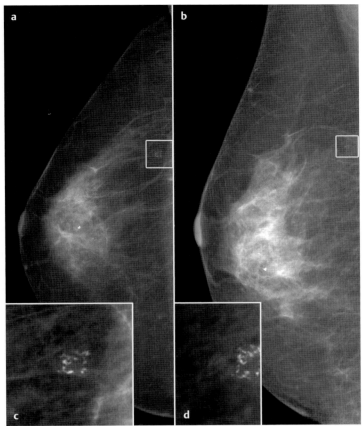

Fig. 5.12 a–d Stereotactic biopsy procedure.
a, b Mammography images. Right CC (**a**). Right LM (**b**). Microcalcifications in lateral aspect of the breast, approx. 10 o' clock.
c, d Magnified detail views. **e–m** See p. 52.

mality guides the procedure. The needle approach, for example, must be chosen such that the target does not lie too close to the proximal skin surface, which might cause problems in creating a vacuum (sample notch not completely in the breast). On the other hand, the target abnormality should not lie too close to the detector/breast support, which could forbid firing the biopsy gun (stroke margin). As a rule, excessively long access paths should be avoided to prevent needle deviation or dislocation of the target lesion.

The target location on mammography may also make it evident that special patient positioning is necessary to access the abnormality. Target abnormalities very near the lateral aspect of the chest wall, for example, might make it advisable to elevate the contralateral side when positioning the patient on the table.

After analysis of the two-view mammography (CC and ML/LM), the physician and technologist select the appropriate plane for breast compression and decide where to place the biopsy window (**Fig. 5.12e, f**). If possible, it is preferable to avoid a needle approach in the upper medial quadrant of the breast (scar in cleavage).

Targeting the abnormality. Obtaining a scout image with adequate visualization and centering of the abnormality in the biopsy window is an essential step in the stereotactic procedure (C-arm is perpendicular to the image receptor = 0°). If the abnormality is not detected in the first scout image, the image must be carefully analyzed to reposition the biopsy window appropriately and then repeat the scout image until a final working image is obtained (**Fig. 5.12g**). Technically, this process is similar to performing a magnification image in which the abnormality must also be depicted in the partial view. Once an appropriate scout image has been obtained, the next procedure step is to acquire two images by pivoting the C-arm to +15° and –15°, forming the stereo pair for calculation of the target depth. It is then critical to accurately identify and mark the same point in both (planar) stereo images with the cursor (**Fig. 5.12h, i**). The unit's computer then calculates the appropriate coordinates and transfers them to the needle guidance system.

Tips and Tricks

Always compare the abnormality depth with the indicated breast thickness. Make sure that the entire sample notch of the vacuum biopsy needle can be placed within the breast. Rule out a subcutaneous position or position too near the detector/breast support (stroke margin).

5

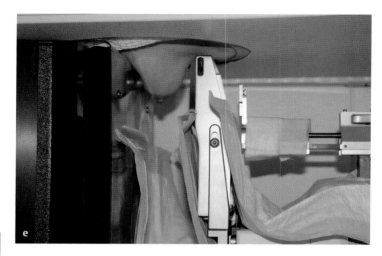

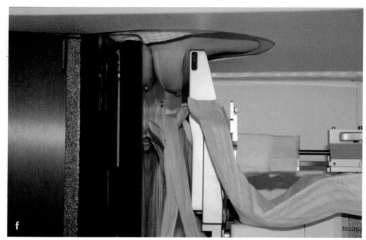

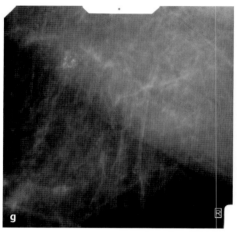

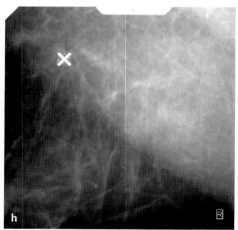

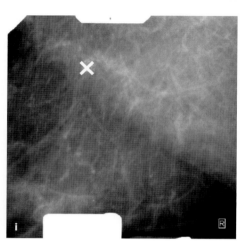

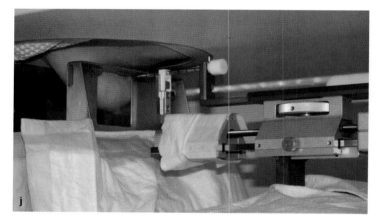

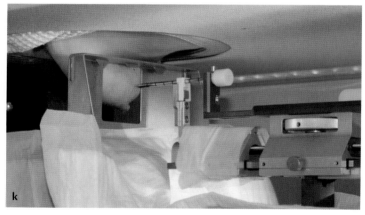

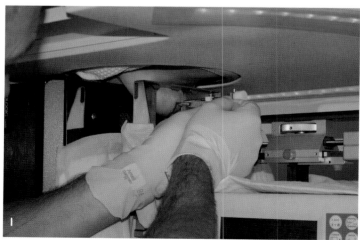

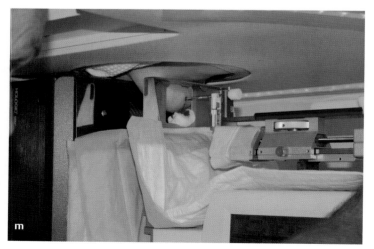

Fig. 5.12e–m

e, f Patient positioning for stereotactic VAB. Positioning in the selected plane for biopsy (**e**). Positioning of biopsy window and immobilization by applying adequate compression (**f**).

g Visualization of microcalcifications.

h, i Appropriate placement of cursors in stereo images.

j, k Calibration of coaxial introduction needle length (**j**) and guidance to calculated x,y position (**k**).

l, m Local anesthesia and nick incision (**l**). Coaxial introduction needle in prefire position (**m**).

n–w See p. 53.

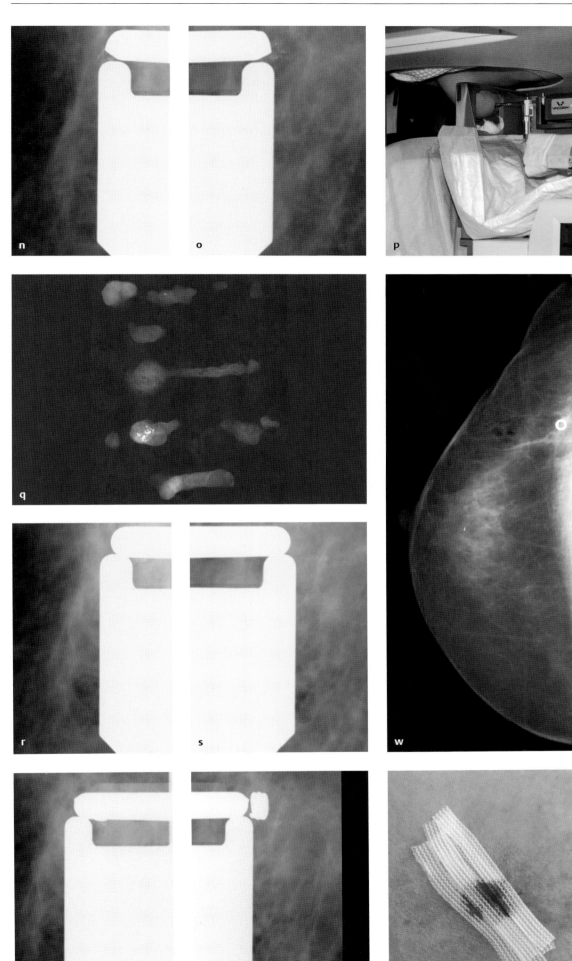

Fig. 5.12n–w
n, o Prefire images.
p Jet-advancement of vacuum biopsy needle and specimen acquisition.
q Specimen radiography.
r, s Postbiopsy images.
t, u Localization coil, placed after biopsy.
v Adhesive strips.
w Mammography in CC projection after biopsy.

5

Needle placement. The extremely expensive sterile working materials should only be opened after the feasibility of performing the intervention is certain. At this time, the patient can be familiarized with the noises she will be hearing during the examination (needle firing, vacuum, and cutting noises). Before beginning the examination on the Lorad stereotactic table, the needle is placed in the needle guide for calibration. After positioning the needle tip in line with the notch and bead sight located in the upper part of the compression plate, calibration is performed (**Fig. 5.12j**). The needle can then be moved to the calculated target coordinates in the x- and y-axes (**Fig. 5.12k**). The needle is carefully advanced toward the skin to indicate the site of needle insertion for disinfection and administration of local anesthesia. Once anesthesia is effected, a small skin incision of approx. 3–5 mm is made to allow smooth passage of the biopsy needle (**Fig. 5.12l**). The biopsy needle is then advanced to the appropriate depth (**Fig. 5.12 m**). Some stereotactic systems signal if the stroke margin falls below the tolerance value when advancing the needle to the appropriate z-coordinate value.

Tips and Tricks

An adequate skin incision of 3–5 mm is important to allow smooth needle advancement and avoid skin drag, which could displace breast tissues and the target lesion.

Prefire stereo images (+15° and –15°) are acquired to ensure correct needle placement and to check for abnormality movement (**Fig. 5.12n, o**). The anterior needle guide should be retracted to prevent superimposition over the area of interest. If the needle position is not correct, the error must be analyzed. If necessary, the target can be marked anew on the last stereo pair, and the coordinate calculations redone.

Sample harvesting. The trigger button is pushed to fire the needle forward only after ensuring that the prefire needle position is correct, the stroke margin is positive, and the anterior needle guide is forward. The direction in which the first samples are harvested is sometimes influenced by the position of the target lesion in relation to the needle. Generally, the sample notch is rotated in the closed position to acquire contiguous samples: e.g., 12, 1, 2, 3, to 11 o'clock. An alternate approach (our philosophy) is 12, 2, 4, 6, 8, and 10 o'clock, then 1, 3, 5, 7, 9, and 11 o'clock (**Fig. 5.12p**). The harvesting of tissue samples normally causes little discomfort. Additional anesthetic can be given through the biopsy or coaxial introduction needle should a patient experience pain.

Good Practice Recommendations[*]

VABs typically use 11- to 9-gauge needles.
When using an 11-gauge needle, ≥ 12 tissue specimens should be acquired. When using larger gauge needles, the volume equivalent number of tissue specimens should be acquired.
[*]European S3 guideline: Early Breast Cancer Detection

If microcalcifications have been biopsied, specimen radiography is performed after acquiring the first 6 or 12 samples (**Fig. 5.12q**). If the target calcifications are detected in the core samples, then this is confirmation of representative sampling. If no calcifications are detected, then the source of error must be located: Was the correct needle selected (Fischer table)? Is the target lesion visible in the postfire stereo images (+15° and –15°)? Can the target lesion be accessed by taking additional samples in the appropriate direction (clock time)? Are microcalcifications visible in the specimen radiography of these additional samples? If not, restarting the examination from the beginning should be considered.

Clip/coil marking. A poststudy stereo image documentation (+15° and –15°) with the needle in place is performed to verify a successful biopsy (**Fig. 5.12r, s**). At least a partial removal of radiographic evidence of the abnormality should be perceptible. If the target lesion has been completely excised, a clip or coil marker should be placed in the biopsy cavity (**Fig. 5.12t, u**). These markers are especially easy to place when the biopsy was performed using a coaxial introduction needle. After removal of the biopsy needle, the clip or coil can be introduced through the coaxial cannula. When using single needle biopsy systems, there are specialized pushers available for each system that release the marker through the side notch.

Tips and Tricks

After releasing the clip or coil into the breast through the side notch of the biopsy needle, rotate the sample notch 180° before removing the needle from the breast. This prevents the marker from getting caught in the notch and being dislocated when withdrawing the needle.

Completion of the intervention. When the intervention has been completed, the needle is removed from the breast. The biopsy area is then compressed using a sterile swab, and the compression plate retracted. Now the patient is allowed to move. Once the table has been lowered, the patient can sit up and leave the stereotactic table.

A reclining chair should be made available to the patient for subsequent compression and cooling of the area for approximately 30 minutes. The resulting vasoconstriction should prevent relevant bleeding i.e., a large hematoma. The cold pack used should be wrapped in a hand towel or cloth for hygienic reasons. To prevent the patient's hand from getting cold, an additional towel can be placed over the cold pack. After approximately 30 minutes of compression, when bleeding has ceased, adhesive skin closure strips and a sterile bandage are applied (**Fig. 5.12v**).

Finally, a postintervention documentation (mammographic images in two orthogonal planes: CC and ML/LM) should be performed (**Fig. 5.12w**).

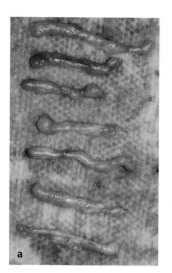
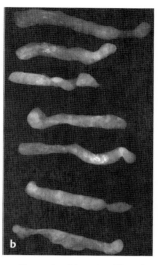
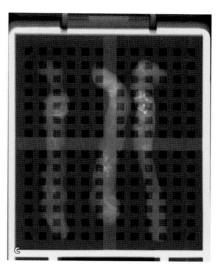
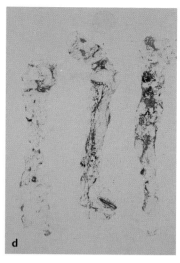

Fig. 5.13a–d Comparison of specimen radiograph with stained histologic section. Biopsy core specimens and specimen radiograph documenting microcalcifications and representative tissue harvesting (**a, b**). Core samples are separated into those with and without microcalcifications. Specimen radiograph of tissue cassette containing biopsy cores with microcalcifications (**c**). Stained histologic specimen. Embedded slice corresponds to specimen radiograph (**d**).

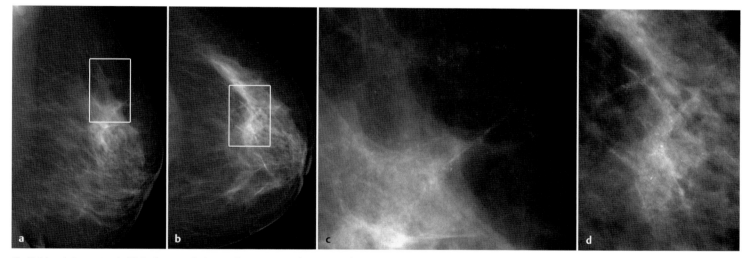

Fig. 5.14a–d Stereotactic VAB of a mass lesion. Left mammography in CC and LM projection (**a, b**). Close-up views (**c, d**): Mass lesion in the upper middle aspect of the left breast with bordering pleomorphic microcalcifications in linear distribution. **e–p** See p. 56.

Specimen radiography of microcalcifications. When the target lesion contains microcalcifications, specimen radiography is an important part of the biopsy procedure. Of all target lesions biopsied by a minimally invasive technique, this is the only case in which the suspicious abnormality biopsied can be demonstrated in an image of the acquired specimens. A specimen radiograph showing target microcalcifications is documentation of correct sample harvesting. To detect even the smallest microcalcifications, magnification specimen radiography should always be performed.

Specimens containing microcalcifications are then placed in separate tissue cassettes from those without microcalcifications for pathologic assessment. To optimize the histologic examination, the specimen radiograph should be submitted to the pathologist along with the specimens because these remain in the same position during embedding. In the age of digital mammography, this data can also be sent to the pathologist via the Internet, or sent along with the specimens on a rewritable data carrier, such as a USB-stick. As a rule, imaging information about the extent and distribution of microcalcifications in the specimens is helpful to the pathologist in detecting these under the microscope (**Fig. 5.13**).

In extremely rare cases, performing a frozen section procedure on specimens acquired by VAB may be justified. It is not, however, recommended for the pathologic assessment of tissue containing microcalcifications because the tissue samples may be lost or rendered noninterpretable due to the mechanical resistance of the calcifications during microtome slicing, possibly resulting in a false-negative histology.

Mass lesions and architectural distortions. Occasionally, stereotactic VAB is performed as part of the diagnostic work-up of mass lesions. Calculation of the mass depth is often problematic if it is not possible to identify a unique point within the abnormality to target in both stereo images (±15°). Marking a recognizable structure on the edge of the mass lesion is recommended in such cases, and then manually move the needle to the mass center after targeting (**Fig. 5.14**).

Architectural distortions can also be subjected to stereotactic VAB for diagnostic work-up. The stereotactic calculation of the

5

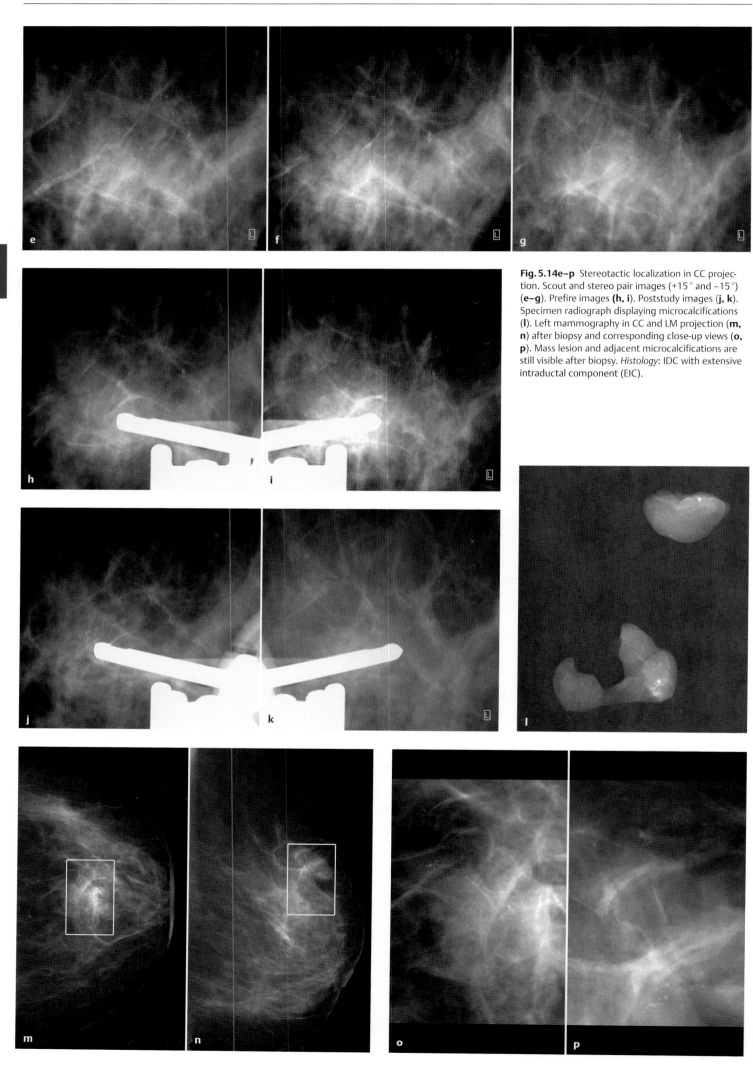

Fig. 5.14e–p Stereotactic localization in CC projection. Scout and stereo pair images (+15° and −15°) (**e–g**). Prefire images (**h, i**). Poststudy images (**j, k**). Specimen radiograph displaying microcalcifications (**l**). Left mammography in CC and LM projection (**m, n**) after biopsy and corresponding close-up views (**o, p**). Mass lesion and adjacent microcalcifications are still visible after biopsy. *Histology*: IDC with extensive intraductal component (EIC).

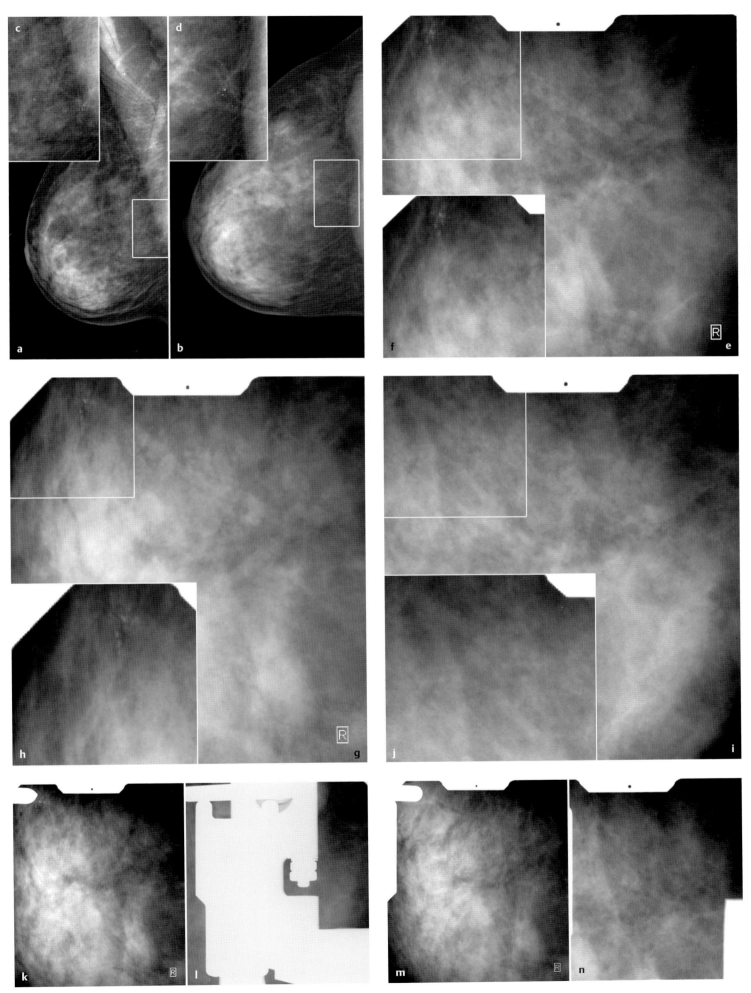

Fig. 5.15a–o Legend see p. 58.

5

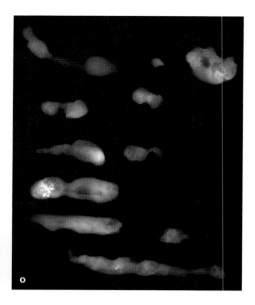

Fig. 5.15a–o Stereotactic calculations based on the 0°- and one stereo (+ or −15°) image ("target on scout"). Right mammography in LM and CC projection (**a, b**). Microcalcifications near the chest wall in close-up views (**c, d**). Scout image (**e**) with close-up view (**f**). −15° stereo image shows microcalcifications (**g**), close-up view (**h**). +15° stereo image shows no microcalcifications (**i**), close-up view (**j**). ± 15° prefire images (**k, l**). −15° and 0° poststudy images reveal complete removal of microcalcifications (**m, n**). Specimen radiograph (**o**).

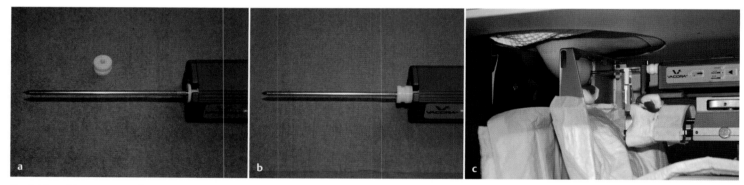

Fig. 5.16a–c Vacora vacuum biopsy needle (Bard Biopsy Systems, Tempe, AZ).
a Spacer ring and biopsy needle.
b Spacer ring in place.

c Biopsy with spacer ring in use.

lesion depth is usually unproblematic for these abnormalities because they contain a distinguishable center, which can easily be targeted in the stereo images.

Problems and solutions. If the needle position does not allow a sufficient stroke margin—the calculated postfire needle tip position is too close to the detector/breast support—then needle advancement can be triggered after retracting the biopsy instrument to a position 2–3 mm before the calculated prefire position. After firing, the needle can then manually be advanced to the correct position.

If the target abnormality is identified in only one of the two stereo images, the stereotactic depth calculations can be based on the one 15° and the 0° image ("target on scout") (**Fig. 5.15**).

If a breast is too thin to accept the biopsy needle excursion from the pre- to the postfire position, i.e., to contain the lateral sample notch and needle tip, there are two options available to allow the intervention to be performed despite this. First, when using the Vacora VAB system, the penetration depth can be reduced by 1 cm by placing a spacer ring onto the needle (**Fig. 5.16**). Consequently, the sample notch is partially within the breast and partially within the coaxial sheath and therefore shortened by 1 cm. The second option is feasible when using the Fischer stereotactic table or the Senographe XR system (GE Healthcare, Chalfont St., Giles, UK) and requires the use of a lateral arm. This allows imaging the abnormality in one projection

and introducing the biopsy needle between the compression plate and the breast support (**Fig. 5.17**). A lateral arm for the Lorad stereotactic table is in development, but has not yet been approved.

The Mammotome biopsy system makes it possible to biopsy abnormalities that lie directly under the skin. The Mammotome sample chamber can be placed so that half is in the breast. The other half can then be covered with a plastic clip-on cover so that the unit can still create a vacuum (**Fig. 5.18**). When performing a biopsy in this way, a greater skin defect should be expected.

When using a dedicated stereotactic biopsy table, if the biopsy window cannot be placed over the abnormality because of its position very near the chest wall, the affected breast and the ipsilateral arm can be placed through the table opening. This is especially helpful for lesions localized in the outer quadrants of the breast. When using the Fischer table, which has an inclined needle approach to the breast, injury to the chest wall is theoretically possible. For this reason, it is especially important to double check whether the intervention is feasible when the patient has been atypically positioned.

Histologic findings and postbiopsy procedure. The stereotactic VAB report should contain details about the size and position of the target abnormality, the size and position of the biopsy defect, as well as the relation between the target abnormality and the

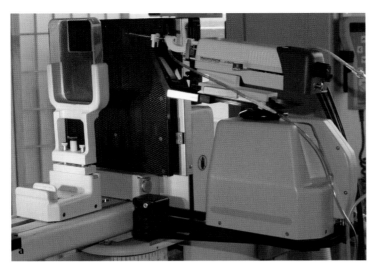
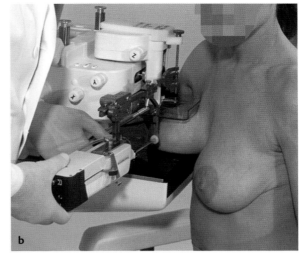

Fig. 5.17a, b Lateral arm.
a Fischer stereotactic table with lateral arm attachment.
b Senograph XR table with lateral arm attachment.

5

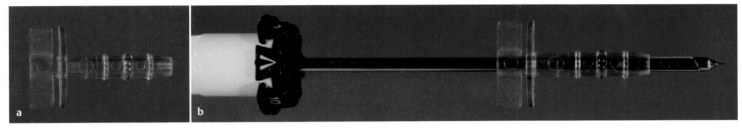

Fig. 5.18a, b Clip-on cover. Plastic clip-on cover for Mammotome biopsy needle (Ethicon Endo-Surgery, Cincinnati, OH) (**a**), in place (**b**).

biopsy cavity. If no residual abnormality can be visualized, its complete removal should be indicated in the report.

An interdisciplinary consultation should be held to correlate imaging with histology after each VAB. When microcalcifications have been biopsied, for example, it is important that these are mentioned in the histology report. If correlation is confirmed, then the biopsy is considered representative. If correlation is questionable, the VAB can be repeated, or an open biopsy performed. An interdisciplinary conference is recommended for planning the follow-up resection for malignancies or borderline findings (e.g., atypical ductal hyperplasia [ADH]).

Tips and Tricks

If there is a discrepancy between the assessment of microcalcifications on mammography and the histologic result, the histology report should be checked for the mention of microcalcifications.

To avoid serious consequences as a result of diagnostic error, it is recommended that a follow-up imaging examination be performed 6 months after every intervention with benign histology.

Good Practice Recommendations: Stereotactic Vacuum-assisted Biopsy**

Indication: To verify breast cancer for better planning before definitive therapy is initiated, as well as to rule out cancer and avoid unnecessary open surgery for findings in the BI-RADS categories 4 and 5.
Procedure:
1. Before beginning a stereotactic VAB, a CC and a strict ML or LM view should be available for exact spatial orientation.

2. The approach for access to the abnormality (e.g., CC, LM, oblique 30°, 45°, 60°) and the stroke margin should be documented (if not already automatically digitally documented).
3. The stereotactic depth calculation should be cross-checked by comparison with the prestudy mammograms. The recorded values are helpful in the case of later stereotactic localization or follow-up resection.
4. VAB of microcalcifications: acquisition of ≥12 tissue cylinders when using an 11-gauge needle. When using a larger caliber needle, the volume equivalent number of tissue cylinders should be harvested. Magnification specimen radiography should be performed. Representative calcifications should be confirmed. If applicable, core samples with microcalcifications should be separated from those without for the pathologist. Poststudy mammograms in two views should be performed.
5. The objective is to acquire representative tissue material from ambiguous abnormalities. If histology reveals invasive malignancy, noninvasive malignancy, or ADH, definitive therapy always includes re-resection by open surgery.
6. The following is required documentation:
   – scout view (0°), stereo pair (+15° and –15°)
   – prefire pair (+15° and –15°)
   – postfire pair (+15° and –15°)*
7. After the biopsy procedure has been completed (or on the following workday at the latest), a poststudy mammogram in two orthogonal views should be performed to confirm correct sampling depth and to provide a basis for preoperative localization if malignancy has been proven.

* *Author's note*: Performing a postfire stereo pair is not necessary under normal circumstances. However, one should not refrain from performing a poststudy stereo pair before removing the biopsy needle if the possibility exists that the radiographic evidence of the target lesion has been completely removed. This information is crucial for deciding on whether or not to place a marker coil/clip.

Procedure description: (± sketch)
Report of compression plane/angle, approach (from medial, lateral, cranial, caudal), needle to detector/breast support distance (stroke margin), and compressed breast thickness.

- Statement about complications, if applicable
- Statement about whether or not biopsy is representative
- Therapy recommendation in dependence upon histology (after consultation/interdisciplinary conference with the pathologist and taking one's own targeting accuracy into account)

Documentation:

- Stereotactic images from two angles without the biopsy needle (stereo pair)
- Stereotactic images from two angles with the biopsy needle before the abnormality (prefire)
- Stereotactic images from two angles with the biopsy needle in the abnormality (postfire)
- Mammography in two orthogonal planes after biopsy

Postbiopsy procedure: For findings in the following pathology reporting categories:

- B1 or B2: Short-term follow-up in 6 months (in special cases earlier)
- B3 or B4: Interdisciplinary conference to decide on the course of action (follow-up, rebiopsy, surgery)
- B5a or B5b: Initiation of appropriate therapy

Documentation and evaluation: Acquisition of data for statistic analysis of all percutaneous biopsies.

- Short-term follow-up after 6 months for all biopsies with benign histology (follow-up mammography is preferably performed at the diagnosing facility)
- Interdisciplinary consultation is required for all ambiguous or discrepant findings

** European S3 guideline: Early Breast Cancer Detection

Checklist: Stereotactic Vacuum-assisted Biopsy

1. Establish indication (supplemental diagnostic procedure?).
2. Mammography in CC and ML projection.
3. Obtain informed consent (in advance).
4. Verify calibration of stereotactic system, set stroke of biopsy instrument (device-specific).
5. Position biopsy window over abnormality and obtain scout image (0°).
6. Identify target.
7. Acquire stereo pair (+15° and −15°) and identify target on at least one stereo image.
8. Target the abnormality for coordinate calculation, transfer coordinates to biopsy platform (confirm feasibility of performing the intervention).
9. Calibrate needle, if appropriate.
10. Disinfect breast skin and administer local anesthesia.
11. Demonstrate biopsy sounds.
12. Skin incision and placement of biopsy needle/coaxial introduction needle.
13. Obtain two prefire images (+15° and −15°, 0° if targeting on scout), correct needle position if necessary.
14. Fire biopsy needle.
15. Obtain tissue samples: ≥ 12 tissue cylinders with 11-gauge needle, or volume equivalent.
16. Perform magnification specimen radiography.
17. If necessary, harvest additional tissue samples after obtaining appropriate +15°,−15°, and/or 0° images for orientation.
18. Obtain postfire images (+15° and −15°, 0° if targeting on scout), if abnormality is completely excised: consider placing marker coil/clip.
19. Remove needle.
20. Release compression device and move patient to reclining chair, apply compression and cool the area.
21. Perform final mammograms in two orthogonal planes.

Core Needle Biopsy

Indications and Goals

Stereotactic large CNB should only be performed in rarely justified exceptional cases, e.g., large, sonographically occult masses. Normally, a 14-gauge needle is used for such cases. When biopsying microcalcifications or an architectural distortion, however, VAB is the method of choice. In special cases, when the lower costs and tissue trauma associated with core biopsy is of importance, it can be considered as an alternative.

Materials

There are several devices available that are specialized for the performance of large core breast biopsies. These consist of a hand piece with a spring mechanism, and a biopsy needle. The biopsy needle consists of an inner needle with a sampling chamber, and an outer cannula with a cutting edge. Devices are available as semi-automatic and fully automatic biopsy guns (see Chapter 7: Materials).

Semi-automatic biopsy needles. The inner stylet of a semi-automatic biopsy gun is manually advanced into the lesion or region of interest after loading the spring mechanism. Some needles provide the choice of a 1-cm or 2-cm penetration depth. By pushing a trigger button, the outer cutting cannula is rapidly advanced, cutting and capturing the specimen tissue, which is then be retrieved from the notch.

Automatic biopsy gun. In contrast to the semi-automatic units described above, these biopsy guns perform the steps after loading the spring mechanism and positioning the needle before the lesion in an automatic one-step operation. Here too, the penetration depth is variable. Fully automatic biopsy guns are available as complete sterile disposable systems, and as reusable systems (handgun) fitted with disposable sterile needles.

Procedure

Targeting the abnormality. The procedure for performing a stereotactic large CNB of a mammographic mass is the same in principle as that for performing a VAB of microcalcifications. To plan the procedure, the exact location of the target abnormality must be known, requiring prestudy mammograms in two orthogonal planes (CC and LM/ML). After verifying the calibration of the stereotactic unit, selecting the appropriate plane for breast compression and the stroke length, the patient is positioned appropriately and the biopsy window placed over the abnormality (**Fig. 5.19a**). Once an appropriate scout image has been obtained, the next procedure step is to acquire the stereo pair in +15° and −15° positions for calculation of the target depth (**Fig. 5.19b, c**). After marking the targets by mouse click in these images, the appropriate coordinates are calculated by the unit's computer. Calculation of the mass depth is problematic because often it is not possible to identify a unique point within the abnormality to target in both stereo images (± 15°). Calcifications within a mass facilitate the process enormously. If none are present, one should mark other recognizable structures, if necessary on the edge of the mass lesion. Later manual adjustment of

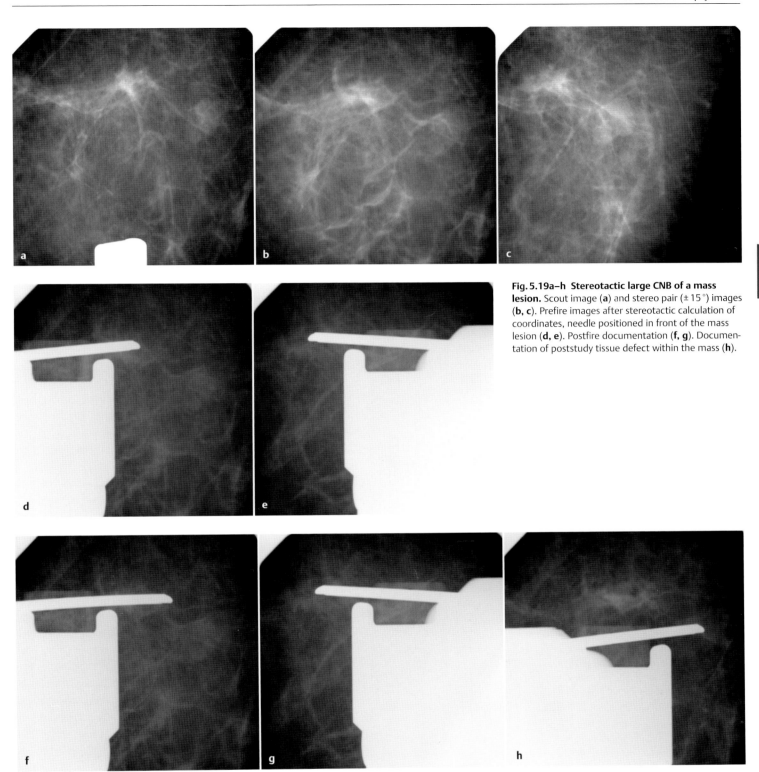

Fig. 5.19 a–h Stereotactic large CNB of a mass lesion. Scout image (**a**) and stereo pair (± 15°) images (**b, c**). Prefire images after stereotactic calculation of coordinates, needle positioned in front of the mass lesion (**d, e**). Postfire documentation (**f, g**). Documentation of poststudy tissue defect within the mass (**h**).

5

the needle position in the x- and y-axes is unproblematic. Once the mass depth has been calculated, then the x-, y-, and z-coordinates are transferred to the needle guidance system.

Needle placement and sample harvesting. If the stroke margin is positive (ample thickness for needle excursion), then the needle guide and coaxial introduction needle can be placed in the respective holders. At this time, the patient can be familiarized with the noise of firing the needle. With some units, the needle length must be calibrated (Lorad stereotactic table). With others, the needle length is calibrated and saved in a computer file (beware of correct needle selection). The needle can then be

moved to the calculated target coordinates in the x- and y-axes, indicating the site where local anesthesia is administered. A small skin incision is performed after skin disinfection. The coaxial introduction needle is then advanced to the appropriate depth (z-position) and prefire stereo images (+15° and –15°) are acquired (**Fig. 5.19 d, e**). If the mass lesion is correctly positioned in front of the needle tip in both images, then the loaded biopsy gun can be placed and secured into the holder and the needle fired into the breast. Postfire images should document that the needle is in the mass lesion (**Fig. 5.19 f, g**). The biopsy needle is then retracted from the breast through the coaxial introduction needle and the sample removed from the notch. The process of

5

sample harvesting is repeated at least four times when biopsying mass lesions. If microcalcifications have been targeted, specimen radiography should verify correct sampling. If no calcifications are visualized in the tissue cores, further sampling is required.

Completion of the intervention. When the intervention has been successfully completed, the coaxial introduction needle is removed from the breast. A poststudy documentation is recommended (**Fig. 5.19h**). The biopsy area is then manually compressed and the compression plate retracted. Now the patient is allowed to move and can sit up and leave the stereotactic table. Subsequent compression with a cold pack is applied for approx. 10 minutes. When bleeding has ceased, adhesive skin closure strips and a sterile bandage are applied.

Fine needle aspiration biopsy. Today, fine needle aspiration biopsy (FNAB) is mainly performed as a therapeutic and diagnostic measure for symptomatic cysts and in the evaluation of suspicious lymph nodes. Because these lesions are easily seen on US, there is no longer an indication for performing a stereotactic FNAB.

Checklist: Stereotactic Core Neeedle Biopsy

1. Establish indication (supplemental diagnostic procedure?).
2. Mammography in CC and ML projection.
3. Obtain informed consent (in advance).
4. Verify calibration of stereotactic system, set stroke of biopsy instrument (device-specific).
5. Position biopsy window over abnormality and obtain scout image (0°).
6. Identify target.
7. Acquire stereo pair (+15° and –15°) and identify target on at least one stereo image.
8. Target the abnormality for coordinate calculation, transfer coordinates to biopsy platform (confirm feasibility of performing the intervention).
9. Place needle guide and coaxial introduction needle in holder (if applicable, calibrate needle).
10. Disinfect breast skin and administer local anesthesia.
11. Demonstrate sound of firing biopsy gun.
12. Skin incision and placement of biopsy needle.
13. Obtain two prefire images (+15° and –15°, 0° if targeting on scout), correct needle position if necessary.
14. Fire biopsy needle.
15. Obtain two postfire images (+15° and –15°, 0° if targeting on scout).
16. Remove biopsy needle and retrieve tissue sample from notch: ≥ four tissue cylinders using 14-gauge needle.
17. If biopsying microcalcifications (rare), perform specimen radiography in magnification technique.
18. Remove coaxial introduction needle.
19. Release compression device, move patient to reclining chair, apply compression, and cool the area (10 minutes).

Stereotactic Localization

The open biopsy of palpable findings can be performed without auxiliary means because the surgeon can feel his way to his goal. Locating a nonpalpable finding intraoperatively, however, is hardly possible without prior marking, i.e., preoperative wire localization. The great majority of mammographic findings subjected to preoperative stereotactic localization are clustered microcalcifications. Most mass lesions can be identified on US and can therefore be localized under US guidance.

Normally, preoperative localization is performed using a hook wire, which is advanced and released from the hollow of the guide cannula once the needle tip is in the correct position. The wire tips have one or more hooks to prevent the wire from being dislocated once released into the breast tissue. This allows the surgeon to selectively remove the targeted area later. A specimen radiograph is performed postoperatively to document the correct excision.

Indications and Goals

As a rule, stereotactic localization is performed on nonpalpable lesions in the BI-RADS category 6 (histologically verified breast carcinoma) that do not have a correlating lesion on US. In special cases, mammographic findings in the BI-RADS categories 4 and 5, rarely also BI-RADS category 3, that do not have a correlating US finding and have not been histologically verified by percutaneous biopsy may be subjected to preoperative wire localization (e.g., multifocal or contralateral breast cancer).

The objective of a preoperative localization is to achieve a sufficient breast resection at the correct location while limiting tissue excision to the necessary extent.

- *Microcalcifications* are a common indication for surgery of nonpalpable findings. They may be a sign of early breast cancer and are usually only detected on mammography.
- *Mass lesions* that are not visible on US are localized mammographically. This can be performed stereotactically.
- The preoperative localization of *mammographic densities* is preferably performed stereotactically. Because a density normally remains visible on the stereo pair (+15° and –15°), its depth can be calculated by this method.
- *Architectural distortions* are usually localized mammographically. The hook wire is placed in the center of such lesions.

The preoperative localization of clips or coils that have been placed during a minimally invasive biopsy is a special case. Such clips/coils are placed, for example, in the biopsy cavity when microcalcifications or mass lesions have been completely removed by VAB. In special situations, lesions detected solely on MR mammography can be marked with a clip/coil for later localization. This can be the case, for example, when suspicious multifocal, multicentric, or contralateral magnetic resonance imaging (MRI) findings are present before neoadjuvant chemotherapy. Otherwise, occult MR mammography lesions can also be marked with a clip or coil to make a preoperative localization later and/or at a distant medical facility without MRI localization equipment available.

Materials

Several preoperative localization wires are available; their advantages and disadvantages should be known to choose optimally. The composition of the breast tissue in which a localization wire is placed is an important factor to consider. It is advisable, for example, to use a double hook wire in fatty breast tissue because it is more securely anchored than a single hook wire. If the patient has a long journey to the medical facility where she will be operated, or surgery is not planned for the day of localization, the placement of a marker clip, coil, or Ariadne's thread hook wire (Invivo Corp., Orlando, FL) is advantageous (see Chapter 7, Instrumentation).

Single-hook wires. Several single hook wires are not repositionable after having been advanced into the breast. Others can be retracted into the guide cannula so that the needle can be redirected to the proper position before advancing the wire again. In some cases, the wire can be advanced to exit the needle in a certain direction, thereby bringing it closer to the target lesion.

Double-hook wires. Double-hook wires are more securely anchored in the breast tissue than single-hook wire configurations. These are therefore less likely to be dislodged from their original position. Advancing a double-hook wire through the guide cannula, however, is associated with higher resistance and one must be careful not to kink the wire.

Procedure

Position of abnormality. Before beginning a stereotactic localization, it is necessary to know the exact position of the abnormality to be localized. This requires access to the mammogram of the affected breast in two orthogonal views (CC and ML/LM). After positioning the patient and selecting the appropriate plane, the biopsy window of the compression plate can be placed over the abnormality. The acquired scout image must show the abnormality adequately centered in the biopsy window (**Fig. 5.20a**). To calculate the abnormality depth, a stereo pair (+ 15 ° and –15 °) is obtained and the abnormality targeted on the unit's monitor (**Fig. 5.20b, c**). The needle is then placed in the holder and guided to the x- and y-coordinates.

Tips and Tricks

Before beginning a localization procedure, make yourself acquainted with the sliding resistance encountered when the localization wire is advanced within the guide needle (advance and retract wire within the needle, outside the breast). Considerable mechanical resistance is perceived, especially when using a double-hook wire. To advance the wire, hold it first just in front of the Luer-Lok stabilizer and advance in small increments of ≤1 cm to avoid kinking the wire. Then hold the stabilizer and push until it butts against the hub of the needle (wire is now released into the breast). Remove Luer-Lok stabilizer and push the wire slightly forward while retracting the guide needle.

Needle and hook-wire placement. It is advisable to apply local anesthesia after skin disinfection when using thicker localization needles (21-gauge and thicker). The needle can then be advanced to the calculated depth (z-coordinate). The correct needle position is checked in +15 ° and –15 ° images (**Fig. 5.20d, e**). The needle tip should be verified within or directly behind the target lesion before advancing the hook wire. When using a repositionable wire, another +15 ° and –15 ° image pair is obtained after the wire is released (**Fig. 5.20f, g**). If correction is necessary, the wire can be retracted into the guide needle and repositioned (**Fig. 5.21**). According to the current guidelines, a localization wire should preferably penetrate, otherwise at least lie within 1 cm of the targeted lesion. Once the wire is in the desired position, the needle can be removed and the final two orthogonal mammographic views performed (**Fig. 5.20i–l**).

Tips and Tricks

If the localization needle does not lie within the target lesion, using a single-hook wire will allow placing the wire closer to the lesion by releasing the wire in the corresponding direction.

A specimen radiography of the excised tissue should be performed promptly to verify correct excision or give the surgeon the opportunity to widen the excision boundaries, if necessary.

Good Practice Recommendations: Stereotactic Localization of Nonpalpable Lesions[*]

Definition: Preoperative hook wire localization of a nonpalpable abnormality. Localizations using marker dye solutions or simple cannulas should only be performed in justified cases.

Indication: To mark nonpalpable abnormalities before open surgery.
- The abnormality must be clearly identifiable.

Localization results: The localization wire should penetrate the target lesion, but not project more than 1 cm past the distal border.
- If the wire does not penetrate the target lesion, then it should lie within 1 cm of the lesion border.
- When localizing a nonmass lesion, several markers/wires can be placed at the surgically relevant borders without adhering to the 1-cm limit.

Localization documentation: Mammograms in two orthogonal planes after localization of mammographic abnormalities (if applicable, ultrasonographic documentation).
1. Description of wire location in relation to the target lesion (± sketch).
2. Documentation of complications.
The surgeon must be informed about points 1 and 2.

Specimen radiography (if applicable, additional specimen sonography).
A specimen radiography should be performed for all nonpalpable, mammographic abnormalities, and all abnormalities containing microcalcifications.
- Performance: with compression. If microcalcifications are expected, use in magnification specimen radiography.
- Specimen radiography of embedded slices, if necessary.
- A specimen sonography can be additionally performed after US-guided localization (permits a prompt communication of specimen findings to the surgeon).

Specimen radiography documentation (if applicable, specimen sonography): Findings and statement.
- The lesion is verified within specimen
  a. and complete excision is certain
  b. and complete excision is uncertain
  c. and only partially excised
- The lesion is definitely not contained within the specimen.
- It is uncertain whether or not the lesion is contained within the specimen.
Specimen radiography findings must be verbally reported to the surgeon intraoperatively. A written report on these findings must be sent to the surgeon postoperatively, and to the pathologist along with the specimen.

Result monitoring after localization: After receipt of histology
- Prepare statement as to whether or not histology is representative.
- If histology is not representative, initiate further postoperative work-up within 14 days: two-view mammography/ stereotactic rebiopsy/ re-excision.
- Case discussion/ interdisciplinary conference.

[*]European S3 guideline: Early Breast Cancer Detection

5

5

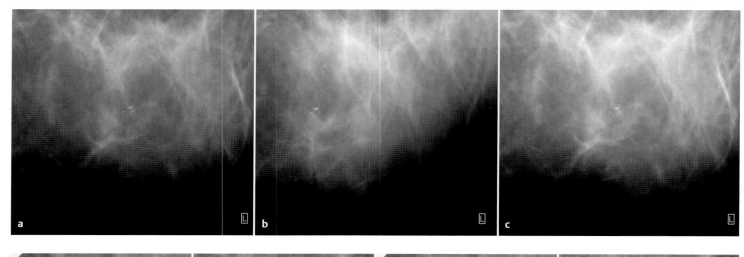

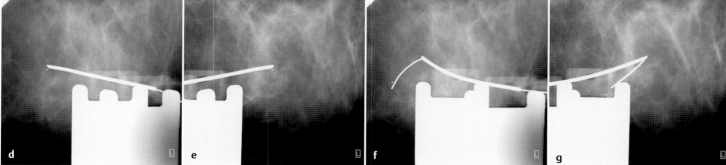

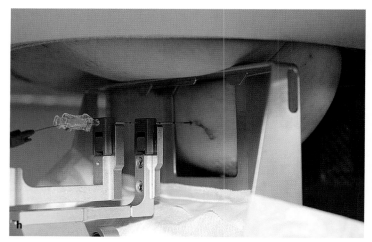

Fig. 5.20a–l Stereotactic localization of clustered microcalcifications in patient with histologically verified breast carcinoma at other location. Scout image 0° (**a**) and stereo pair (± 15°) images (**b, c**). Prefire images after stereotactic calculation of coordinates, needle positioned in microcalcification cluster (**d, e**). Documentation after release of localization wire (**f, g**). Localization needle in holder of stereotactic unit (**h**). Poststudy mammography in CC and LM views with close-up view of hook wire overlapping microcalcifications, note mass lesion in lateral aspect of breast (**i–l**). *Histology*: mass = IDC, microcalcifications = sclerosing adenosis.

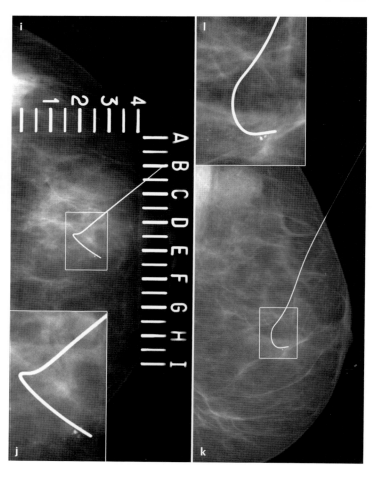

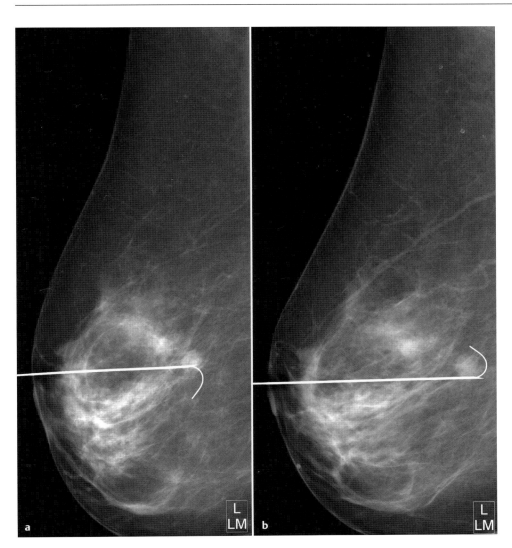

Fig. 5.21a, b Closer approach to target lesion by repositioning single-hook wire.
a Suboptimal wire localization.
b Optimal wire position.

5

Checklist: Stereotactic Wire Localization

1. Mammography in CC and ML projection, if not already available.
2. Verify calibration of stereotactic system.
3. Position biopsy window over abnormality.
4. Obtain scout image (0°) and identify target.
5. Acquire stereo pair (+15° and –15°).
6. Target the abnormality and transfer coordinates to biopsy platform.
7. Place localization needle in holder and move to calculated x- and y-position.
8. Disinfect breast skin and administer local anesthesia.
9. Advance needle to calculated depth (z-coordinate).
10. Obtain two stereo images (+15° and –15°, 0° if targeting on scout), correct position if necessary.
11. Release wire.
12. When placing repositionable wire, obtain two stereo images (+15° and –15°, 0° if targeting on scout), correct position if necessary.
13. Remove cannula.
14. Release compression device and allow patient to move.
15. Perform final mammograms in two orthogonal planes.

5

Problems and Causes of Error

If the abnormality to be biopsied is too close to the detector/breast support, then the stroke margin is negative and the needle will exit the backside of the breast if fired, causing injury to the skin and possibly to the detector. To make the biopsy feasible, the breast can be repositioned in the opposite direction (e.g., craniocaudal/caudocranial) or in a different plane.

If the prefire position of the needle tip is not correctly in front of the targeted abnormality, then the abnormality can be retargeted on these images and the needle repositioned after retraction of the needle into the subcutaneous tissues (see Problem Case 4, p.82). Because the error is often only in millimeters, a new skin incision is not usually required. Multidirectional vacuum-assisted devices allow some leeway in the accuracy of needle placement as the biopsy chamber can be rotated in the direction of the abnormality.

If the abnormality lies directly in the skin plane, the sample chamber can be placed so that only half is in the breast. The other half can then be covered with a plastic clip-on cover so that the unit can still create a vacuum (Mammotome system, **Fig. 5.18**). When performing a biopsy in this way, a greater skin defect should be expected. As an alternative, primary surgery with local anesthesia or in general anesthesia may be considered in these cases. Because the abnormality is located directly under the skin, a simple preoperative marking of the skin with a permanent felt-tip pen after stereotactic localization is sufficient (see Problem Case 5, p.83). Just as for other stereotactic biopsies, specimen radiography is obligatory.

If a suspicious mammographic finding is not distinguishable in the stereotactic images, then open surgery after free-hand localization is performed to obtain a histologic specimen.

A specific problem can arise when performing a stereotactic intervention using the Fischer stereotactic unit. In the course of planning the intervention, the biopsy needle to be used must be selected in a computer program list. If the wrong needle having a different length or throw is selected, then the stereotactic calculation of the z-coordinate will be incorrect.

In the case of an extremely small breast, breast positioning on a dedicated stereotactic system can sometimes be especially difficult or even impossible. If, in addition, scars and/or edema after radiotherapy are present, compressing and fastening the breast in position is even more difficult. In such cases, performing an intervention can be attempted using a diagnostic mammography unit and a compression paddle with a coordinate system. A free-hand VAB can be performed after appropriate placement of the coordinate system (**Fig. 5.22**).

Scar tissue formation is rare after VAB. Due to the accompanying granulomatous reaction, contrast enhancement may be seen on MR mammography. When microcalcifications have been biopsied and demonstrated in the specimen radiograph, it is likely that a new density will be due to scar tissue formation. If this is questionable, a short-term follow-up in 6 months may be indicated (**Fig. 5.23**).

In the course of patient positioning for a stereotactic intervention, it is important to take comfort and patient mobility into account. Especially when performing a biopsy on older patients who sometimes suffer from osteoporosis, pressure on the ribs should be avoided.

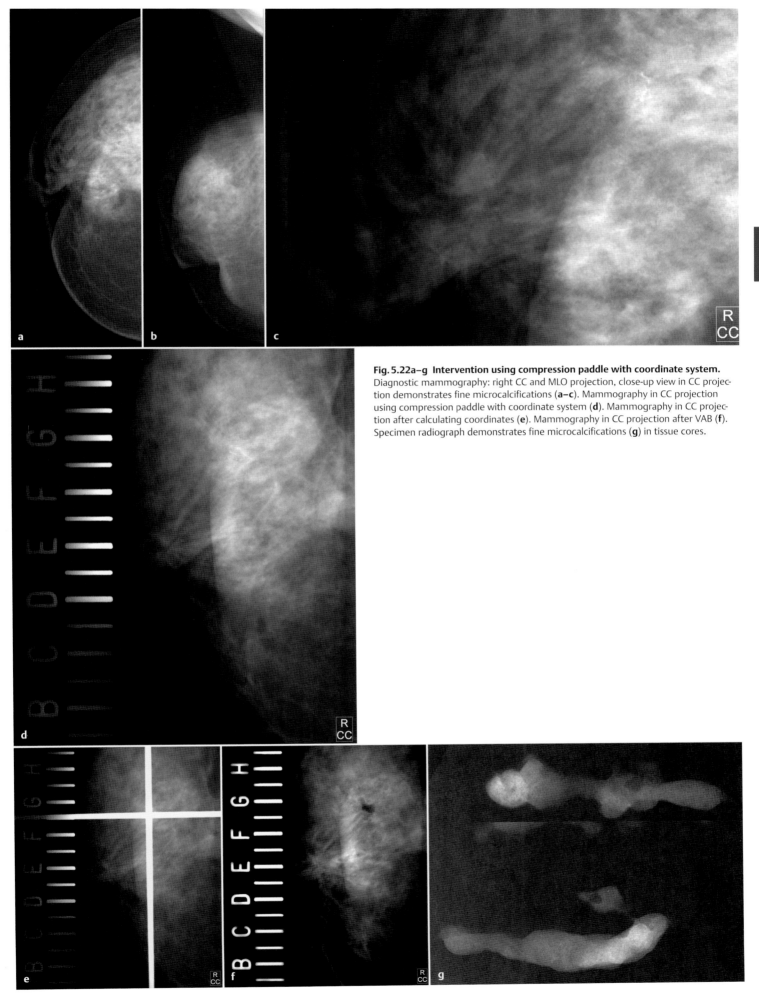

Fig. 5.22a–g Intervention using compression paddle with coordinate system.
Diagnostic mammography: right CC and MLO projection, close-up view in CC projection demonstrates fine microcalcifications (**a–c**). Mammography in CC projection using compression paddle with coordinate system (**d**). Mammography in CC projection after calculating coordinates (**e**). Mammography in CC projection after VAB (**f**). Specimen radiograph demonstrates fine microcalcifications (**g**) in tissue cores.

5

5

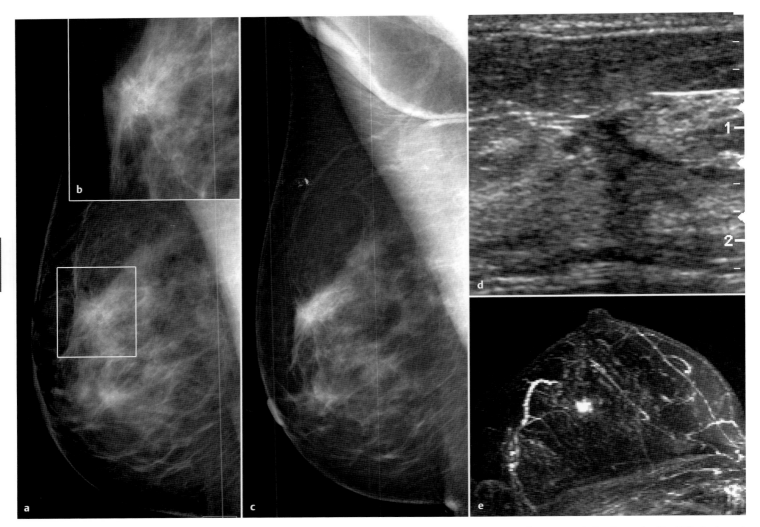

Fig. 5.23a–e Scar tissue formation after VAB. Mammography in MLO projection with close-up view (**a, b**). Depiction of a new mass lesion 6 months after VAB of microcalcifications on mammography in MLO projection (**c**), US (**d**), and MR mammography (**e**). *Histology*: granulomatous mastitis after VAB.

Stereotactic Cutting Biopsies

Coramate mammo biopsy system. The Coramate biopsy system (Siemens, Berlin/Munich, Germany) collects tissue by a rotational cutting technology on a cutting helix. With the aid of a coaxial introduction needle, the cutting cannula is advanced up to the target lesion. The metal cutting helix then screws itself into the abnormality. The tissue sample can be harvested from inside the cutting helix after removing the needle from the breast using a release element. To perform a further biopsy, the coaxial introduction needle must first be moved to a different position.

ABBI (advanced breast biopsy instrumentation). The ABBI system (United States Surgical Corporation, Norwalk, CT) was introduced as a diagnostic and therapeutic instrument in the 1990s. With the development of the less traumatic VAB systems at the end of the 1990s, implementation of the ABBI system has been increasingly limited to therapeutic indications. The objective of this surgical technique is to remove an intact, nonpalpable breast carcinoma under image guidance.

The system is used in combination with stereotactic imaging equipment. After localization of the target abnormality, a wire is guided into the lesion to anchor it. Next, a narrow tube with a cutting cannula is inserted into the breast, using the wire as a guide. The core specimen of breast tissue containing the lesion and wire is then removed. The diameter of the cutting cannula can be selected between 5, 10, 15, 20, and 30 mm. The ABBI procedure requires the removal of a significant portion of normal breast tissue between the skin and the lesion. Once the cutting cannula has reached the desired depth and the lesion is within the tissue cylinder, a looped high-frequency (HF-) cautery wire is used to remove the core specimen (**Figs. 5.24** and **5.25**). The skin defect then requires suturing. Because this technique has a high rate of incomplete tumor removal or inadequate tumor-free margins (> 50 % re-resections for tumors < 10 mm), it has not gained widespread acceptance.

SiteSelect breast biopsy device. Like the ABBI-system, the SiteSelect breast biopsy device (SiteSelect Medical Technologies, Pharr, TX) is another minimally invasive diagnostic instrument used in combination with stereotactic imaging equipment. After wire localization of the target abnormality, a retractable stylet cutting blade is used to slice through and separate the healthy breast tissue without removing it. A coring cannula is then used to cut around the sample to be taken and moved forward until it is in the healthy tissue distal to the lesion. The cannula can be chosen in diameters of 5, 10, 15, and 20 mm. A cutting garrote wire slices the tissue distal of the lesion, which can then be removed through the widened incision. The skin then requires suturing.

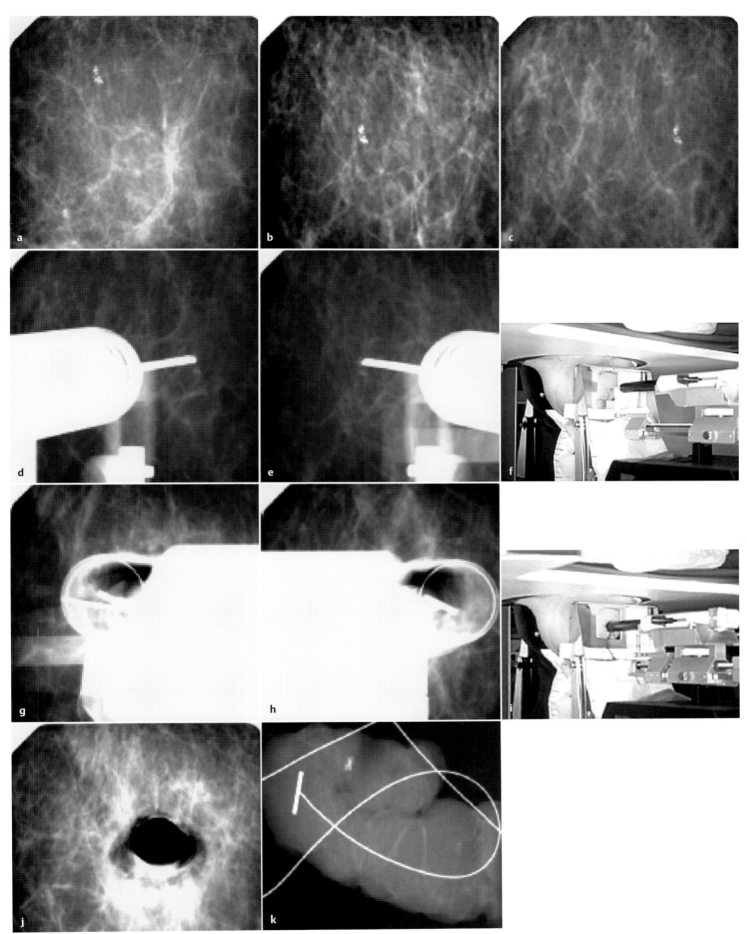

5

Fig. 5.24a–k Stereotactic ABBI biopsy (United States Surgical Corporation, Norwalk, CT).
a Scout image showing clustered microcalcifications.
b, c Stereo images (±15°)

d–f ±15° images after insertion of needle into the abnormality.
e–i ±15° images showing cauterization wire.
j Postbiopsy image.
k Specimen radiograph with microcalcifications.

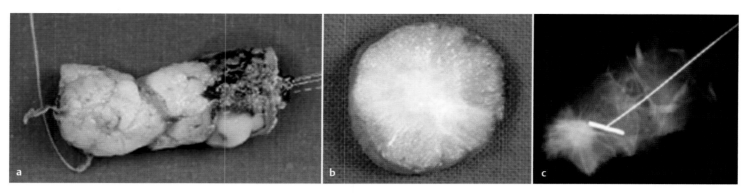

Fig. 5.25a–c ABBI tissue cylinder (United States Surgical Corporation, Norwalk, CT).
a Resection cylinder after ABBI biopsy of a mass lesion.
b Cross section of tissue cylinder.
c Specimen radiograph.

Data in Current Literature

Data pertaining to stereotactic biopsy is usually concerned with the diagnostic work-up of microcalcifications. Studies varied from those that histologically verified findings that had been classified in the BI-RADS category 5 only, and those concerned with abnormalities in the BI-RADS categories 3, 4, and 5. Most biopsies were performed using the vacuum-assisted technique. Comparison to core biopsies showed that the VAB technique achieves a higher accuracy and reduces the false-negative rate. **Table 5.3** lists reference articles pertaining to stereotactic large core and vacuum-assisted breast biopsies. Studies performed by the following working groups have earned special mention: Libermann (New York, NY), Pfarl (Vienna, Austria), Siegmann (Tübingen, Germany), Kettritz (Berlin, Germany), and Diebolt (Frankfurt, Germany).

A synopsis of the existing data indicates that the average quota of malignant to benign findings after stereotactic biopsy is approximately 2 : 3 (40% malignant results) with an accuracy of 96%. Using the VAB technique, the false-negative rate is 1–2%. With experienced personnel, the time required to perform a VAB is 30–45 minutes (table-time). The rate of relevant complications averaged 2%.

Table 5.3 Current literature pertaining to stereotactic core and vacuum-assisted breast biopsies

Work group	Liberman	Liberman	Pfarl	Siegmann	Kettritz	Dieboldt
Year	1998	2001	2002	2003	2004	2005
No. of patients	80	89	325	132	485	58
No. of biopsies	112	105	332	166	500	61
Gauge	11	14*/11	11	11	11	8
No. of specimens	14	7/16	n. s.	26	>20	13
Calcifications	100%	100%	52%	91%	100%	100%
Mass lesion/Density	0%	0%	34%	8%	0%	0%
Calcifications + mass lesion	0%	0%	14%	1%	0%	0%
Malignant	33%	80%	64%	23%	32%	30%
Borderline	11%	10%	5%	4%	2%	7%
Benign	56%	10%	31%	73%	66%	63%
Accuracy	95%	n. s.	93%	99%	n. s.	95%
False-negative	1%	7%	2%	2%	0.4%	0%
Time expenditure (11 gauge)	n. s.	n. s.	n. s.	57 min	n. s.	n. s.
Time expenditure (10 gauge)	n. s.	n. s.	n. s.	n. s.	n. s.	n. s.
Time expenditure (9 gauge)	n. s.	n. s.	n. s.	n. s.	n. s.	29 min
Complication rate	<3%	n. s.	n. s.	18%[†]	1.8%	3.5%

* Twenty-five 14-gauge core biopsies + 17 14-gauge VABs
† Included hematomas >2 cm diameter
Abbreviation: n. s., not specified.

Clinical and Problem Cases

Clinical Case 1: Stereotactic Vacuum-assisted Biopsy of a Mass Lesion (Fig. 5.26)

5

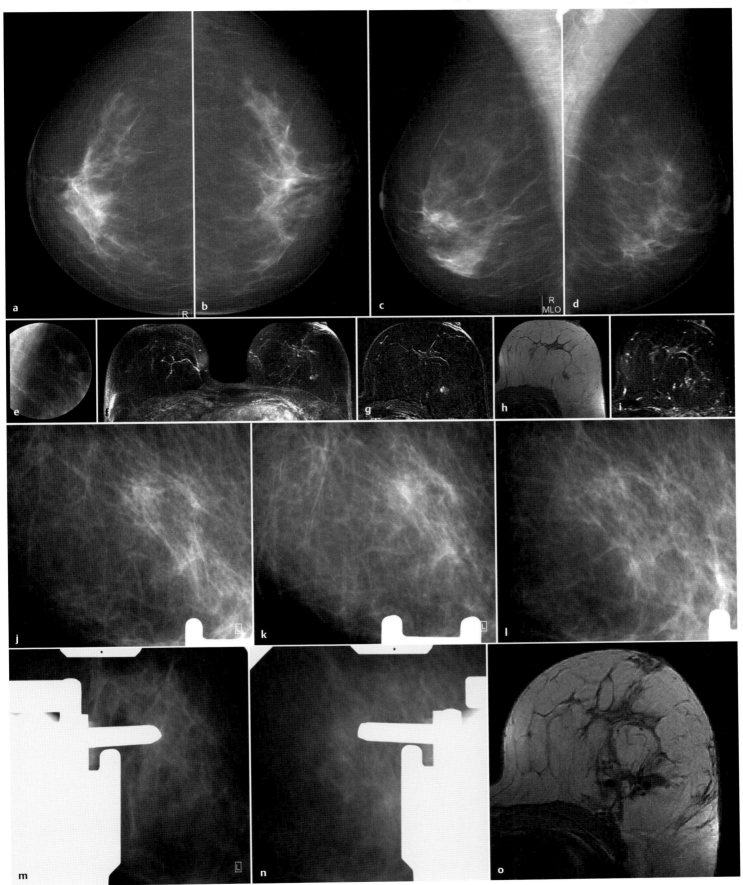

Fig. 5.26a–o Stereotactic VAB of a mass lesion. Bilateral digital mammography in CC and MLO projection showing ill-defined mass in left upper outer quadrant (**a–d**). Spot compression from left MLO view (**e**). MR mammography: subtraction maximum intensity projection (MIP) image (**f**). MR mammography: subtraction image (**g**), precontrast T1-weighted image (**h**), T2-weighted image (**i**). Stereotactic localization: scout image (**j**), stereo pair (±15°) (**k, l**). ±15° prefire images (**m, n**). Post-study MR mammography: T1-weighted image (**o**). *Histology*: invasive lobular breast carcinoma.

Clinical Case 2: Bifocal Vacuum-assisted Biopsy of Microcalcifications (Fig. 5.27)

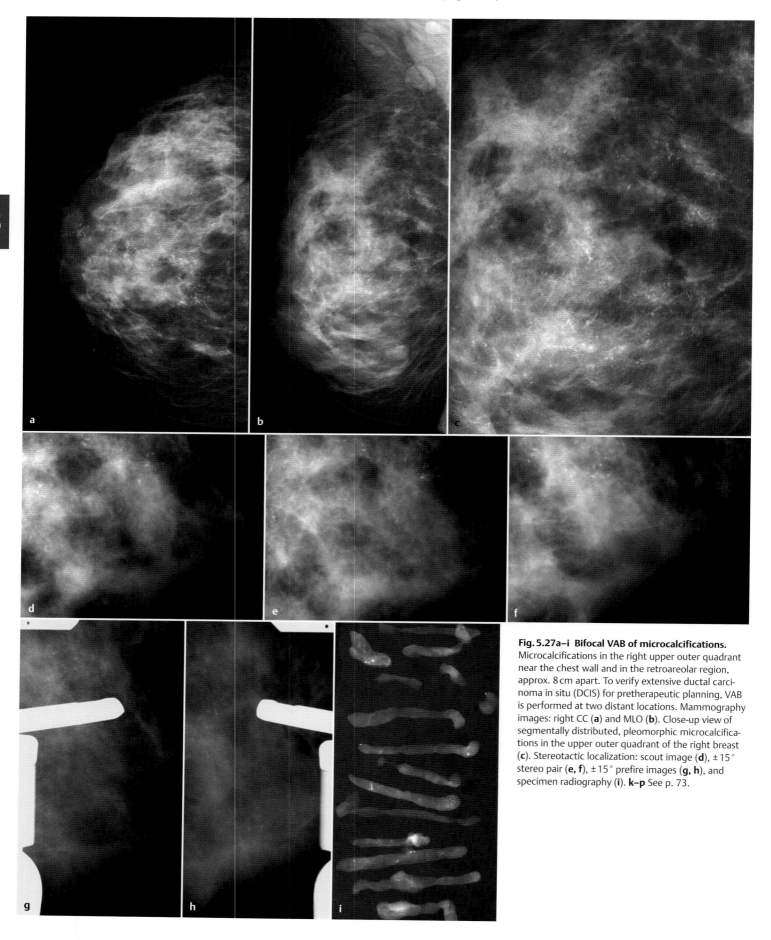

Fig. 5.27a–i Bifocal VAB of microcalcifications.
Microcalcifications in the right upper outer quadrant near the chest wall and in the retroareolar region, approx. 8 cm apart. To verify extensive ductal carcinoma in situ (DCIS) for pretherapeutic planning, VAB is performed at two distant locations. Mammography images: right CC (**a**) and MLO (**b**). Close-up view of segmentally distributed, pleomorphic microcalcifications in the upper outer quadrant of the right breast (**c**). Stereotactic localization: scout image (**d**), ±15° stereo pair (**e, f**), ±15° prefire images (**g, h**), and specimen radiography (**i**). **k–p** See p. 73.

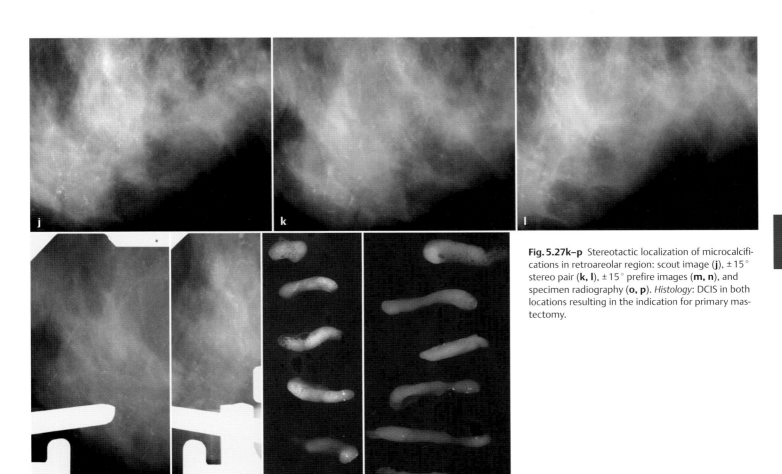

Fig. 5.27 k–p Stereotactic localization of microcalcifications in retroareolar region: scout image (**j**), ±15° stereo pair (**k, l**), ±15° prefire images (**m, n**), and specimen radiography (**o, p**). *Histology*: DCIS in both locations resulting in the indication for primary mastectomy.

Clinical Case 3: Free-hand Localization of Coil Marker (Fig. 5.28)

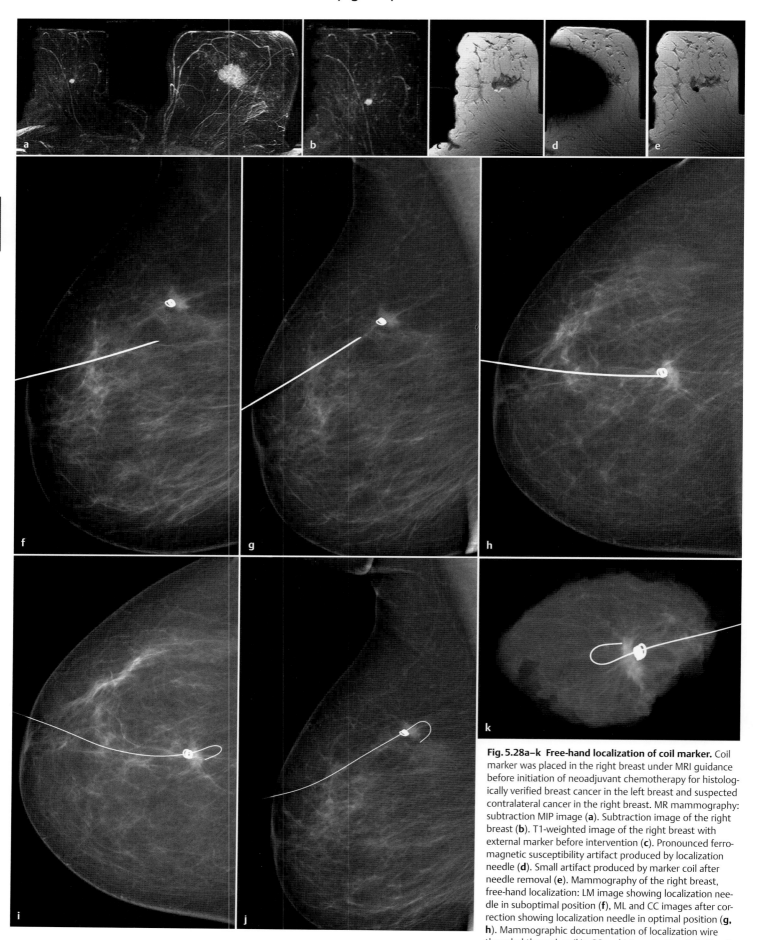

Fig. 5.28a–k Free-hand localization of coil marker. Coil marker was placed in the right breast under MRI guidance before initiation of neoadjuvant chemotherapy for histologically verified breast cancer in the left breast and suspected contralateral cancer in the right breast. MR mammography: subtraction MIP image (**a**). Subtraction image of the right breast (**b**). T1-weighted image of the right breast with external marker before intervention (**c**). Pronounced ferromagnetic susceptibility artifact produced by localization needle (**d**). Small artifact produced by marker coil after needle removal (**e**). Mammography of the right breast, free-hand localization: LM image showing localization needle in suboptimal position (**f**), ML and CC images after correction showing localization needle in optimal position (**g, h**). Mammographic documentation of localization wire threaded through coil in CC and ML projection (**i, j**). Specimen radiography (**k**). *Histology*: contralateral IDC in the right breast.

Clinical Case 4: Stereotactic Vacuum-assisted Biopsy of an Architectural Distortion (Fig. 5.29)

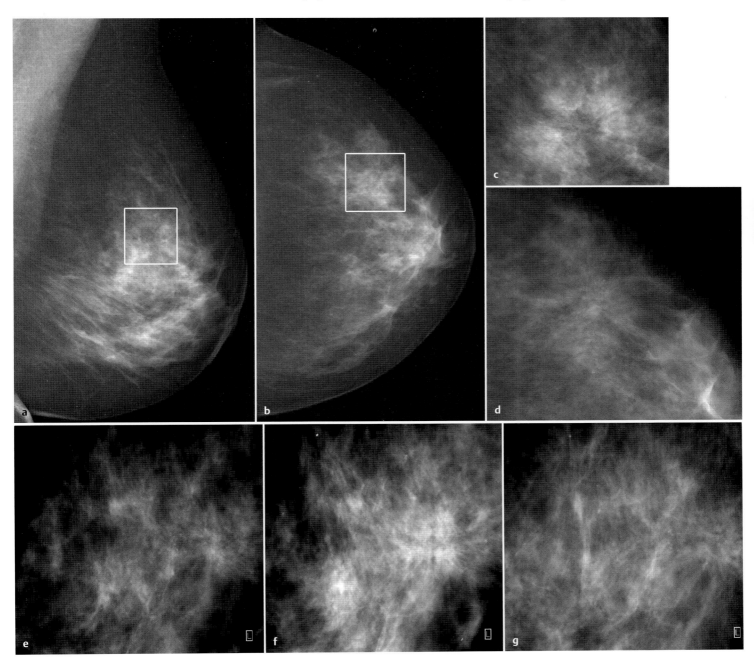

Fig. 5.29a–g Stereotactic VAB of an architectural distortion. Mammography of the left breast in LM and CC projections (**a, b**). Close-up view in LM and CC projections (**c, d**). Architectural distortion at the lateral aspect of the left breast, 9 o'clock. Stereotactic localization: scout image (**e**), ±15° stereo pair (**f, g**). **h–n** See p. 76.

5

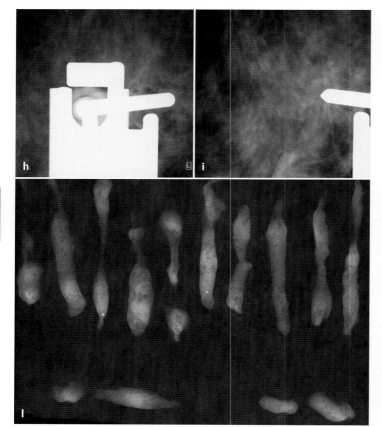

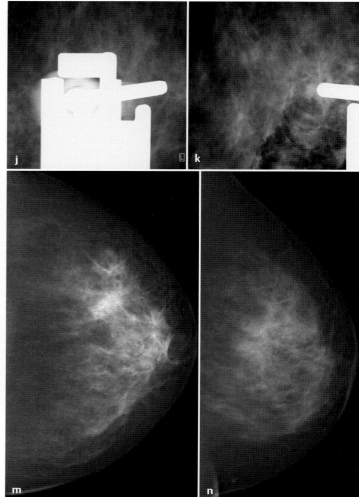

Fig. 5.29h–n Stereotactic localization: prefire images (**h, i**) and postfire images (**j, k**). Specimen radiography demonstrates a few microcalcifications (**l**). Mammographic poststudy documentation in CC and ML projection (**m, n**). *Histology*: radial scar with DCIS.

Clinical Case 5: Stereotactic Vacuum-assisted Biopsy of an Intraductal Papilloma (Fig. 5.30)

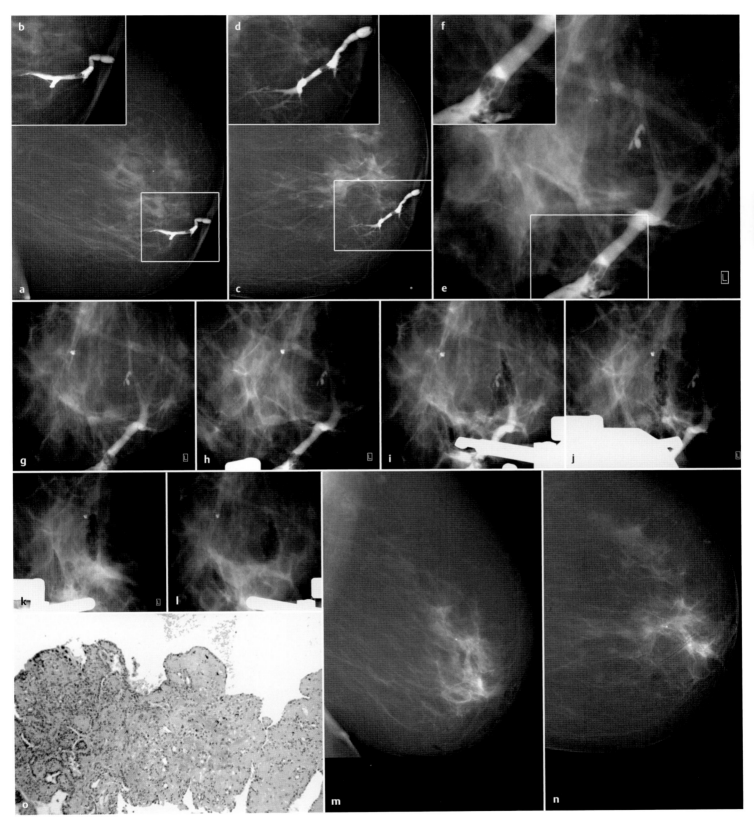

5

Fig. 5.30a–o Stereotactic VAB of an intraductal papilloma. Galactography of the left breast in LM and CC projections with respective close-up views (**a–d**): intraductal filling defect in medial duct. Stereotactic localization: scout image and close-up view after galactography (**e, f**), and ± 15° stereo pair (**g, h**). Biopsy needle is posi-tioned above the intraductal filling defect (**i, j**). ± 15° poststudy images (**k, l**). Mammographic poststudy documentation in ML and CC projection (**m, n**). *Histology*: intraductal papilloma (**o**).

5

Problem Case 1: Stereotactic Vacuum-assisted Biopsy with Atypical Patient Positioning (Fig. 5.31)

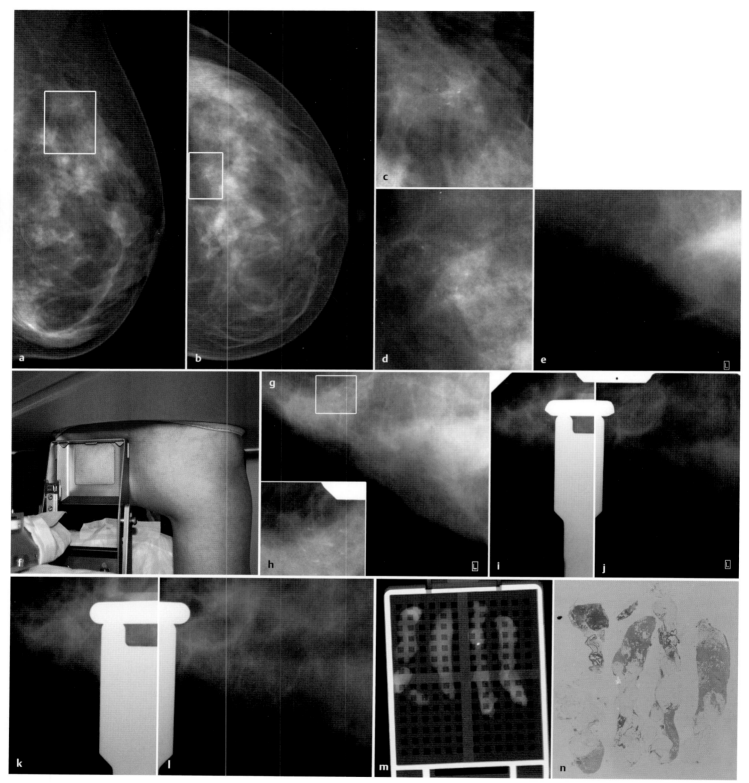

Fig. 5.31a–n Stereotactic VAB with atypical patient positioning. Mammography of the left breast in LM and CC projections (**a, b**). Close-up view in LM and CC projections (**c, d**): microcalcifications near the chest wall at 1 o'clock, 9 cm from the nipple. Stereotactic localization: 0 ° scout image without demonstration of microcalcifications (**e**). Atypical patient positioning by lowering the ipsilateral arm through the table opening (**f**). Repeat scout image now demonstrates the target microcalcifications (**g**), close-up view (**h**). Prefire images (**i, j**). Postfire images (**k, l**). Specimen radiography demonstrates calcifications in core biopsies (**m**). Corresponding stained histologic specimen (**n**). *Histology*: sclerosing adenosis.

Problem Case 2: Dislocation of Marker Clip after Stereotactic Vacuum-assisted Biopsy of a Mass Lesion (Fig. 5.32)

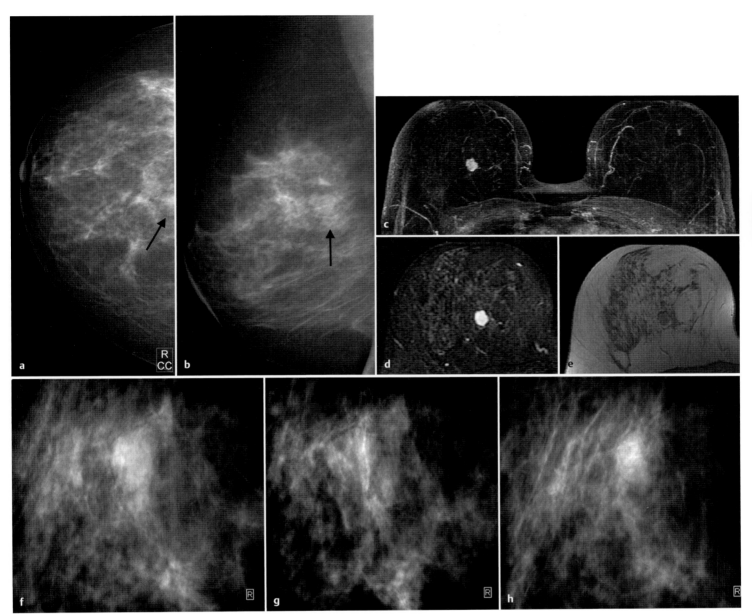

5

Fig. 5.32a–h Dislocation of marker clip after stereotactic VAB of a mass lesion. Mammography of the right breast in CC and LM projections (**a, b**) demonstrating a smoothly bordered mass lesion in the central portion of the breast (arrows). MR mammography: subtraction maximum intensity projection (MIP) image (**c**), sub- traction slice image (**d**), and T1-weighted image (**e**) demonstrate correlating lobu- lated mass lesion. Stereotactic localization: scout image (**f**), ± 15° stereo pair (**g, h**). **i–r** See p. 80.

5

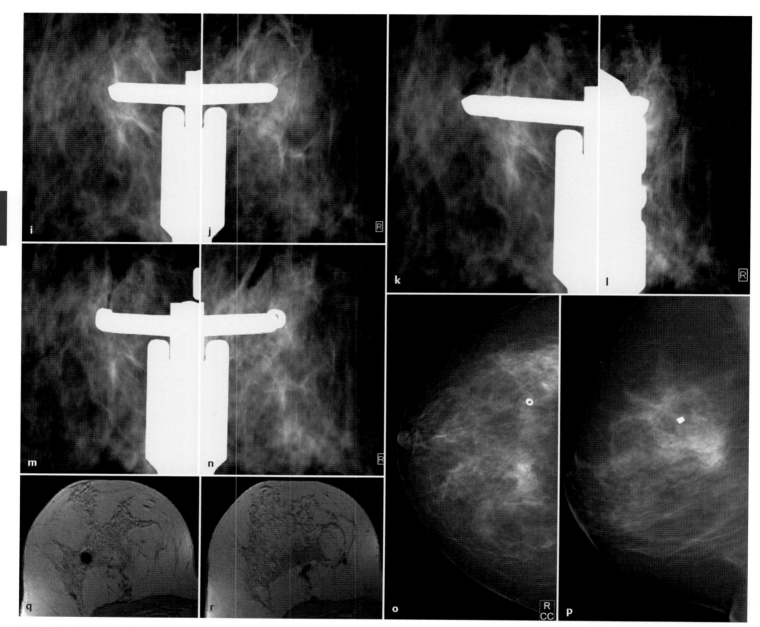

Fig. 5.32i–r Pre- and postfire images (**i–l**). Stereo images after releasing coil into biopsy cavity (**m, n**). Mammographic poststudy documentation in CC and ML projection demonstrates coil laterally displaced (**o, p**). T1W image shows coil artifact laterally of the target lesion (**q**), and biopsy cavity on medial side of the target lesion (**r**). *Histology*: fibroadenoma.

Problem Case 3: Nonvisualization of Microcalcifications: Alternative MRI-guided Localization (Fig. 5.33)

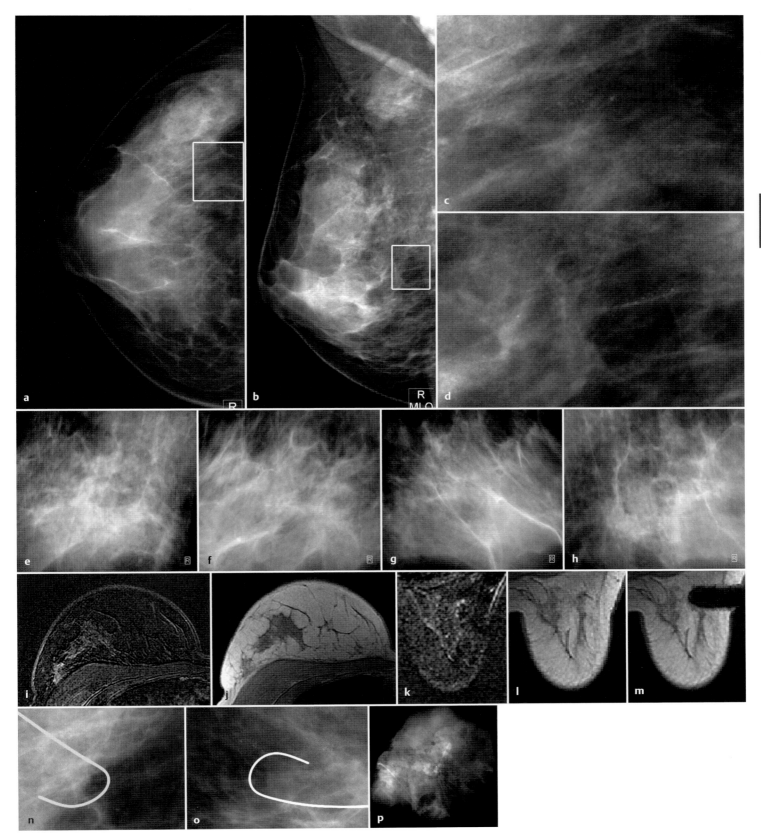

5

Fig. 5.33a–p Nonvisualization of microcalcifications: alternative MRI-guided localization. Mammography of the right breast in CC and MLO projections demonstrate new, monomorphic, linearly distributed microcalcifications (**a, b**). Close-up view in CC and MLO projections (**c, d**). Microcalcifications could not be identified on repeated scout images (**e–h**). MR mammography: subtraction image shows segmental enhancement corresponding to microcalcifications in the outer aspect of

the right breast (**i**). Corresponding T1-weighted precontrast image (**j**). MRI-guided localization: subtraction image (**k**), T1W image without (**l**) and with localization wire (**m**). Close-up views of mammographic poststudy documentation in CC and ML projection demonstrate microcalcifications (**n, o**). Specimen radiograph (**p**). *Histology*: DCIS.

Problem Case 4: Correction of Needle Position during Stereotactic Vacuum-assisted Biopsy (Fig. 5.34)

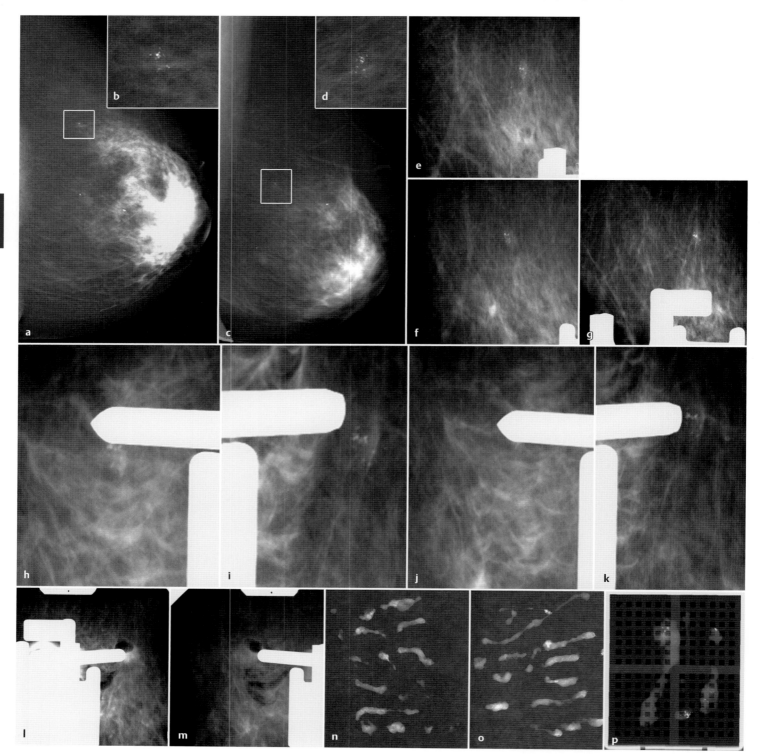

Fig. 5.34a–p Correction of needle position during stereotactic VAB. Mammography of the left breast in CC and LM projections (**a, b**) showing clustered microcalcifications at 2 o'clock. Close-up view in CC and LM projections (**c, d**). Stereotactic localization: scout image (**e**), ± 15° stereo pair (**f, g**). Prefire images show incorrect needle position (**h, i**). Prefire images after correction show clustered microcalcifications on lateral side of needle (**j, k**). Postfire images demonstrate complete removal of target microcalcifications (**l, m**). Specimen radiography (**n–p**). *Histology*: fibrocystic adenosis.

Problem Case 5: Stereotactic Skin Marking of Subcutaneous Microcalcification Cluster (Fig. 5.35)

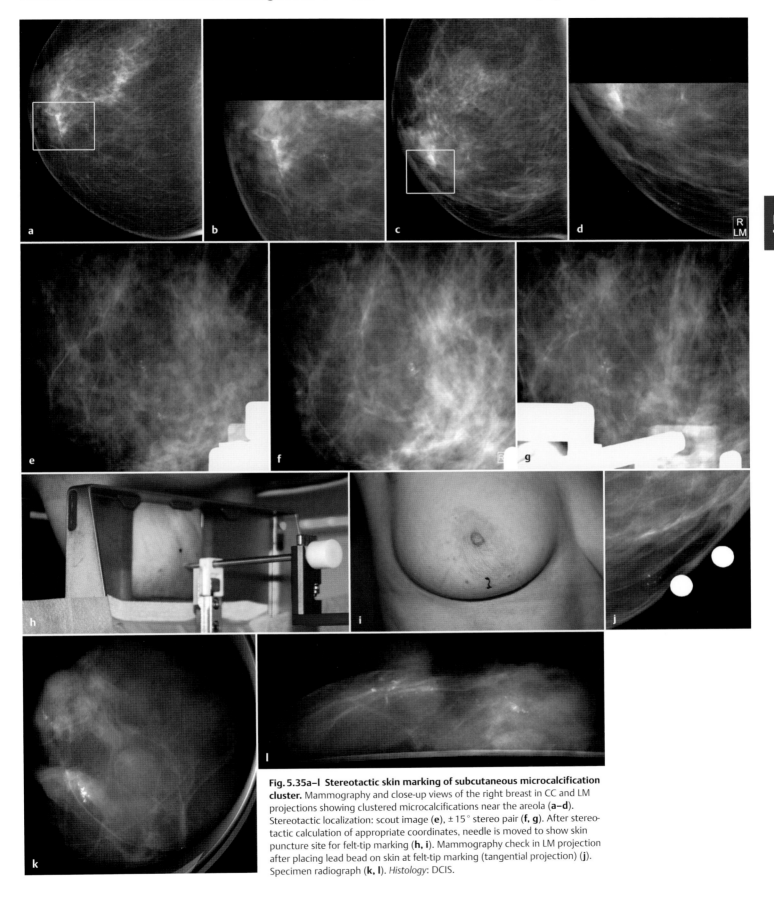

Fig. 5.35a–l Stereotactic skin marking of subcutaneous microcalcification cluster. Mammography and close-up views of the right breast in CC and LM projections showing clustered microcalcifications near the areola (**a–d**). Stereotactic localization: scout image (**e**), ± 15° stereo pair (**f, g**). After stereotactic calculation of appropriate coordinates, needle is moved to show skin puncture site for felt-tip marking (**h, i**). Mammography check in LM projection after placing lead bead on skin at felt-tip marking (tangential projection) (**j**). Specimen radiograph (**k, l**). *Histology*: DCIS.

Further Reading

Berg WA, Campassi C, Langenberg P, Sexton MJ. Breast Imaging Reporting and Data System: inter- and intraobserver variability in feature analysis and final assessment. AJR Am J Roentgenol 2000;174(6):1769–1777

Burnside ES, Ochsner JE, Fowler KJ, et al. Use of microcalcification descriptors in BI-RADS 4th edition to stratify risk of malignancy. Radiology 2007;242 (2):388–395

Ciatto S, Bonardi R, Ravaioli A, et al. Benign breast surgical biopsies: are they always justified? Tumori 1998;84(5):521–524

Hanna WC, Demyttenaere SV, Ferri LE, Fleiszer DM. The use of stereotactic excisional biopsy in the management of invasive breast cancer. World J Surg 2005;29(11):1490–1494, discussion 1495–1496

Jacobs TW, Byrne C, Colditz G, Connolly JL, Schnitt SJ. Radial scars in benign breast-biopsy specimens and the risk of breast cancer. N Engl J Med 1999;340(6):430–436

Kettritz U, Morack G, Decker T. Stereotactic vacuum-assisted breast biopsies in 500 women with microcalcifications: radiological and pathological correlations. Eur J Radiol 2005;55(2):270–276

Liberman L, Gougoutas CA, Zakowski MF, et al. Calcifications highly suggestive of malignancy: comparison of breast biopsy methods. AJR Am J Roentgenol 2001;177(1):165–172

Liberman L, Abramson AF, Squires FB, Glassman JR, Morris EA, Dershaw DD. The breast imaging reporting and data system: positive predictive value of mammographic features and final assessment categories. AJR Am J Roentgenol 1998;171(1):35–40

Markopoulos C, Kakisis J, Kouskos S, Kontzoglou K, Koufopoulos K, Gogas J. Management of nonpalpable, mammographically detectable breast lesions. World J Surg 1999;23(5):434–438

Müller-Schimpfle M, Wersebe A, Xydeas T, et al. Microcalcifications of the breast: how does radiologic classification correlate with histology? Acta Radiol 2005;46(8):774–781

Osuch JR, Reeves MJ, Pathak DR, Kinchelow T. BREASTAID: Clinical results from early development of a clinical decision rule for palpable solid breast masses. Ann Surg 2003;238(5):728–737

Pfarl G, Helbich TH, Riedl CC, et al. Stereotactic needle breast biopsy: Diagnostic reliability of various biopsy systems and needle sizes. [Article in German] Rofo 2002;174(5):614–619

Philpotts LE, Shaheen NA, Carter D, Lange RC, Lee CH. Comparison of rebiopsy rates after stereotactic core needle biopsy of the breast with 11-gauge vacuum suction probe versus 14-gauge needle and automatic gun. AJR Am J Roentgenol 1999;172(3):683–687

Pisano ED, Gatsonis C, Hendrick E, et al; Digital Mammographic Imaging Screening Trial (DMIST) Investigators Group. Diagnostic performance of digital versus film mammography for breast-cancer screening. N Engl J Med 2005;353(17):1773–1783

Schulz KD, Albert US. Stufe 3 Leitlinie Brustkrebsfrüherkennung in Deutschland. Munich: Zuckschwerdt; 2003

Siegmann KC, Wersebe A, Fischmann A, et al. Stereotactic vacuum-assisted breast biopsy—success, histologic accuracy, patient acceptance and optimizing the BI-RADSTM-correlated indication. [Article in German] Rofo 2003;175(1):99–104

Spencer NJ, Evans AJ, Galea M, et al. Pathological-radiological correlations in benign lesions excised during a breast screening programme. Clin Radiol 1994;49(12):853–856

5

6 MRI-guided Interventions

U. Fischer

MR Mammography

Significance

After mammography and ultrasound (US), magnetic resonance imaging (MRI) of the breast is the third diagnostic imaging technique used in the diagnostic work-up of breast findings. In contrast to the other techniques, MRI primarily gives information on the vascularization of intramammary structures. Because malignant tumors typically have an increased vascularization attributed to tumor neoangiogenesis, this phenomena can be visualized in the slice images acquired after administration of a contrast medium to differentiate between benign and malignant findings of the breast.

Numerous studies substantiate that magnetic resonance (MR) mammography is clearly superior to other imaging modalities in the detection of invasive breast cancers. Furthermore, first studies show that MRI using HR methods is also superior in the detection of intraductal tumors. Currently, MRI of the breast has a sensitivity of approx. 85–95%. The specificity achieved by working groups performing MR mammography with a high technical and procedural quality is approx. 90%.

Indications

In general, the performance of contrast-enhanced MR mammography is expedient when less costly examination techniques such as mammography and US are of limited diagnostic value. This is primarily the case when breast tissue is mammographically dense (American College of Radiology [ACR] density types III and IV) and inhomogeneous on US. Several studies have shown, however, that even when breast tissue is not dense, mammographically occult carcinomas can be detected by MR Mammography.

Generally accepted indications for the performance of MR mammography are preoperative local staging of patients with a lesion highly suspicious of malignancy (BI-RADS 5; Breast Imaging Reporting and Data System—classification system according to the ACR), or with a proven malignancy after percutaneous biopsy (BI-RADS 6). The relevant questions to be answered in this constellation refer to the tumor size; the presence of an extensive intraductal component (EIC); a multifocal, multicentric, and/or contralateral tumor. In addition, MRI provides important criteria for the differentiation between scar tissue and a malignant tumor. Numerous studies have also documented the great value of MR mammography for women with an increased risk of developing breast cancer (e.g., BRCA [breast cancer] gene mutation carriers). In fact, MRI of the breast is now considered the most important examination technique for these women because it has been found to be superior to all other imaging modalities in detecting breast cancer. Other reasonable indications for performing MR mammography include the monitoring of patients undergoing neoadjuvant chemotherapy, and the search for a primary tumor in cases of CUP syndrome (cancer of unknown primary). Ultimately, MR mammography is regularly used as a problem solver when an ambiguous finding cannot be resolved by mammography and a breast US examination. Apart from these indications relating to tumor detection and visualization, an MRI examination without the administration of contrast material is the most reliable examination technique for the diagnostic work-up of prosthesis complications.

A modern strategy in breast diagnostics is the "Göttinger Optipack." It is the combination of a bilateral digital mammogram in mediolateral oblique (MLO) projection with a contrast-enhanced MR mammography. This combination has the highest sensitivity for the detection of breast cancer at the lowest possible radiation exposure. It is (if one does not take the cost into account) the ideal strategy in the early diagnosis of breast cancer.

Technique and Methodology

Equipment. MR mammography is preferably performed in a whole-body magnet with a field strength of 1.5 T. Systems with lower field strengths no longer satisfy the quality requirements for a high-resolution breast examination. Positive reports have also been published pertaining to the use of 3.0-T magnets. A breast MRI examination is performed using a dedicated, 4- or 8-channel phased array surface coil made to fit the breast form. To perform a breast intervention, an open coil that allows access to the breast from the lateral and/or medial aspect, or from the cranial aspect, is required. In addition, open breast coils allow good immobilization of the breast by using integrated compression devices during a diagnostic MR mammography examination.

Contrast material. MRI measurements are performed using T1-weighted gradient echo (GE) sequences, which have a great sensitivity for paramagnetic contrast materials. Measurements are typically performed before and repeatedly after intravenous (IV) administration of an appropriate MRI contrast material in the cubital vein. The amount of contrast material required (e.g., gadopentetate dimeglumine) is 0.1 mmol/kg body weight (BW). In addition to the T1-weighted sequences, water-sensitive sequences (e.g., T2-weighted, turbo spin echo [TSE], T2-weighted inversion recovery [IR]) should be performed with identical slice positioning before performing the contrast-enhanced dynamic measurements.

Minimum and preferred requirements. To attain a high-quality, contrast-enhanced MR mammography, standardized methods and techniques must be employed. **Table 6.1** lists the minimal requirements and the currently preferred parameters used for performing a high-standard MR mammography.

Table 6.1 Examination parameters for the performance of contrast-enhanced MR mammography: Minimum requirements and the currently preferred protocol*

Criteria	Minimum requirement	Optimal settings
Technique	2D/3D	2D/3D
Spatial resolution: slice thickness	≤4 mm/slice	≤3 mm/slice
Spatial resolution: matrix	256 × 256	512 × 512
Temporal resolution	<2.5 minutes/sequence	<2 minutes/sequence
TE	In phase	In phase
FOV	350	350

* Recommended by the "AG Mammadiagnostik" of the German Radiology Association, 2003.

Abbreviations: TE = echo time; FOV = field of view.

Time of examination performance.

In premenopausal women, MR mammography should be performed in the second week of the menstrual cycle (less optimally in the third week). The first and fourth week of the menstrual cycle should be avoided. In certain cases (e.g., local pretherapeutic MRI-staging of women with a lesion in the BI-RADS category 6), however, a prompt examination without consideration of the menstrual cycle is indicated. The interpretation of MR mammography examinations performed on postmenopausal women should take hormone replacement therapy into account.

Terminology

Essentially, three types of contrast enhancement are differentiated in the analysis of MR mammography findings (**Fig. 6.1**).

Foci. Foci are spotty or blotchy enhancing breast areas up to 5 mm in diameter. A bilateral, symmetric, focal enhancement pattern within the parenchyma is often a physiologic finding, representing enhancement within the breast lobuli. It is usually a harmless and normal finding, and therefore does not necessitate short-term follow-up. However, a single focus or multiple foci seen near a malignant lesion have a higher probability of representing a carcinoma or satellite lesions.

Mass lesions. Mass lesions are space-occupying, three-dimensional (3D) findings with increased vascularization and a diameter over 5 mm. Interpretation of such lesions takes multiple characteristics into account, including morphologic and hemodynamic criteria (see Göttingen Score).

Nonmass lesions. Nonmass lesions of the breast are characterized by a diffuse uptake of contrast material, which typically respects lipomatous structures. The differential diagnosis includes:

- an inflammatory process
- a radial scar
- a malignant process (ductal carcinoma in situ [DCIS], invasive lobular carcinoma)
- normal findings

Evaluation Criteria

Evaluation criteria are essentially divided into morphologic and dynamic criteria. With the increasing spatial resolution of modern MR equipment, however, morphologic criteria are attaining greater importance (**Table 6.2**). The dynamics of contrast enhancement is differentiated into a so-called early or initial, and late phase or postinitial.

Initial phase. The first 3-minute period after contrast administration constitutes the initial dynamic phase. The so-called initial signal increase ($S_{initial}$) is calculated as the percentage of signal increase (maximum signal S_{max} within the first 3 minutes after contrast administration) in relation to the initial signal in the precontrast image ($S_{precontr}$). Typically, the initial signal increase is classified as slight, moderate, or strong. The quantitative assignment of the percentage signal increase to one of these classes is dependent upon the examination technique and methodology (e.g., contrast material dose, field strength, 2D- or 3D-measurement technique) and must therefore be adjusted based on the user.

$$S_{initial} = (S_{max} - S_{precontr}) / S_{precontr} \times 100 \; [\%]$$

Late phase. The late or postinitial phase constitutes the period between the third minute after contrast administration and the end of the dynamic measurements, typically 8 minutes after contrast administration. The postinitial signal behavior takes the

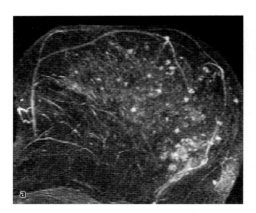
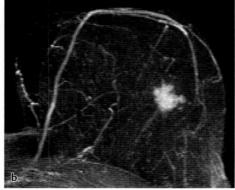
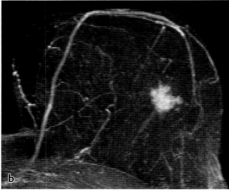

Fig. 6.1a–c Various types of contrast-enhancement in MR mammography.
a Foci (adenosis).

b Mass lesion (IDC).
c Nonmass lesion (ILC).

maximum signal within the first 3 minutes and the final signal (S_{final}) after 8 minutes into account. If the signal intensity value between these measurements increases (>10%), then the postinitial signal behavior is described as a *continuous increase*. If the signal intensity value between these measurements decreases (>10%), then the postinitial signal behavior is described as having a *wash-out effect*. When the signal intensity values remain relatively constant (<10% difference), then this is considered to be a postinitial plateau (**Fig. 6.2**).

$$S_{postinitial} = (S_{final} - S_{max}) / S_{max} \times 100 \ [\%]$$

Morphologic criteria. Morphologic criteria are especially applied to the evaluation of mass lesions. The most important criteria include shape, margins, and internal enhancing pattern (**Table 6.2**, **Fig. 6.3**). Nonmass lesions, however, also display different morphologic characteristics which should be used for their description (**Fig. 6.4**).

No single feature alone, however, can determine the assessment of an ambiguous finding. In fact, the application of multiple diagnostic criteria in the evaluation of MR mammography findings has been shown to significantly increase the specificity of this method. The Göttingen Score (**Tables 6.3** and **6.4**), for example, is a scoring method developed to facilitate the assessment of MR mammography mass lesions. By evaluating several diagnostic criteria, a lesion can be assigned a point score, which can then be translated to a MR mammography BI-RADS category (**Tables 6.4** and **6.5**).

Furthermore, a description of the internal enhancement pattern can also be applied to help assess a lesion. These include nonenhancing internal septations, enhancing internal septations, and a central enhancement (**Fig. 6.3e**). Nonenhancing internal septations (dark septations) are typical for myxoid fibroadenomas and represent non- or slightly enhancing fibrotic strands within the tumor, i.e., an additional criterion for benignity. Enhancing internal septations and central enhancement within a ring enhancement are indicative of proliferative changes within the tumor. They are more likely a sign of malignancy.

6

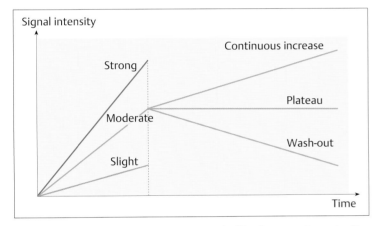

Fig. 6.2 Diagnostic criteria in MR mammography kinetic curves. Dynamic criteria in the initial and postinitial phases.

Table 6.2 Morphologic criteria for enhancing mass lesions

Criteria	Description
Shape	Round, oval (more likely benign)
	Irregular (more likely malignant)
Margins	Well circumscribed (more likely benign)
	Indistinct (more likely malignant)
Internal contrast enhancement pattern	Homogeneous (more likely benign)
	Inhomogeneous (unspecific)
	Ring enhancement (more likely malignant)

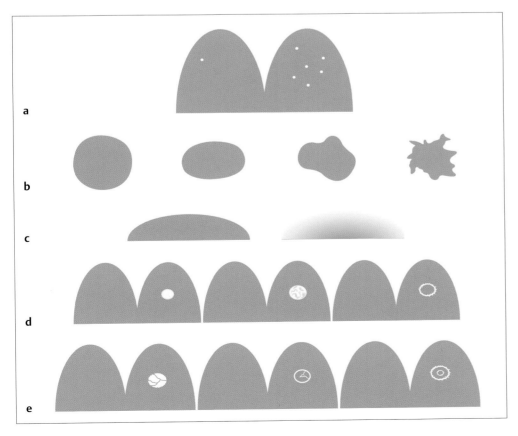

Fig. 6.3a–e Foci and mass lesions.
a Focus/foci (up to 5-mm diameter).
b Mass lesion—shape: round, oval, lobulated, irregular (from left to right).
c Mass lesion—margins: well circumscribed (left), indistinct (right).
d Mass lesion—enhancement pattern: homogeneous, inhomogeneous, ring enhancement (from left to right).
e Mass lesion—internal septations: nonenhancing septations, enhancing septations, central enhancement (from left to right).

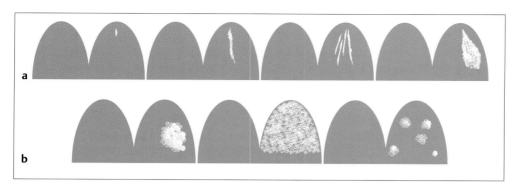

Fig. 6.4a, b Nonmass lesions.
a Focal, linear, dendritic, segmental enhancement (from left to right).
b Regional, diffuse, multiple enhancements (from left to right).

Table 6.3 Göttingen Score for the evaluation of mass lesions in MR mammography

Criteria	No points	1 point	2 points
Shape	Round, oval	Irregular	–
Margins	Well circumscribed	Indistinct	–
Enhancement pattern	Homogeneous	Inhomo-geneous	Ring enhancement
$S_{initial}$	<50%	50–100%	>100%
$S_{postinitial}$	Continuous increase	Plateau	Wash-out

Table 6.4 Assignment of MR mammography BI-RADS category to a mass according to it's Göttingen Score

Total points	MR mammography BI-RADS category
0–1	MR mammography BI-RADS 1
2	MR mammography BI-RADS 2
3	MR mammography BI-RADS 3
4–5	MR mammography BI-RADS 4
6–8	MR mammography BI-RADS 5

Table 6.5 Categorization of MRI findings according to MR mammography BI-RADS categories*

Category	Assessment	Examples	Carcinoma-risk	Consequence
0	Incomplete	Strong early bilateral enhancement pattern without circumscribable pathologic abnormality (MR mammography density type 4)	Not known	Additional imaging evaluation
1	Negative	Normal findings without an enhancing lesion, e.g., MR mammography density type 1 (Göttingen score: 0–1 points)	0%	No additional evaluation required
2	Benign finding(s)	Simple cyst, lymph node, fibrotic fibroadenoma, oil cyst, scar (Göttingen score: 2 points)	0%	No additional evaluation required
3	Probably benign finding	Myxoid fibroadenoma (Göttingen score: 3 points)	<2%	Targeted second-look US (knowing lesion location and size), otherwise short-term follow-up** after an appropriate interval (typically 6 months), in indicated cases MRI-guided VAB
4	Suspicious abnormality	Hypervascularized, indistinct mass (Göttingen score: 4–5 points)	4A: 2–30% 4B: 30–60% 4C: 60–90%	Percutaneous biopsy for histologic evaluation, typically MRI-guided VAB (if no correlating lesion is found on mammography or US)
5	Highly suggestive of malignancy	Hypervascularized mass with ring enhancement and postinitial wash-out (Göttingen score: 6–8 points)	90–100%	Percutaneous biopsy for histologic evaluation, typically MRI-guided VAB (if no correlating lesion is found on mammography or US)
Overall BI-RADS 6†	Pathologically verified breast cancer by CNB or VAB	Independent of MR mammography imaging findings	100%	Initiation of appropriate definitive therapy

* from: Fischer, U., Baum, F.: Diagnostische Interventionen der Mamma. Georg Thieme Verlag, 2008.
** Size increase or development of suspicious features at follow-up examination results in an upgrading of the BI-RADS category. Stability of solid lesion features and size results in downgrading the BI-RADS category.
† Note: At the end of the diagnostic chain (clinical exam, mammography, US, MR mammography, percutaneous biopsy), the final diagnosis is stated in the medical report and given an overall BI-RADS category 1–6.

Particularities of MRI-guided Interventions

Materials. MRI-guided interventions must accommodate the special conditions encountered during an MRI scan. This pertains especially to the extremely strong magnetic field, which prohibits the use of customary ferromagnetic materials (**Fig. 6.5**). Biopsy and localization grids, post and pillar systems, biopsy equipment, as well as all materials inserted into the breast (coils, clips, wires) must be made of MRI-compatible materials, usually plastics or titanium- and nickel-based alloys (**Fig. 6.6**). These alloys cause only slight susceptibility artifacts and can therefore be distinctly seen. On the other hand, they do not cause a significant interference during imaging, and therefore do not mask relevant findings and fine structures.

The degree of signal extinction caused by susceptibility artifacts is dependent upon the composition of the materials used, and upon the examination parameters (among other factors). In comparison to GE sequences, for example, T1-weighted SE sequences have a lower response to contrast materials and require a longer examination time. They show significantly less interfering signal alterations and are therefore well suited for the final documentation of localization materials in the breast.

Localization fixtures must also be made of MRI-compatible materials without ferromagnetic substances, which cause interference in the acquired images. Plexiglas materials have proven suitable for this purpose because they can be adequately processed and can withstand a large amount of material stress. In addition, all utensils must meet the appropriate hygienic requirements.

Diagnostic time slot. Another special condition encountered during MRI-guided interventions concerns the detection of ambiguous breast findings: the depiction of hypervascularized findings after IV contrast administration is usually only possible within a time interval of a few minutes. The target finding must be clearly identified within this time slot (**Fig. 6.7**). All the following steps of an intervention are performed later, when the target lesion can generally no longer be differentiated from the surrounding, now also enhancing healthy breast tissue. If the target lesion cannot be identified within the diagnostic time slot, or a relevant displacement of breast tissue takes place in the course of the intervention procedure, then the intervention must be discontinued. Generally, the repeat intervention procedure can be performed on the following day at the earliest.

6

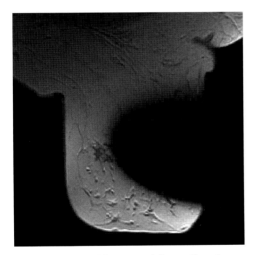

Fig. 6.5 Unacceptable susceptibility artifact. Strong signal extinction due to use of inappropriate ferromagnetic needle in MRI intervention.

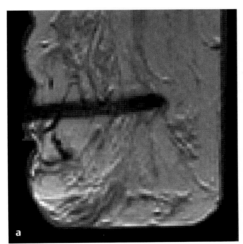

Fig. 6.6a, b Acceptable and optimal susceptibility.
a Needle shows acceptable signal extinction in GE sequence image.
b Very slight susceptibility artifact and more precise depiction of the same needle in a spin-echo (SE) sequence image.

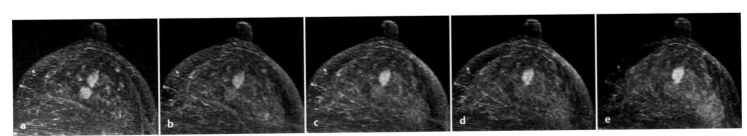

Fig. 6.7a–e Diagnostic time slot during MR mammography. Different perfusion patterns of two adjacent mass lesions: dorsal mass = carcinoma, ventral mass = fibroadenoma. Early enhancement of both lesions (**a**). Wash-out in the carcinoma during the second and third measurement (**b–c**) (limited time frame for visualization = approx. 3 minutes). Increasing enhancement within the fibroadenoma during entire examination sequence (**a–e**).

MRI-guided Vacuum-assisted Biopsy: Diagnostic Procedure

Indications and Objective

The main indication for the performance of MRI-guided biopsy is the diagnostic work-up of a suspicious finding on MR mammography (MR mammography BI-RADS category 4 or 5) that has no clearly correlating clinical or other image modality finding. Occasionally, an MRI-guided biopsy can be performed for the diagnostic work-up of a finding in the category MR mammography-BI-RADS 3. This is indicated when the patient wishes a definitive diagnosis, or to rule out multicentricity and/or bilateral breast cancer if the patient has a BI-RADS 5 finding at another location.

The purpose of an MRI-guided percutaneous biopsy is to attain a definitive histopathologic diagnosis of ambiguous MRI findings by obtaining representative tissue samples. Thus, it has a diagnostic, and not a therapeutic objective, and does not normally aim to remove the ambiguous finding completely. Small intraductal papillomas, however, are the exception. Here the complete removal by VAB with a therapeutic objective can be a reasonable alternative to surgery. The procedural strategy in this context requires that the harvested samples be systematically harvested and arranged for pathologic study in a structured manner.

Patient Positioning

MRI-guided interventions are performed with the patient lying in the prone position and the breast hanging freely inside the surface coil. If the target is accessed from the lateral aspect of the breast, then the opposite breast can also hang inside the surface coil. If the target is accessed from the medial aspect of the breast, then the opposite breast must be positioned outside the surface coil. The patient's head may be positioned to one side, or preferably face down because this usually causes less cervical complaints. Earplugs or music headphones can increase patient com-

fort in this situation. In the face-down position, it is also possible to create a free view by means of an integrated mirror optic (**Fig. 6.8a**). Based on the coil design, the arms may be positioned above the head or alongside the body. When positioning the arms alongside the body, use a bathrobe belt to maintain the arms' positioning (**Fig. 6.8b**). Position the patient's legs and feet comfortably, and ensure an agreeable room temperature.

Materials

Surface coils and localization equipment. The performance of MRI-guided VAB requires use of an open breast surface coil, which allows access to the breast from the lateral, medial, and/or CC direction. In addition, special needle guide attachments that allow the exact and reliable localization of the puncture coordinates in the x- and y-axes must be used. These are available as biopsy and localization grid systems (some of which can be angled), and continuously variable targeting and puncture systems (post and pillar) (**Fig. 6.9**). Breast surface coils with ventral breast access are not recommended for performing vacuum-assisted interventions.

Puncture equipment. At present, there are three functional systems available for performing MRI-guided VABs: **Fig. 6.10** depicts their clinical applications.

Procedure

Once the indication for MRI-guided percutaneous biopsy has been ascertained in a diagnostic MR mammography examination, the intervention steps are performed as shown in **Fig. 6.11**.

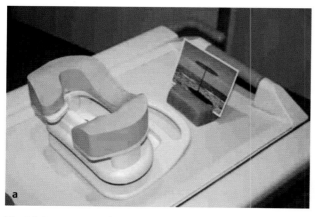 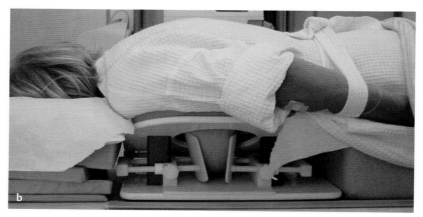

Fig. 6.8 Positioning and comfort during MR mammography examination.
a Head support with integrated mirror optic.
b Patient positioned with arms in relaxed position, hanging in belt loop.

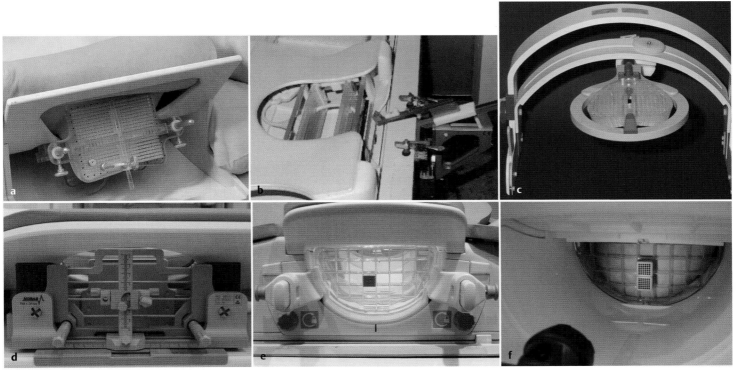

Fig. 6.9a–f Dedicated MRI-compatible puncture equipment.
a Open breast surface coil with Plexiglas attachment containing multiple puncture channels (Phillips Healthcare, Amsterdam, the Netherlands). Patient lies in oblique position.
b Dedicated unilateral open intervention coil with puncture equipment mounted on edge of examination table (Siemens, Berlin/Munich, Germany).

c Commercial shoulder flex coil with integrated, gadolinium solution-filled puncture components mounted on a C-arm (self-construction; Göttingen University, Germany).
d–f Open diagnostic breast surface coil (GE Healthcare, Chalfont St., Giles, UK): Lateral puncture attachment with post and pillar targeting equipment (Noras MRI Products, Hochberg, Germany) (**d**). Lateral biopsy and localization grid (Noras MRI Products) (**e**). Medial biopsy and localization grid (Noras MRI Products) (**f**).

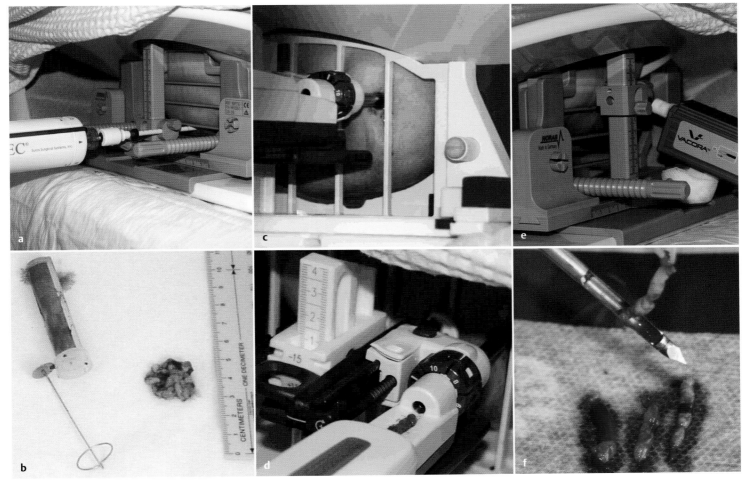

Fig. 6.10a–f Various needle systems for MRI-guided VAB.
a ATEC biopsy system with appropriate coaxial introduction needle (Suros Surgical Systems, Inc., Indianapolis, IN).
b Retrieval of tissue samples from specimen retrieval chamber.
c Mammotome biopsy system with appropriate coaxial introduction needle (Ethicon Endo-Surgery, Cincinnati, OH).

d Consecutive retrieval of tissue samples from specimen collection window.
e VACORA biopsy system with appropriate coaxial introduction needle (Bard Biopsy Systems, Tempe, AZ).
f Specimen retrieval from biopsy notch.

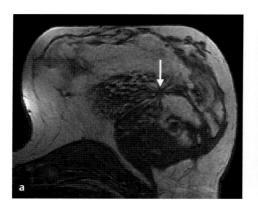

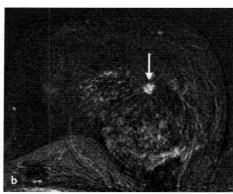

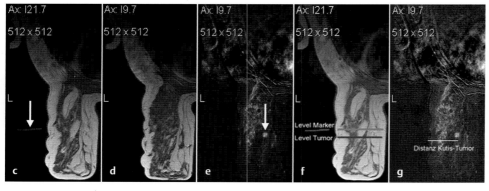

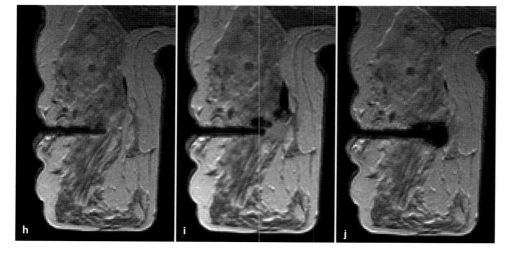

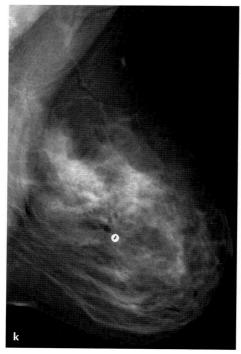

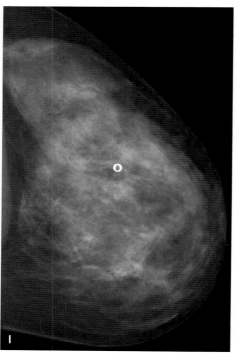

Fig. 6.11a–l Procedure steps performed during MRI-guided VAB. Diagnostic MR mammography shows suspicious lesion in the left breast. Precontrast image (**a**). Subtraction image (**b**) (arrows). After positioning the patient for the performance of MRI-guided VAB, an external marker (arrow) with a high signal intensity in the T1-weighted measurements (e.g., containing oil or gadolinium) is placed on the puncture device at the estimated lesion position to serve as the zero-point for calculations (**c**). Contrast-enhanced MR mammography is performed prior to VAB. The T1-weighted precontrast image shows the external marker in slice image "Ax I 21.7" (arrow) (**c**). The target lesion (arrow) is identified in the subtraction image of slice "Ax I 9.7" (**e**). The corresponding T1-weighted precontrast image (**d**) is used for comparison with check images during biopsy. The puncture coordinates (x- and y-axes) must now be calculated taking the arbitrary zero-point into consideration, and the depth (z-axis) measured in the appropriate slice. In the case presented here, the puncture site lies 12 mm cranially (y-axis) of the zero-point: the external marker is in slice image "Ax I 21.7," the target lesion is in slice "Ax I 9.7" (**c, e**), the puncture position is thus moved this difference of 12 mm in the cranial direction. In the x-axis, the puncture position must be moved ventrally the distance between the level of the marker and the level of the target lesion (10 mm) (**f**). The depth of the lesion is marked on the monitor from the skin to the lesion and calculated by the computer (**g**). It is prudent to perform a check MR mammography (T1-weighted series) before puncture and after moving the external marker to the calculated x- and y-coordinates. After disinfection of the skin and application of local anesthesia at the calculated puncture site, the coaxial introduction needle is inserted to the calculated depth (if necessary, perform nick incision). The position of the coaxial introduction needle is checked by performing an MRI T1-weighted series after replacing the puncture stylet with a MRI-compatible mandrin (**h**). If necessary, correct position and perform an additional position-check.

Once the correct position has been achieved, the biopsy needle is inserted into the coaxial introduction cannula and the specimens are harvested using a vacuum-assisted technique. After the harvesting of specimens is completed, the biopsy needle is removed and another MRI check is performed with the MRI-compatible mandrin in place (**i**). The additional administration of contrast material at this point is optional. The acquired images should be evaluated to ascertain whether the target lesion has been completely or incompletely removed, or possibly missed. If necessary, further tissue samples should be harvested. It is optional, but sometimes prudent, to place a marker coil/clip in the biopsy cavity through the coaxial introduction cannula (**j**).

Finally, the coaxial introduction needle can be removed, and the biopsy site compressed, cooled, and bandaged. A postbiopsy mammogram in craniocaudal and mediolateral projection should be performed for documentation (**k, l**).

Checklist: MRI-guided Vacuum-assisted Biopsy

1. Establish indication.
2. Confirm that there is no correlating finding on mammography and/or (second-look) US.
3. Obtain informed consent (in advance).
4. Position patient comfortably in an open breast surface coil with a biopsy option.
5. Choose the appropriate puncture equipment (grid, post and pillar).
6. Position external marker at estimated target position (arbitrary zero-point).
7. Perform dynamic MR mammography examination with image subtraction.
8. Identify target.
9. Calculate appropriate x-, y-, and z-coordinates.
10. Move external marker to appropriate puncture site and perform MRI check.
11. Disinfect breast skin and administer local anesthesia; if necessary, perform a nick incision.
12. Introduce coaxial introduction needle.
13. Perform MRI check of needle position in relation to target lesion and correct position, if necessary.
14. Demonstrate biopsy sounds.
15. Obtain tissue samples: ≥12 tissue samples with 11-gauge needle, or volume equivalent.
16. Perform MRI check of biopsy cavity position in relation to target lesion (possibly with additional contrast administration).
17. If necessary, harvest additional tissue samples.
18. Consider placing marker coil/clip.
19. Remove coaxial introduction needle.
20. Release breast from puncture device while applying compression to puncture site. Move patient to reclining chair, apply compression, and cool puncture site.
21. Perform final mammograms in two orthogonal planes.

Postbiopsy MRI check with contrast administration. It is important to perform an MRI check of the biopsy cavity during the course of or after concluding a diagnostic intervention. This can be performed with or without the additional administration of contrast material, depending on the target lesion. An MRI check without contrast administration is usually sufficient to confirm the biopsy cavity location in relation to nonmass lesions. In the case of a mass-like enhancement, a contrast-enhanced MRI check to document the partial (**Fig. 6.12**) or complete (**Fig. 6.13**) removal of the target lesion is recommended. Knowledge of the exact location of residual tumor areas will also facilitate the directed harvesting of further tissue samples when required. When performing a contrast-enhanced MRI check, keep in mind that there is a potential for bleeding into the biopsy cavity, and this should not be confused with residual tumor in the subtraction image (**Fig. 6.14**).

6

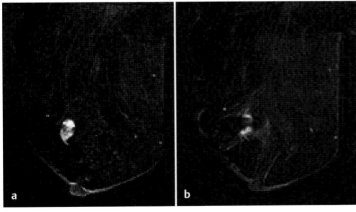

Fig. 6.12a, b Partial removal of enhancing lesion. a Ambiguous oval mass before MRI-guided VAB. **b** Periinterventional contrast enhanced MR mammography check after harvesting 12 tissue samples. Documentation of a partial removal from the center of the target lesion.

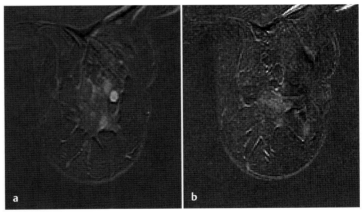

Fig. 6.13a, b Complete removal of enhancing lesion. a Primary finding on MR mammography shows mass lesion in the left breast before MRI-guided VAB. **b** Contrast-enhanced MR mammography check after harvesting nine tissue samples (8 gauge) shows no more contrast enhancement as confirmation of complete removal.

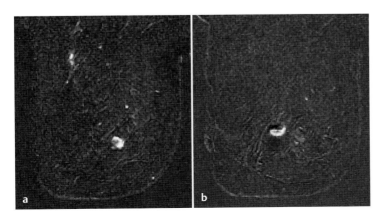

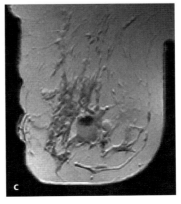

Fig. 6.14a–c False residual tumor.
a Hypervascularized mass lesion in diagnostic MR mammography before MRI-guided VAB.
b Contrast-enhanced MR mammography check (subtraction image) after harvesting 12 tissue samples shows signal-intense structure that could possibly be falsely interpreted as residual tumor.
c In direct comparison with the T1-weighted examination, the signal-intense structure seen in the subtraction image can be localized within the biopsy cavity and represents contrast-containing blood (jet effect).

Procedure: Contrast-enhanced MR mammography is performed with the localization equipment positioned on the affected side to reproduce the target lesion necessary for the MRI-guided biopsy.

- If the target lesion is not, or only questionably, reproduced then the intervention should be discontinued and a short-term follow-up examination in 6 months recommended.
- If the target lesion is clearly identified, then the puncture coordinates (x-, y-, and z-axes) are calculated. The calculated puncture site is marked with an external marker (e.g., oil-containing), and a MRI-check is performed without additional contrast administration.
- If the marker position is incorrect, then a new calculation is performed and the marker position corrected. If the marker position is correct, then the skin is disinfected and local anesthesia is administered (if necessary, a skin nick incision). The coaxial introduction needle is positioned (e.g., using the metal puncture stylet) to the appropriate depth (z-axis). The correct position is dependent upon the VAB system being used.
- The puncture stylet is replaced by a MRI-compatible mandrin and the position of the coaxial introduction needle is checked by performing an MRI T1-weighted series without contrast. If the position is incorrect, then a new calculation is performed and the needle is repositioned and rechecked. If the position is correct, then MRI-compatible mandrin is removed and replaced with the VAB needle.
- Tissue samples are then harvested in a contiguous manner with the VAB needle by rotating the biopsy notch. Twelve or more tissue samples should be obtained, which is the equivalent of one complete rotation around the clock time positions (1 to 12 o'clock). When appropriate, an MRI check can be performed during the intervention to confirm the representative position of the biopsy cavity or to redirect further sampling.
- Perform a postinterventional MRI check (when indicated with contrast administration, e.g., mass lesions) as a final confirmation of representative tissue sampling (target size is reduced, target is no longer detected, the biopsy cavity position is representative). If necessary, further sampling should be performed.
- Place a marker coil/clip in the biopsy cavity through the coaxial introduction cannula (optional). Confirm (without contrast) intramammary coil position with MRI.
- Remove the coaxial introduction needle. Compress and cool puncture channel. Apply a compression bandage.
- Optional: Perform postbiopsy mammograms in CC and ML projection for the topographic localization of the biopsy cavity, or to document the coil position for the planning of future surgery.

Report: Was the target finding reproducible (yes/no)?

- Position of target finding (quadrant, clock-time position, distance from the skin)
- Vacuum needle caliber (e.g., 11-gauge, 9-gauge)
- Number of tissue samples primarily harvested (if applicable, secondary harvesting)
- Documentation of relevant complications

Documentation: MR image of target finding (subtraction image)

- MRI of coaxial introduction needle position (prefire)
- MRI of biopsy cavity or of VAB needle position after biopsy
- Optional: MRI check with additional contrast administration
- Optional: Mammography in CC and ML projection

Quality criterion: Complete or partial removal of the lesion to be histologically verified by MRI-guided percutaneous biopsy.

Postbiopsy procedure: For findings in the following pathology reporting categories:

- B1 or B2: Short-term MRI follow-up in 6 months (in special cases earlier)
- B3 or B4: Interdisciplinary conference to decide on the course of action (e.g., MRI follow-up, rebiopsy, surgery)
- B5a or B5b: Initiation of appropriate therapy

* German Radiology Association's Breast Diagnostics Working Group 2007

Tips and Tricks

Second-look US. Before performing an MRI-guided VAB of an ambiguous finding that does not have a correlating finding on the primary clinical, mammographic, or ultrasonographic examination, a second-look US should always be performed (**Fig. 6.15**). Knowing the exact location, size, and configuration of the MRI finding, it is sometimes possible to identify a corresponding lesion on US, making it amenable to the much simpler and less-expensive US-guided CNB. If it is not possible to attain a conclusive diagnosis in this way, then a MRI-guided intervention should always be performed. In this context, it is sometimes desirable to confirm that the biopsied US finding definitely correlates with the suspicious MRI-finding. In such cases, it is possible to place a manually removable localization wire (e.g., Homer Mammalok) into the biopsy region after US-guided biopsy and establish correlation in a MRI examination. For this purpose, a T1-weighted series without administration of contrast material is usually sufficient.

Biopsy without contrast material. MRI findings that have a distinct signal intensity and characteristic morphology in the T1-weighted-precontrast or T2-weighted image can often be identified and biopsied without the administration of contrast material (**Fig. 6.16**). It must be kept in mind, however, that under biopsy conditions, the greater and altered breast compression can result in a distortion of the original shape and make identification more difficult. The administration of contrast material remains a viable option.

Puncture through lesion. The exact, primary placement of the biopsy needle within the target finding is not always possible due to the great differences in the consistency of internal breast structures. This makes corrections of the needle depth necessary. It is preferable to primarily place the needle deeper into the breast and correct the position by pulling it back out the appropriate distance (easier to control), than to place the needle primarily too superficially and have to push it deeper (possible further displacement of structures during correction) (**Fig. 6.17**).

Long intramammary needle path. Occasionally, it is not possible to access subcutaneous lesions by the shortest, direct approach. If the biopsy needle is inserted too deeply, the lesion will be missed. If the biopsy needle is not inserted deeply enough, the notch will not be completely within the breast and will suck in air and not create the necessary vacuum. In such cases, it is necessary to perform the intervention with an approach from the opposite side of the breast, i.e., taking a long path through the breast. To avoid penetrating or painfully irritating the skin with the needle tip, it is recommended to choose a biopsy needle with a rounded tip. The difficulties experienced in a long approach to a target finding are also encountered when biopsying findings near the chest wall (**Fig. 6.18**).

Small mass lesions. When biopsying small lesions (e.g., ≤10 mm diameter), it can be advantageous to position the biopsy needle a few millimeters ventrally or dorsally of the lesion and selectively harvest tissue samples in the direction of the lesion while applying increasing pressure in this direction by either tilting the needle, or moving the needle toward the lesion in a parallel fashion (unidirectional biopsy with post and pillar system). Proceeding in this way, the lesion is sucked into the biopsy notch and cannot repeatedly slip away and elude being biopsied, as is conceivably possible when biopsying a hard lesion and proceeding in the usual way (rotating the biopsy notch) (**Fig. 6.19**). This unidirectional procedural method results in better immobilization of small, firm lesions, especially when located within "soft" lipomatous tissue.

Cyst aspiration. If there are large simple breast cysts along the expected biopsy path, then these should be percutaneously aspirated before contrast administration. Otherwise, puncturing the cyst(s) during the intervention can cause substantial breast tissue displacement (**Fig. 6.20**).

Aspiration of a postbiopsy hematoma and coil placement. Once a marker coil or clip has been placed within the biopsy cavity, no further attempts should be made to aspirate a postbiopsy hematoma through the coaxial introduction cannula. Occasionally, this can lead to aspiration and removal of the marker coil/clip (**Fig. 6.21**).

Compression using a swab. After removing the coaxial introduction needle, the puncture site can be compressed using a sterile swab. This facilitates removing the compression unit of the biopsy fixture while avoiding bleeding from the puncture site (**Fig. 6.22**).

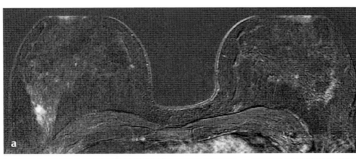

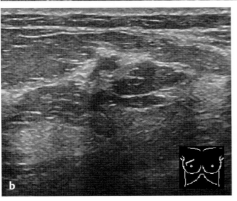
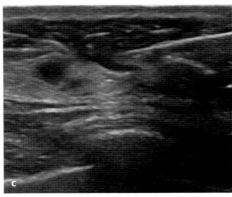
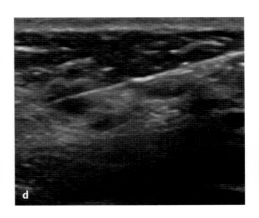

Fig. 6.15a–d Second-look US. Hypervascularized mass lesion of 6-mm diameter in the lateral aspect of the right breast on MR mammography (subtraction image) (**a**). The primary clinical, mammographic, and ultrasonographic examinations were without pathologic findings. Directed, second-look US revealed a vague correlating finding (**b**). A tentative US-guided CNB was performed: pre- and postfire documentation (**c, d**). *Histology*: IDC.

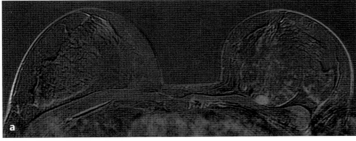
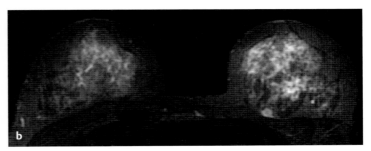

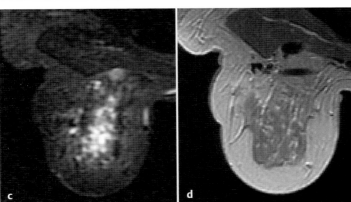

Fig. 6.16a–d MRI-guided intervention without contrast administration. Diagnostic MR mammography (subtraction image) reveals a hypervascularized mass lesion in the upper inner quadrant of the left breast (**a**). The target lesion shows a high signal intensity in the T2-weighted image (**b**). T2-weighted and postbiopsy T1-weighted images acquired during MRI-guided biopsy (**c, d**). *Histology*: mucinous carcinoma.

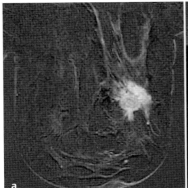
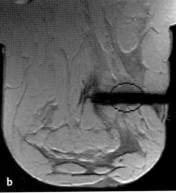
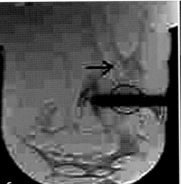
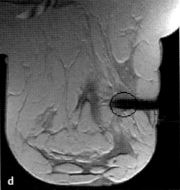

Fig. 6.17a–d MRI-guided intervention with primary deep placement of biopsy needle. Subtraction image depicts suspicious hypervascularized lesion (**a**). T1-weighted image shows coaxial introduction needle with MRI-compatible mandrin (**b**). The position of the coaxial introduction needle tip is approx. 1 cm too deep and must be corrected (**c**). The MRI check now shows the coaxial introduction needle tip in the center of the target lesion (**d**).

6

6

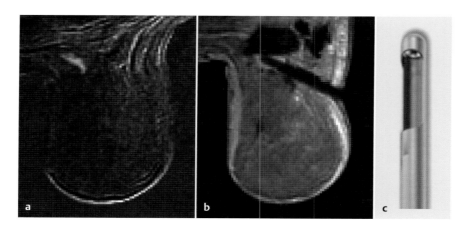

Fig. 6.18a–c Rounded biopsy needle tip for MRI-guided VAB of findings near the skin and chest wall. Subtraction image of a hypervascularized finding near the chest wall that should preferably be accessed from the opposite side of the breast, using a biopsy needle with a rounded tip (**a**). Postbiopsy T1-weighted image after harvesting 12 tissue samples. Biopsy cavity position confirms representative sampling (coaxial introduction needle in place) (**b**). VAB needle with rounded tip (**c**).

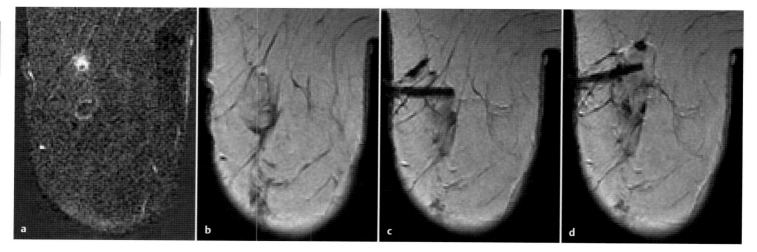

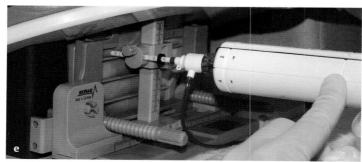

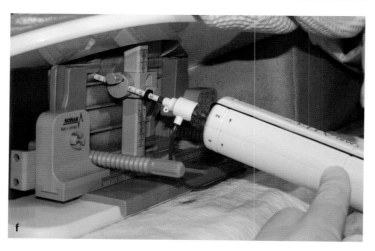

Fig. 6.19a–f Unidirectional sample harvesting during MRI-guided VAB of small mass lesion. Subtraction image of small target lesion in the left breast (**a**). T1-weighted postcontrast image (**b**). The coaxial introduction needle is inserted horizontally into the breast with the tip placed on the ventral side of the target lesion (**c**). Tissue samples are harvested unidirectionally with the biopsy notch opening toward the chest wall. The T1-weighted image shows the end position of the coaxial introduction needle after harvesting 12 samples (**d**). Start position of biopsy equipment (**e**). End position after completion of the intervention (**f**). *Histology*: fat necrosis.

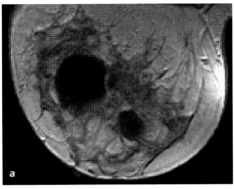

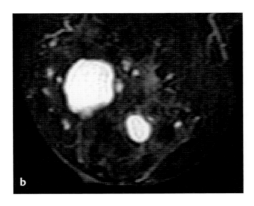

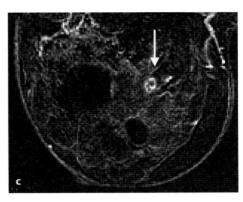

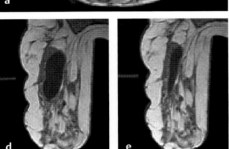

Fig. 6.20a–e Cyst aspiration before contrast administration during MRI- guided intervention. Diagnostic MR mammography reveals a suspicious mass lesion with ring-enhancement in the right breast and a large simple cyst in the expected biopsy path.
a T1-weighted precontrast image.
b T2-weighted image.
c Subtraction image with arrow marking suspicious lesion.
d T1-weighted precontrast, preintervention image before cyst aspiration.
e T1-weighted precontrast, preintervention image after maximum possible fluid aspiration.

6

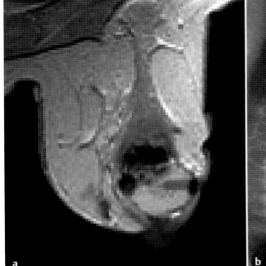

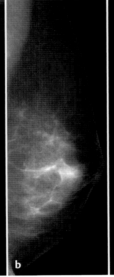

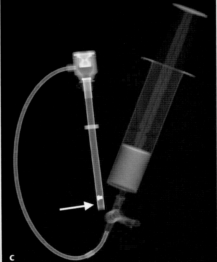

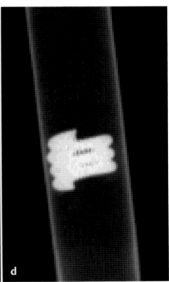

Fig. 6.21a–d Unintentional coil removal during aspiration of postbiopsy hematoma.
a T1-weighted image after MRI-guided VAB and coil placement.

b Subsequent aspiration of hematoma. Postbiopsy mammography shows no coil in biopsy cavity.
c X-ray photograph of coaxial introduction needle shows coil within the cannula (arrow).
d Magnified partial view of coil.

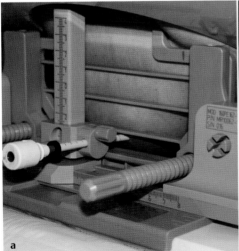

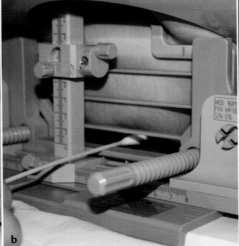

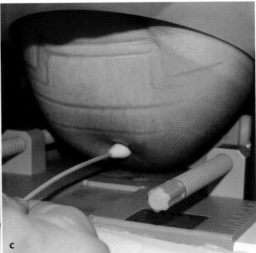

Fig. 6.22a–c Compression of puncture site with sterile swab.
a Clinical situation after concluding sample harvesting shows breast with biopsy compression device and coaxial introduction needle in place.

b Swab is used to compress puncture site after removal of coaxial introduction needle.
c Compression device is easily removed without excess bleeding from puncture site.

6

Computer-aided Interventional Guidance Systems

Several companies have developed software programs that perform real-time calculations of needle insertion coordinates (x-, y-, and z-axes) to aid the performance of MRI-guided interventions of the breast. In principle, all systems calculate the target coordinates in relation to a reference point, and then report the puncture position to which the needle must be moved and the depth of insertion (three dimensions). At present, there are three systems available:

- SureLoc, Confirma Europe, Berlin, Germany (**Fig. 6.23**)
- DynaLOC, Invivo Corp., Orlando, FL (**Fig. 6.24**)
- MICS-MIA (MICS = MR Mammography Intervention Coil System, MIA = Mammography Intervention Aid), Machnet BV, Eelde, the Netherlands (**Fig. 6.25**)

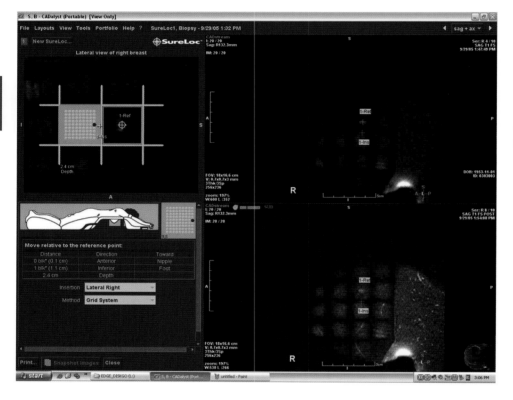

Fig. 6.23 Computer-aided coordinate calculation for MRI-guided interventions (SureLoc, Confirma Europe Inc., Berlin, Germany). Computer display after calculation of puncture coordinates for MRI-guided intervention using the grid method. The Sure-Loc report indicates the appropriate position in the grid stabilization plate into which the block needle guide is to be moved (in relation to the reference block), and the appropriate channel for needle insertion within the block needle guide (here: the 9th horizontal and 5th vertical channel).

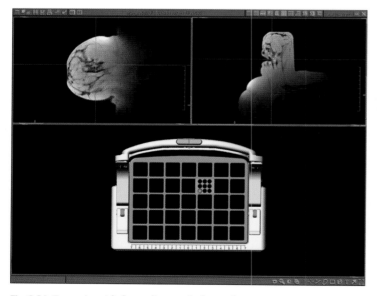

Fig. 6.24 Computer-aided coordinate calculation for MRI-guided interventions (DynaLOC, Invivo Corp., Orlando, FL). Computer display after calculation of puncture coordinates for MRI-guided intervention using the grid method. In this example, the needle block guide is to be inserted into the 5th horizontal, 2nd vertical grid compartment. The needle is then to be inserted into the lower left needle channel within the block guide.

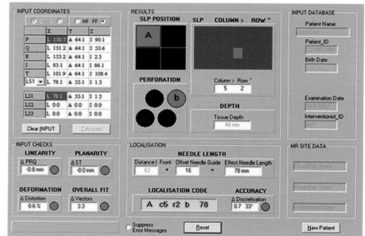

Fig. 6.25 Computer-aided coordinate calculation for MRI-guided interventions (MICS-MIA, Machnet BV, Eelde, the Netherlands). Computer display after calculation of puncture coordinates for MRI-guided intervention using the grid method. In this example, the needle block guide is to be inserted into the 5th horizontal, 3rd vertical grid compartment. The needle is then to be inserted into the upper right needle channel within the block guide. MICS = MR Mammography Intervention Coil System, MIA = Mammography Intervention Aid.

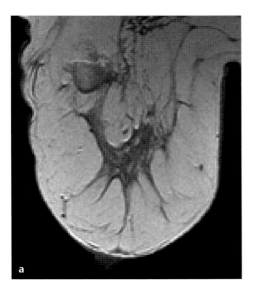

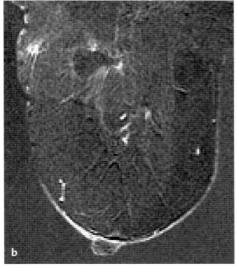

Fig. 6.26a,b MR mammography examination 1 week after VAB.
a T1-weighted precontrast image shows circumscribed hematoma 1 week after VAB.
b Subtraction image after contrast administration shows discrete enhancement at the hematoma borders.

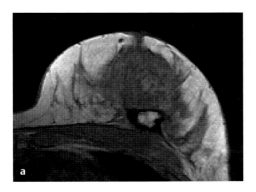

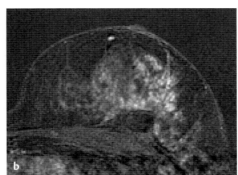

Fig. 6.27a,b Persisting hematoma 6 months after VAB.
a T1-weighted precontrast image shows hematoma in organization 6 months after VAB.
b Subtraction image shows physiologic enhancement of parenchymal tissues after contrast administration. No significant enhancement is seen in direct proximity to the hematoma.

6

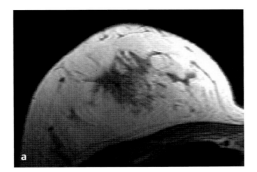

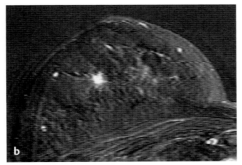

Fig. 6.28a,b Persistant reactive hyperemia in scar area after VAB. The T1-weighted precontrast image shows a focal architectural distortion 6 months after VAB (**a**). Subtraction image after contrast administration shows highly suspicious enhancement in the center of the former biopsy cavity (**b**). *Histology:* lymphocytic inflammation without signs of malignancy.

Follow-up

Biopsy cavity. It can normally be assumed that a biopsy cavity will remain identifiable over a period of days to weeks after VAB. Usually, the tissues surrounding the hematoma will show very little if any contrast enhancement after a few days (**Fig. 6.26**). Occasionally, however, the hematoma (**Fig. 6.27**) and/or a contrast enhancement (**Fig. 6.28**) may remain visible for several months.

Short-term follow-up 6 months after vacuum-assisted biopsy with benign histology. When the results of a VAB are histologically benign, a short-term follow-up is recommended 6 months after biopsy. This is especially important when the histologic results are incongruous with image findings. If the follow-up examination shows that the target lesion is smaller in size or no longer identifiable, then the biopsy can be assumed to be representative and further examinations are recommended in normal intervals (**Figs. 6.29** and **6.30**). If the target lesion appears unchanged in size and configuration, then it remains unclear as to whether or not the lesion was correctly sampled. Because the lesion size has not increased, however, it can usually be assumed that it is a benign lesion. Despite this, a further follow-up examination in 6–12 months is recommended in this situation (**Fig. 6.31**). If the follow-up examination shows that the target lesion has increased in size during the 6-month interval, then the images documenting the MR-guided biopsy procedure should be carefully reviewed to decide whether this development is more likely the result of reactive changes accompanying a prolonged wound healing, or whether the target was missed on biopsy and the lesion is presumably a malignancy (**Fig. 6.32a–e**). If it is deduced that prolonged wound healing is the likely cause of the image development, then another short-term follow-up in 6 months is indicated (**Fig. 6.32f**). If a failed biopsy is assumed, then a renewed percutaneous biopsy or an open biopsy should be discussed.

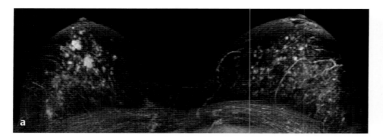

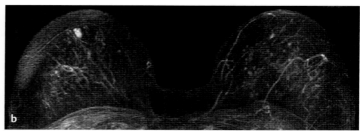

Fig. 6.29a, b Biopsied lesion is no longer identifiable in follow-up 6 months after VAB.
a Numerous bilateral foci and two hypervascularized mass lesions in the right breast on diagnostic MR mammography.

b The larger, centrally located lesion was proven benign on histology. In the follow-up MR mammography 7 months later, the biopsied lesion is no longer identifiable, a sign of complete removal by VAB. The ventral lesion is unchanged.

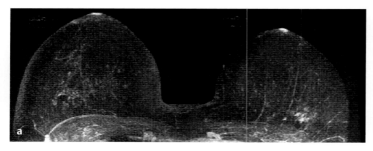

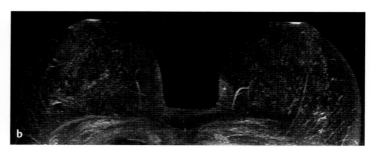

Fig. 6.30a, b Regression of biopsied finding in follow-up 6 months after VAB.
Initial MR mammography (subtraction maximum intensity projection[MIP]) shows regional nonmass enhancement in the lower outer quadrant of the left breast (**a**). MRI-guided VAB revealed focal mastitis (pathologic category: B2). The follow-up

MR mammography shows near normalization of the biopsied finding after 6 months (**b**). Note: In this specific case, it is irrelevant whether the regression is due to the biopsy or to the normal healing process. A malignancy can be ruled out In both cases.

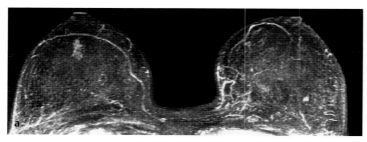

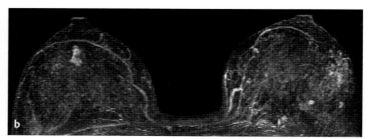

Fig. 6.31a, b Biopsied lesion is unchanged in follow-up 18 months after VAB.
Diagnostic MR mammography shows a nonmass hypervascularization in the right retromamillary region (**a**). MRI-guided VAB revealed a finding of benign histology. The patient did not show up for the recommended 6-month follow-up examination.

The next MR mammography was performed 18 months later and revealed that the finding was completely unchanged (**b**), possibly an indication that the lesion had been missed. Due to the stability of the lesion over 18 months, there is no indication for a rebiopsy.

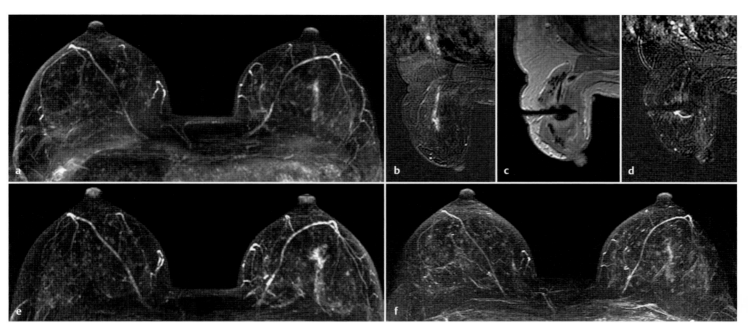

Fig. 6.32a–f Progression of biopsied finding in follow-up 6 months after VAB.
Initial MR mammography (subtraction MIP) shows a linear enhancement in the central aspect of the left breast (**a**). MRI-guided VAB revealed adenosis without signs of malignancy. The documentation images during VAB show that tissue samples were acquired in the ventral portions of the linear enhancement (subtraction image: **b**; T1-weighted image with coaxial introduction needle in place after biopsy: **c**; subtraction image after additional contrast administration: **d**). The follow-up MR mammography shows an increase in vascularization, especially in the ventral portion of the biopsied finding after 6 months (**e**). After careful consideration, no rebiopsy was performed, and another follow-up MR mammography 6 months later now showed a regression of the linear enhancement (**f**).

6

MRI-guided Vacuum-assisted Biopsy: Clinical and Problem Cases

Clinical Case 1: MRI-guided Vacuum-assisted Biopsy of Ambiguous Mass Lesion (Fig. 6.33)

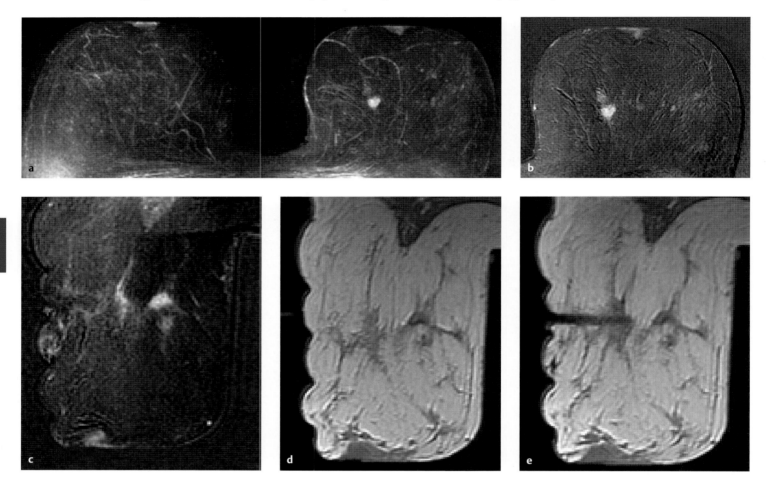

Fig. 6.33a–e   MRI-guided VAB of ambiguous mass lesion. Diagnostic MR mammography performed in woman with dense breast parenchyma (ACR density type IV, BI-RADS 1) and no pathologic findings on breast US. Subtraction MIP (**a**). Subtraction slice image of left breast shows suspicious hypervascularized lesion (**b**).

The lesion is clearly reproduced in the image documentation before MRI-guided VAB (subtraction image: **c**; T1-weighted precontrast image: **d**). T1-weighted image shows exact prefire placement of coaxial introduction needle (VACORA biopsy system; Bard Biopsy Systems, Tempe, AZ) (**e**). *Histology:* IDC (B5b).

Clinical Case 2: MRI-guided Vacuum-assisted Biopsy of Ambiguous Nonmass Enhancement (Fig. 6.34)

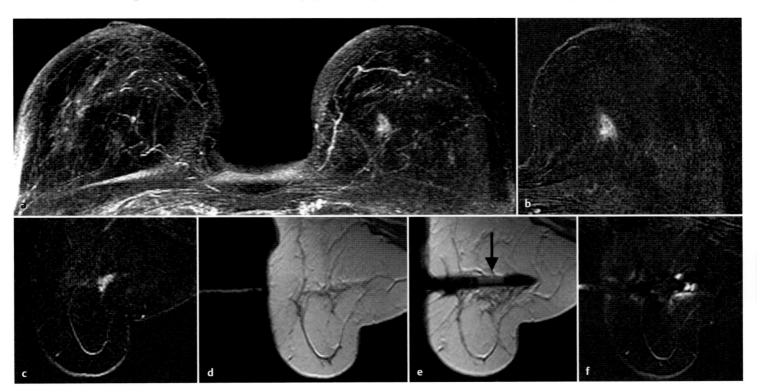

6

Fig. 6.34a–f MRI-guided VAB of ambiguous nonmass enhancement. Diagnostic MR mammography shows ambiguous focal nonmass enhancement in the central portion of the left breast (MR mammography BI-RADS 4). Subtraction MIP (**a**). Subtraction slice image of left breast (**b**). The lesion is clearly reproduced in the image documentation before MRI-guided VAB (subtraction image) (**c**). T1-weighted image check shows correct placement and direction of external marker after calcu-lated adjustment (**d**). T1-weighted image documentation shows exact placement of biopsy needle and sampling notch (arrow) in the center of the target finding (Mammotome biopsy system; Ethicon Endo-Surgery, Cincinnati, OH) (**e**). Final sub-traction image documentation after additional contrast administration (**f**). *Histology*: radial scar (B3).

Clinical Case 3 (Special Situation): Simultaneous MRI-guided Vacuum-assisted Biopsy of Bifocal Suspicious Findings

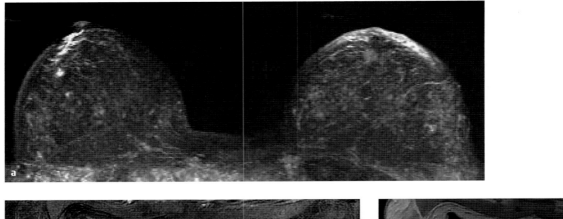

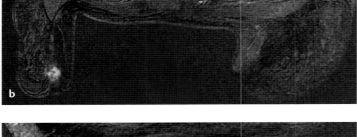

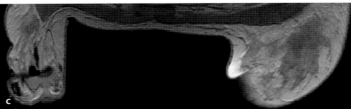

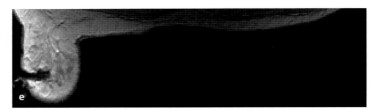

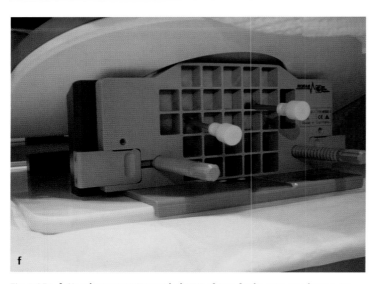

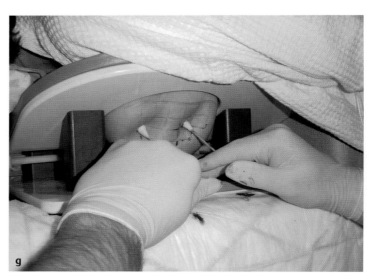

Fig. 6.35a–f Simultaneous MRI-guided VAB of two findings in one breast. Diagnostic MR mammography shows two suspicious findings in the left upper inner quadrant and caudally at 6 o'clock. Subtraction MIP (**a**). Primary VAB of the more suspicious lesion in the upper inner quadrant (subtraction slice image: **b**; T1-weighted postbiopsy image: **c**). Second VAB of the lesion in the caudal aspect (sub- traction slice image: **d**; T1-weighted postbiopsy image: **e**). Clinical situation after concluding sample harvesting shows breast with lateral biopsy and localization grid and both coaxial introduction needles in place (**f**). *Histology*: upper inner lesion: IDC (B5b). Caudal breast lesion: DCIS (B5a).

A simultaneous percutaneous biopsy of bifocal findings within one breast is generally possible. When doing so, the more suspicious of the lesions should be biopsied first, in case the intervention must be prematurely discontinued. It is also important to perform the interventions using a separate sterile intervention set for each lesion so that cell material is not seeded from one location to the other, and so that the harvested tissues are not contaminated (**Fig. 6.35**).

Tips and Tricks

The use of a biopsy and localization grid is recommended when performing simultaneous VABs of unilateral, bifocal lesions because it allows both puncture sites to be selected independently. The vacuum-assisted biopsies should also be performed in coaxial technique. After completion of the first biopsy, the mandrin can be inserted into the coaxial introduction cannula and left in place while performing the second biopsy, avoiding excess bleeding from the first site.

Clinical Case 4 (Special Situation): Simultaneous MRI-guided Vacuum-assisted Biopsy of Bilateral Suspicious Findings (Fig. 6.36)

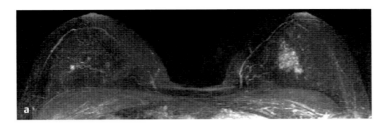

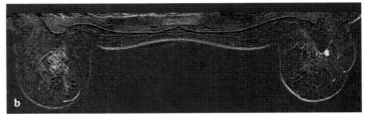

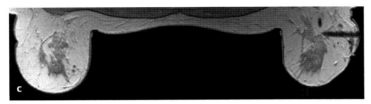

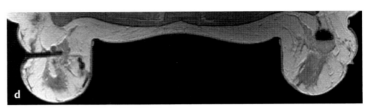

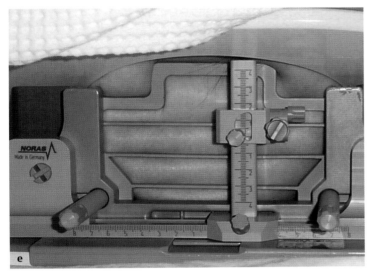

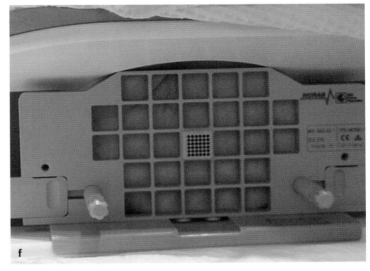

6

Fig. 6.36a–f Simultaneous MRI-guided VAB of bilateral findings. Diagnostic MR mammography shows a suspicious mass in the right breast (MR mammography BI-RADS 5) and an ambiguous focal nonmass enhancement in the left breast (MR mammography BI-RADS 4). Subtraction MIP (**a**). To perform a VAB of both lesions, a post and pillar biopsy attachment was used on the right, more suspicious lesion, and a biopsy and localization grid attachment on the left (**e, f**). Subtraction slice image showing both lesions (**b**). VAB on the right (**c**). VAB on the left. Coaxial introduction needle on the right is still in place (**d**). *Histology*: right lesion: DCIS (B5a). Left lesion: ductal hyperplasia (DH) with atypia (B3).

Tips and Tricks

When performing simultaneous VABs of bilateral lesions, a biopsy and localization grid is often used on one side, and a post and pillar biopsy attachment on the other. An intervention set often contains one of each of these biopsy attachments so that it is not necessary to purchase an additional attachment. Again, the VABs should also be performed in coaxial technique so that the coaxial introduction needle can be left in place while performing the second biopsy, avoiding excess bleeding from the first site.

Clinical Case 5 (Special Situation): MRI-guided Vacuum-assisted Biopsy of a Suspicious Finding near a Breast Prosthesis (Fig. 6.37)

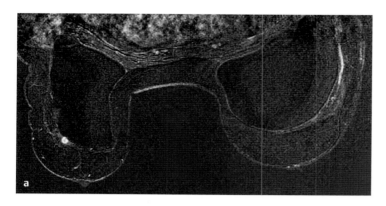

Fig. 6.37a–f MRI-guided VAB of a suspicious finding near a breast prosthesis. Personal history of breast cancer in the right breast 16 years ago, treated by mastectomy and implant-based reconstruction. At that time, the patient opted for an augmentation of the left breast. The diagnostic MR mammography shows a suspicious finding directly adjacent to the left prosthesis (no image). The hypervascularized lesion is clearly reproduced in the image documentation before MRI-guided VAB (subtraction image) (**a, b**). The coaxial introduction needle is angled parallel to the prosthesis surface (**c**). The biopsy needle was introduced so that the sample notch was directed toward the prosthesis and eight tissue samples were harvested unilaterally in this direction. T1-weighted postbiopsy scan with coaxial introduction needle in place (**d**). *Histology* revealed a tubular carcinoma (B5b). Preoperative MRI-guided localization using an Ariadne-thread hook wire (**e**). Mammographic image shows the coil in projection over the breast prosthesis (digitally processed image) (**f**). *Final histology*: tubular carcinoma pT1a, pN0, G1.

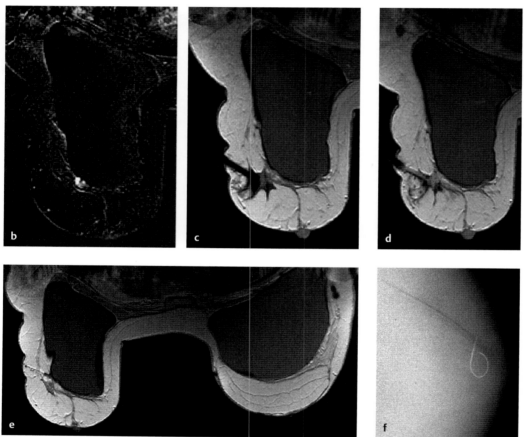

Tips and Tricks

Never choose a puncture direction toward the prosthesis. Always look for a biopsy approach that allows tangential needle placement so that the lateral sampling notch can be directed toward the prosthesis surface for unilateral sample harvesting.

Problem Case 1: Target Lesion Cannot Be Reproduced under MRI-guided Intervention Conditions

Occasionally, the lesion that is to be biopsied cannot (can no longer) be seen in the contrast-enhanced MR mammography examination performed before a planned MRI-guided VAB. In the literature, this is described as the case in 0–2% of cases. The main cause is the intraindividual fluctuation of contrast enhancement in benign breast changes (**Fig. 6.38**). In all cases, however, it is important to ensure that no other causes come into question

(e.g., incomplete imaging of the breast [**Fig. 6.39**], failed contrast injection [check: contrast visible in intramammary veins and internal mammary artery], artifacts). For forensic reasons, a diagnostic MR mammography examination should be performed in the identical menstrual cycle phase shortly after a MRI-guided VAB has been discontinued due to failed lesion visualization.

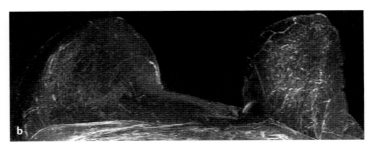

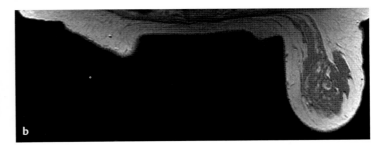

Fig. 6.38a, b Target lesion cannot be reproduced due to intraindividual contrast uptake fluctuations. The diagnostic MR mammography shows a bilateral fine patchy enhancement pattern with a small, indistinct focus in the central portion of the left breast (**a**). The lesion cannot be reproduced in the contrast-enhanced

MR mammography examination performed before planned MRI-guided VAB the following day (**b**). The shape of the left breast is altered by the biopsy compression plate. The biopsy was abandoned and a short-term follow-up examination in 6 months recommended.

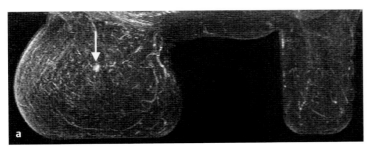

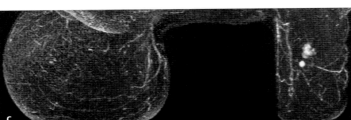

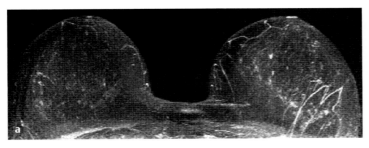

Fig. 6.39a–d Target lesion cannot be reproduced because its position is outside the imaged breast. The contrast-enhanced MR mammography examination performed before planned MRI-guided VAB fails to show a known suspicious lesion in the cranial aspect of the right breast (subtraction MIP) (**a**). Note: the lesion in the caudal aspect of the left breast (arrow) is known to be unchanged over several years. The first cranial T1-weighted image slice shows a significant amount of parenchyma as an indication that the cranial aspect of the right breast is not adequately imaged (**b**). In the contrast-enhanced MR mammography examination

performed before planned MRI-guided VAB the following day, the breast was carefully positioned to include the cranial aspect of the right breast in the image slices. Now the right lesion is clearly reproduced in the subtraction MIP (**c**). Note: now the benign lesion in the caudal aspect of the left breast is no longer visualized due to its position outside the imaged portion of the breast. The first cranial T1-weighted image slice now shows subcutaneous fat indicating that the image slices begin above the parenchyma (**d**).

6

Problem Case 2: Unfavorable Lesion Location

The performance of a percutaneous MRI-guided VAB can be especially difficult or impossible when the breast is very small, the parenchyma is very atrophied, or when the lesion is located in the axillary tail or in the medial aspect of the breast. It is generally important to pay special attention to the positioning of the patient, taking the lesion position into account, so that the target lesion can be most easily accessed. In rare cases, it may be necessary to repeat the examination on the following day if the lesion position is found to be unfavorable on the primary examination (**Fig. 6.40**). Otherwise, it may be necessary to perform an open biopsy after wire localization, which is often feasible despite an unfavorable lesion position.

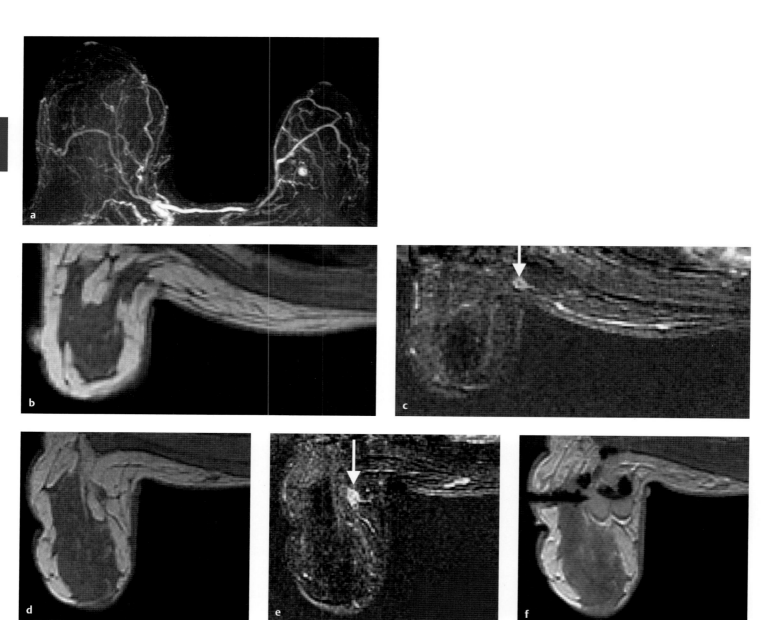

Fig. 6.40a–f Successful intervention after repositioning of the patient because of unfavorable lesion localization in the primary examination. The diagnostic MR mammography examination shows an ambiguous mass in the lower inner quadrant of the right breast (examination performed at an external medical facility: subtraction MIP) (**a**). The contrast-enhanced MR mammography examination performed before MRI-guided VAB shows the target lesion (arrow) in an unfavorable position in the medial breast fold (T1-weighted precontrast image: **b**, subtraction image **c**). In the contrast-enhanced MR mammography examination performed before MRI-guided VAB the following day, the breast was carefully positioned by pulling the lower medial aspect further into the compression device and shows a more favorable lesion position (arrow) (T1-weighted precontrast image: **d**, subtraction image: **e**). T1-weighted postbiopsy documentation verifies complete removal of target lesion (biopsy cavity in representative position, coaxial introduction needle in place) (**f**). *Histology*: IDC (B5b).

Problem Case 3: Impeded Direct Access—Angulated Access

Independent of the biopsy equipment used the direct approach to the target lesion may be impeded by a portion of the biopsy compression attachment (e.g., Plexiglas bar) (**Fig. 6.41**). In these situations alternative, angled approaches with the puncture site adjacent to the impeding obstacle must be considered and appraised.

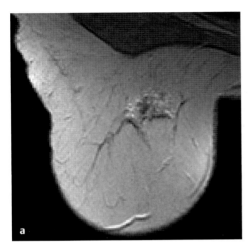
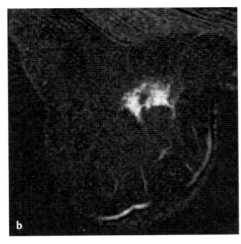

Fig. 6.41a–i **The direct biopsy approach is hindered by biopsy equipment.** T1-weighted postcontrast image (**a**) and subtraction image (**b**) show a nonmass lesion in the left breast. After repositioning the external marker according to the calculated target coordinates, it is evident that a Plexiglass bar (arrow) will prevent needle access to the skin at this site. A puncture site above the bar was chosen and the coaxial introduction needle was angled appropriately (**c**). VAB using the ATEC biopsy system (Suros Surgical Systems, Inc., Indianapolis, IN) (**d**). T1-weighted image documentation of coaxial introduction needle with MRI-compatible mandrin tip positioned within target lesion (**e**). T1-weighted postbiopsy documentation after harvesting 12 tissue samples (**f**). Subtraction image verifies partial removal of target lesion (**g**). Comparison of subtraction MIP images before (**h**) and after (**i**) biopsy. *Histology*: invasive lobular carcinoma (ILC) (B5b).

6

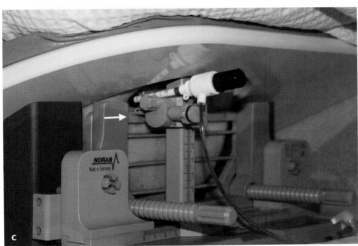
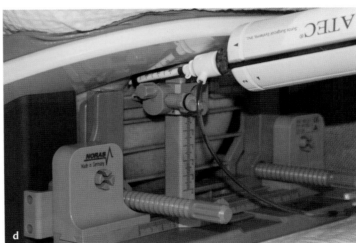

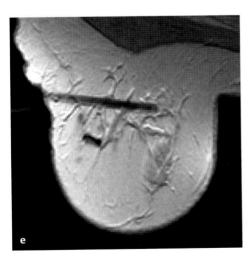
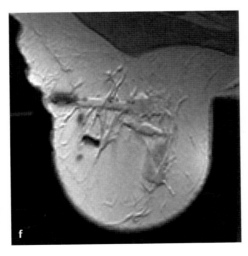
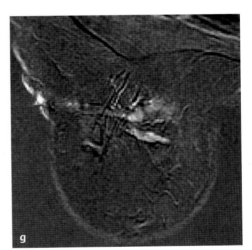

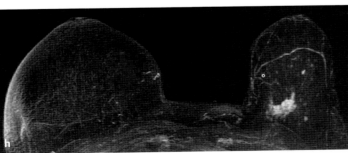
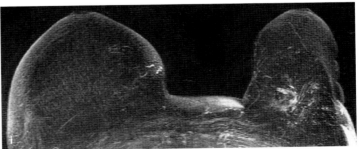

6

Problem Case 4: Displacement of Target Lesion

If a patient is restless (**Fig. 6.42**), or the breast is insufficiently compressed (**Fig. 6.43**) during the performance of a VAB, then the target lesion may become displaced before the intervention is completed. In such cases, it is important that the displacement is noticed, and that the situation be reappraised as to whether the intervention can be continued by orientating oneself according to anatomic structures (e.g., nipple, parenchymal structures), or whether the intervention should be discontinued and repeated at a future date after eliminating the cause.

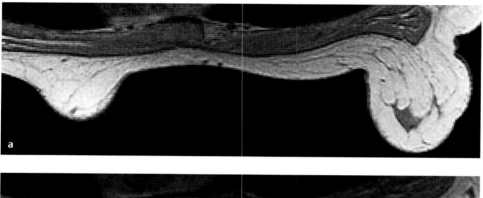

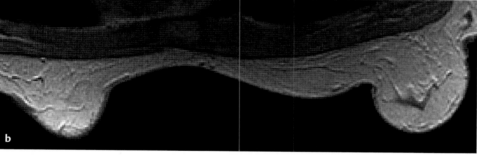

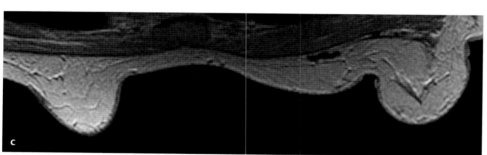

Fig. 6.42a–c Displacement of the target lesion by patient movement.
T1-weighted image at the beginning of the MR mammography examination performed before planned MRI-guided VAB of a left lesion (**a**). Identical image slice after IV contrast administration shows significant displacement of parenchymal structures in the left breast and an increase of the subcutaneous fat tissue volume medial of the left breast due to the breast slipping out of the compressed position (**b**). The additional dynamic measurements show an increasing displacement of the left breast (**c**). The intervention was discontinued due to the unstable lesion position.

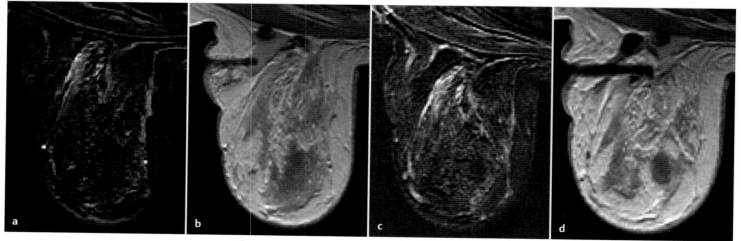

Fig. 6.43a–d Displacement of the target lesion by a hematoma. Regional enhancement in the left breast near the chest wall (subtraction image) (**a**). Tissue harvesting was not representative due to the medial displacement of the enhancing region by a hematoma that developed during biopsy (T1-weighted image) (**b**). The intervention was repeated the following day. The subtraction image shows the regional enhancement and the lateral hematoma (**c**). The T1-weighted image now shows the coaxial introduction needle within the enhancing region (representative tissue sampling) (**d**).

Problem Case 5: Erroneous Adjustment of the Needle Position

The inaccurate placement of the biopsy needle is usually the result of an erroneous calculation of puncture coordinates, or an incorrect realization of the necessary adjustments from the arbitrary zero-point (**Fig. 6.44**). The mistake can usually be rectified easily by simply removing the biopsy- or coaxial introduction needle and reinserting it at the appropriate position. As a rule, the correct position of the puncture site should be checked by performing a T1-weighted measurement after adjusting the external marker position and before application of local anesthesia.

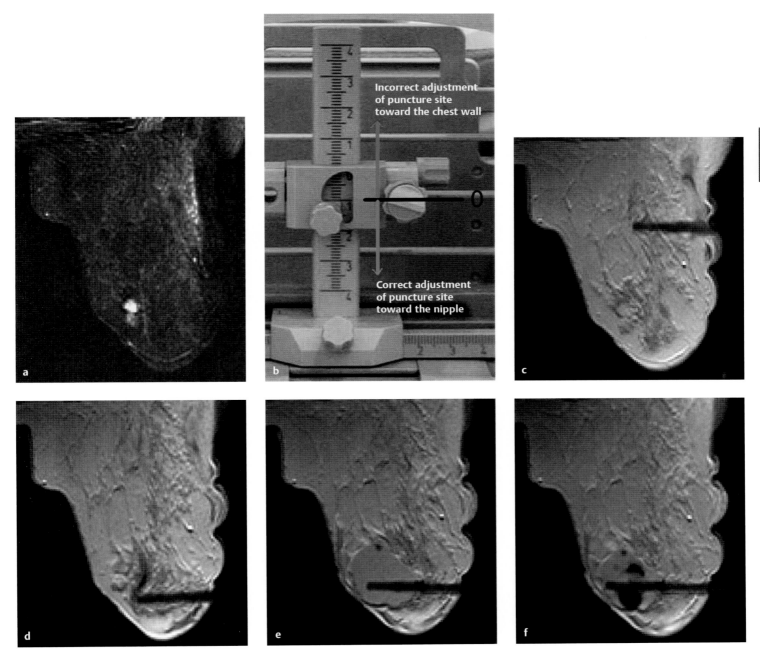

Fig. 6.44a–f Inaccurate placement of the coaxial introduction needle. MRI-guided VAB of an ambiguous mass in the medial aspect of the left breast (subtraction image) (**a**). Calculated puncture coordinates indicate that the puncture site is 25 mm toward the nipple in relation to the zero-point (**b**). The incorrect realization of this adjustment by moving the puncture site 25 mm toward the chest wall on the post and pillar attachment resulted in an inaccurate breast puncture (**c**). Biopsy was performed after removing the coaxial introduction needle and correcting the position. T1-weighted prebiopsy documentation of correct coaxial introduction needle position (**d**). T1-weighted documentation of biopsy cavity (**e**), and coil placement (**f**). *Histology*: fibroadenoma.

MRI-guided Core Needle Biopsy/ Fine Needle Aspiration Biopsy

MRI-guided Core Needle Biopsy

Diagnostic MRI-guided biopsies should preferably be performed as VABs. With this procedural approach, the harvesting of representative tissue samples is achieved with the greatest reliability. The smaller caliber core biopsies should only be performed in justified exceptional cases. Possible exceptions, among others, where a MRI-guided CNB might be justified are:

- unfavorable target location
- increased risk of excessive bleeding
- large tumor size
- ipsilateral secondary lesion

When performing a simultaneous ipsilateral VAB and CNB, the smaller lesion should be biopsied using the VAB technique (**Figs. 6.45** and **6.46**).

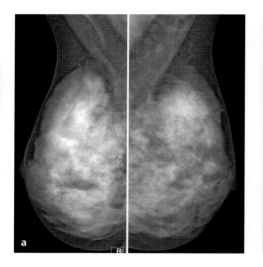
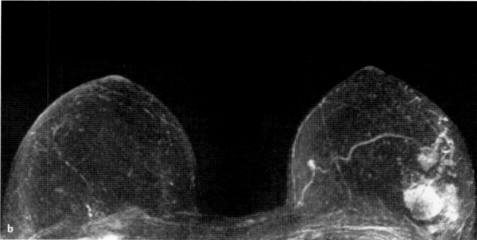

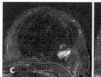

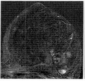

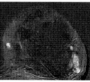

Fig. 6.45a–c   MRI-guided VAB in combination with CNB. Bilateral, diagnostic mammography in mediolateral oblique (MLO) projection shows extremely dense breast tissue, ACR density type IV (**a**). The supplementary diagnostic MR mammography reveals a large hypervascularized lesion in the lateral aspect of the left breast with an extent in the CC dimension of 6 cm (subtraction MIP) (**b**). Documentation of the tumor extent in the subtraction slice images (consecutive presentation of every second slice image, i. e., every 5 mm, from the cranial tumor images on the left to the caudal images on the right) (**c**). MRI-guided VAB was performed at the lower lateral tumor site (**c**: second image from the right). MRI-guided 14-gauge CNB was performed 2 and 3 cm cranially of the VAB site (**c**: sixth and eighth image from the right). *Histology*: tubular breast cancer in all biopsy specimens.

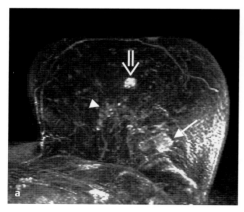
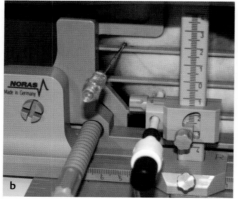
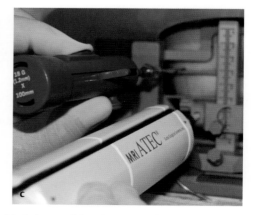

Fig. 6.46a–c   MRI-guided VAB in combination with CNB. A highly suspicious lesion in the lower outer quadrant of the left breast was biopsied under US guidance and revealed invasive breast cancer (BI-RADS 6). The pretherapeutic MR mammographic local staging examination shows the index tumor (single arrow) and revealed a second mass lesion in the cranial aspect of the left breast at 12 o'clock (double arrow), as well as a nonmass lesion (arrowhead) in the upper inner quadrant of the left breast (subtraction MIP) (**a**). The second mass lesion was biopsied in MRI-guided vacuum-assisted technique, and then the nonmass lesion in CNB technique. Clinical situation at the conclusion of both procedures showing the breast with biopsy compression fixture and both coaxial introduction needles in place (**b**). Clinical situation showing the Angiomed core biopsy needle (Angiomed GmBH, Karlsruhe, Germany) and the ATEC biopsy needle (Suros Surgical Systems, Inc., Indianapolis, IN) in place (**c**). *Histology*: mass lesion = fibroadenoma, nonmass lesion = fibrosis.

MRI-guided Fine Needle Aspiration Biopsy

Because of the high rate of false-negative results, an FNAB is not recommended to attain a definitive diagnosis of solid MRI lesions. In justified cases, however, an FNAB can be performed to obtain liquid intramammary samples, e.g., during an MRI-guided intervention performed for other reasons (**Fig. 6.47**).

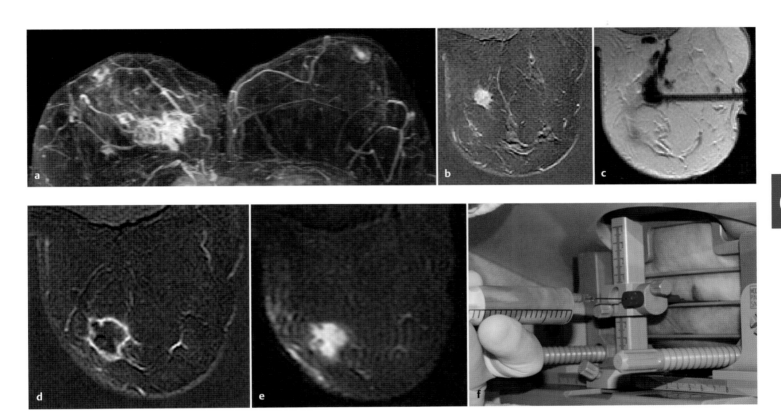

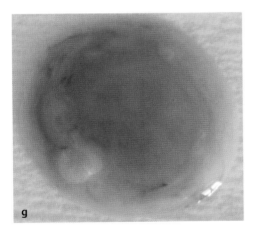

Fig. 6.47a–g MRI-guided VAB in combination with fine needle aspiration. The diagnostic MR mammography shows an index lesion highly suspicious of malignancy in the lower inner quadrant of the right breast, as well as a second lesion suspicious of an abscess in the cranial aspect of the right breast (ring enhancement and high signal intensity in the T2-weighted series). Subtraction MIP performed at an external medical facility (**a**). MRI-guided VAB of the index tumor: subtraction image showing index tumor (**b**) and T1-weighted prebiopsy image with coaxial introduction needle in place (**c**). Reproduction of second lesion cranially of the index tumor in the subtraction image (**d**), and the T2-weighted image (**e**). MRI-guided fine needle aspiration of this lesion (**f**) and withdrawal of pus (**g**). *Histology*: abscessing mastitis. *Cytology*: pus.

6

Data in the Current Literature

Currently, there are only a few reports concerning MRI-guided vacuum-assisted breast interventions. Some of these discuss the development and presentation of MRI-compatible targeting equipment. Older publications pertaining to sample harvesting are concerned primarily with the performance of CNBs, whereas more recent publications are increasingly dealing with the results of MRI-guided VABs. A synopsis of the existing data indicates that the accuracy rate and the time expenditure of MRI-guided VABs is in the same range as that of stereotactic VABs.

Table 6.6 lists the relevant data derived from reference articles published to date, as well as the results acquired in the Women's Health Care Center Göttingen from 2004 to 2007. Studies performed by the following working groups have earned special mention: Schrading, Kuhl (Bonn, Germany), Libermann (New York, NY), Viehweg (Dresden, Germany), Orel (Philadelphia, PA), Lehman (Seattle, WA), Perlet (Munich, Germany; multicenter study), and the Women's Health Care Center Göttingen (Göttingen, Germany).

A synopsis of the existing data indicates that the average quota of malignant to benign findings after stereotactic biopsy is approx. 1 : 3 (25% malignant results) with an accuracy of >98%. Experienced work groups required 30–45 minutes (MRI table-time) to perform an MRI-guided VAB. The rate of relevant complications averaged <1%.

Table 6.6 Current literature pertaining to MRI-guided core- and vacuum-assisted breast biopsies

Work group	Schrading, Kuhl	Liberman	Viehweg	Orel	Lehmann	Perlet	Women's Health Care Center Göttingen
Year	2007	2005	2007	2006	2005	2006	2008
No. of patients	200	106	39	75	28	538	365
No. of biopsies	316	112	53*	85	38	538	389
Gauge	10.9	9	11	9	9	11	10.9
No. of specimens	n. s.	approx. 12	>20	n. s.	>n. s.	20	approx. 15
Malignant	43%	25%	26%	61%	37%	27%	27%
Borderline	5%	20%	4%	21%	5%	3%	13%
Benign	52%	55%	70%	18%	58%	70%	60%
Accuracy	99%	97%	100%	98%	100%	96%	99%
Target not reproduced	n. s.	12%	12%	n. s.	n. s.	16%	6.8%
Time expenditure (11 gauge)	–	–	approx. 60 min	–	–	70 min	–
Time expenditure (10 gauge)	62 min	–	–	–	–	–	46 min
Time expenditure (9 gauge)	34 min	33 min	–	30–60 min	–	38 min	39 min
Complication rate	3%	5.3%	n. s.	0%†	0%	<1%	<1%

* Including eight wire localizations
† No major complications
Abbreviations: n. s., not specified

MRI-guided Vacuum-assisted Biopsy: Therapeutic Objective

MRI-guided VAB can be performed as a therapeutic procedure for small borderline lesions. This is especially true for papillomas, which have a potential for malignant transformation. Because it is recommended that borderline lesions be excised and MRI-guided VAB can excise small lesions completely as an outpatient procedure, it is an alternative to open biopsy (**Fig. 6.48**).

Surgical excision is, however, mandatory after percutaneous VAB of breast cancer (**Fig. 6.49**). If no residual tumor tissue is found on pathology because the malignant lesion has been com-

pletely removed by VAB, then there are often problems in defining the pT (pathologic stage of primary tumor) classification. Ultimately, because the tumor stage is relevant for therapy planning, it must be defined by the measurements made in the initial imaging studies in such cases. In this context, MR mammography has been shown to have the highest precision in depicting the tumor size in comparison to the other imaging modalities.

The declaration of the tumor size (T-stage) for carcinomas that have been completely removed by VAB should be stated as "pbT." The letters "pb" designate that the T-stage has been defined by image measurements due to complete removal on percutaneous biopsy.

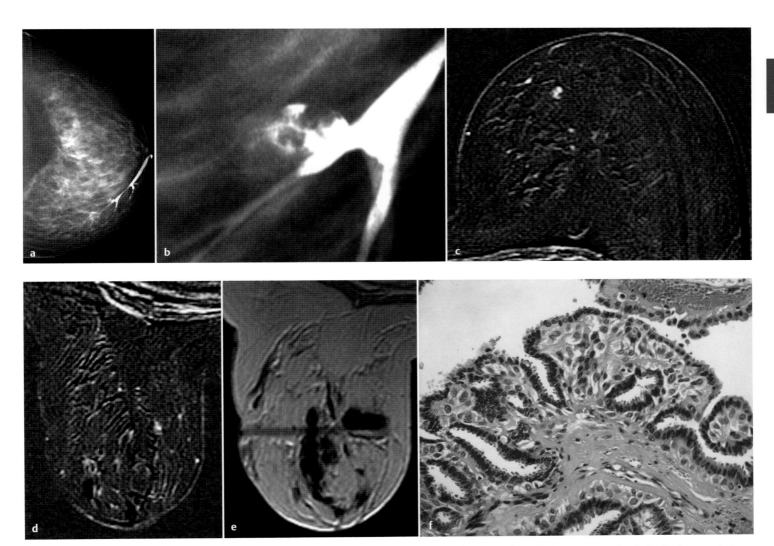

Fig. 6.48a–f MRI-guided vacuum-assisted papilloma removal. Diagnostic imaging of patient with bloody discharge. Two mL of contrast material was injected into the appropriate left milk duct. Galactography shows a filling defect in a paraductal cyst due to an intracystic proliferation, focal ductectasia, and abrupt duct truncation (**a**). Magnified partial view in CC projection (**b**). The HR-MR mammography shows a 5-mm hypervascularized lesion, corresponding to the finding on galactography (subtraction image) (**c**). Unambiguous reproduction of lesion to be excised on the subtraction image (**d**). T1-weighted documentation after vacuum-assisted excision (12 tissue samples) (**e**). *Histology*: papilloma is completely removed (**f**).

6

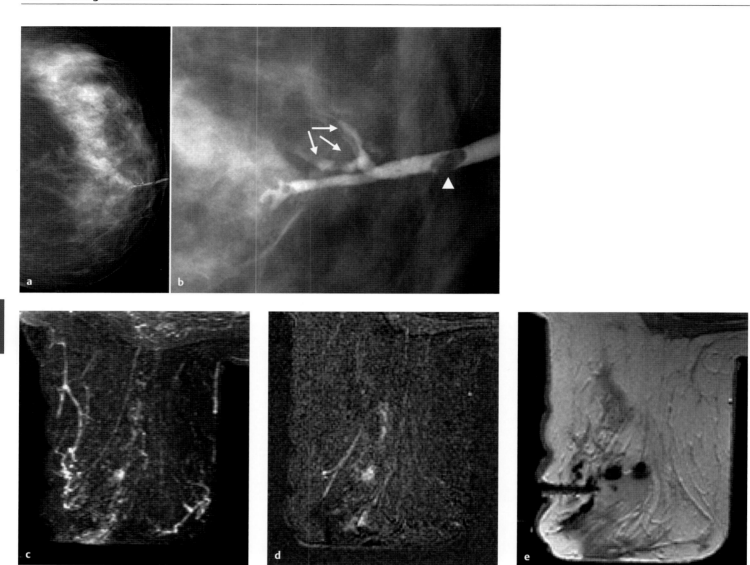

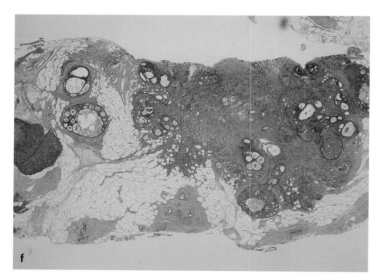

Fig. 6.49a–f   MRI-guided VAB with complete removal of breast carcinoma.
Diagnostic imaging of patient with bloody discharge from one milk duct. Galactography shows a straight milk duct of normal diameter with a focal spreading of small ductal branches and associated intraductal filling defects (arrows). In addition, one sees an artificial filling defect in the retromamillary region (arrowhead) (**a**). Magnified partial view in CC projection (**b**). MR mammography shows a 6-mm hypervascularized lesion, corresponding to the finding on galactography (subtraction MIP) (**c**). MRI-guided VAB was planned to completely excise the lesion thought to be a papilloma. Subtraction image during intervention (**d**). T1-weighted postbiopsy documentation of complete excision (**e**). *Histology* unexpectedly revealed an IDC (B5b) (**f**). Surgical excision of the biopsy cavity showed no pathologic evidence of residual carcinoma. Final classification: IDC pbT1b (pb = percutaneous biopsy, see text).

MRI-guided Localization

Indications and Objectives

MRI-guided localizations are primarily performed preoperatively in cases when the MRI-lesion to be excised cannot be clinically palpated or detected with other imaging techniques. In addition, coil/clips markers can be placed under MRI-guidance to mark the relevant borders of a tumor before neoadjuvant chemotherapy.

The aim of a preoperative MRI-guided localization is to provide the surgeon with markers for optimal orientation during surgery. This is necessary to accomplish the objectives of completely excising the suspicious, and usually histologically verified lesion with an adequate tumor-free safety margin (R0 resection), while limiting the excision volume to the necessary extent to attain optimal cosmetic results.

Positioning

MRI-guided interventions are classically performed with the patient lying in the prone position and the breast hanging freely inside the surface coil. It is, however, possible to perform interventions with the patient in an oblique or supine position. When the breast is accessed from the lateral aspect, the contralateral breast can also be positioned within the breast surface coil. When the breast is accessed from the medial aspect, the contralateral breast must be positioned outside the coil's target volume. During the intervention, the patient's head may be positioned to one side, or preferably face down; this usually causes less cervical complaints (**Fig. 6.50**). Based on the coil design, the arms may be positioned above the head or alongside the body. When positioning the arms alongside the body, use a bathrobe belt to maintain the arms' positioning (**Fig. 6.51**). Position the patient's legs and feet comfortably, and ensure an agreeable room temperature.

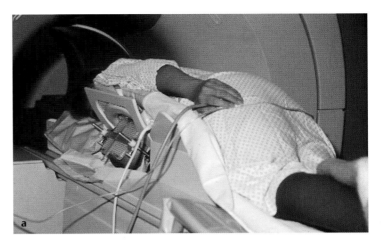

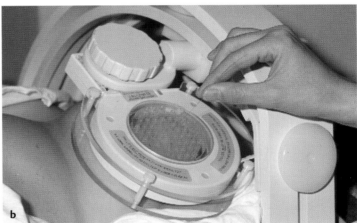

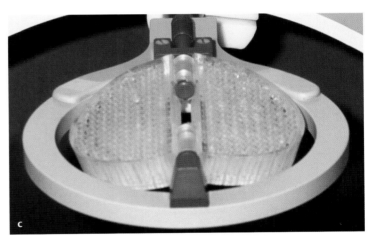

Fig. 6.51a–c Alternative patient positioning for MRI-guided lesion localization.
a Patient in oblique position with a puncture device (Phillips Healthcare, Amsterdam, the Netherlands).
b Patient in supine position with puncture attachment (Göttingen model type I) integrated into an eye/ear surface coil in place.
c Göttingen model type II consists of two puncture components that can be angled and are integrated into a shoulder-flex coil.

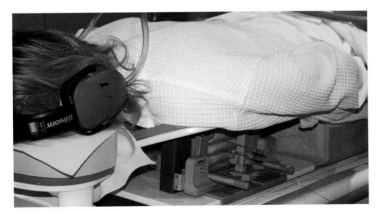

Fig. 6.50 Standard patient positioning for MRI-guided lesion localization.
Patient in the prone position, the arms alongside the body and face down with forehead on head support. Clinical situation after placement of two localization wires (breast surface coil: MRI device, post and pillar attachment; Noras MRI Products, Hochberg, Germany).

Materials

Localization wires and markers. Several MRI-compatible wires, as well as coil and clip markers are available for use when performing MRI-guided preoperative localizations (**Figs. 6.52** and **6.53**). These are typically alloys with a high titanium and nickel content. Because they only have minor ferromagnetic properties, the susceptibility artifacts that they cause produce a signal extinction that can be distinctly seen without masking relevant findings and fine structures. Examples of the most important materials are presented below in T1-weighted GE images (**Figs. 6.52** and **6.53**).

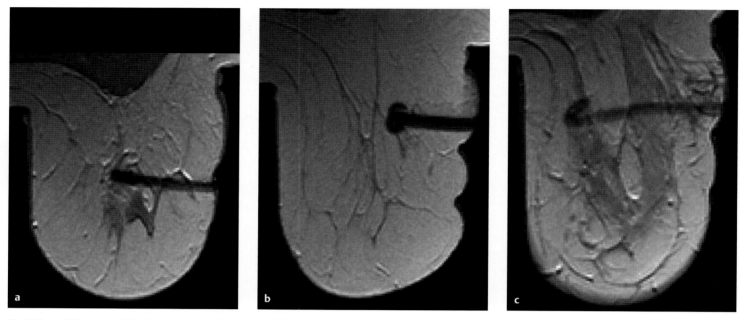

Fig. 6.52a–c   MR images of localization wires. T1-weighted GE images showing signal extinction caused by a localization hook wire (**a**), a double hook wire (**b**), and a J-wire (**c**).

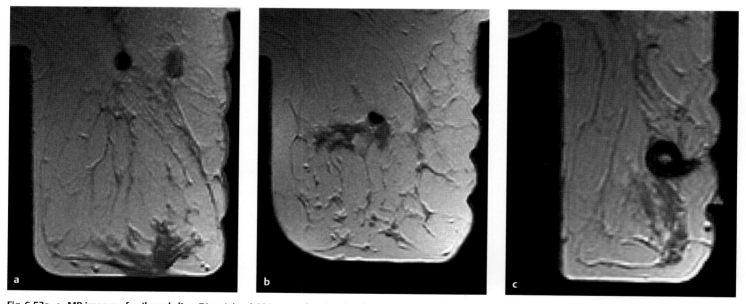

Fig. 6.53a–c   MR images of coils and clips. T1-weighted GE images showing signal extinction caused by a coil marker (**a**), a clip marker (**b**), and a threaded coil (**c**).

Quality Control: MRI-guided Preoperative Localization

Guidelines*

Indications: MR mammography findings that must be subjected to open biopsy and have no correlating finding on clinical examination or in other imaging techniques (mammography, US).

Equipment: MRI unit with at least 1.0 T
- open breast surface coil allowing access to the breast
- MRI-compatible localization equipment
- MRI-compatible marker equipment:
  - wire (preferred for localizations performed immediately before surgery)
  - coil, clip marker (preferred when the final localization is performed at a different medical facility, or at a later time)
  - cutaneous marker (only used for subcutaneous lesions—relatively rare)

Procedure: Contrast-enhanced MR mammography is performed with the localization equipment positioned on the affected side to reproduce the target lesion for the MRI-guided localization.
- If the target lesion is not reproduced, or is only questionably reproduced, and the lesion is not histologically proven to be a carcinoma, then the intervention should be discontinued and a short-term follow-up examination in 6 months is recommended.
- If the target lesion is unequivocally identified, then the puncture coordinates (x-, y-, and z-axes) are calculated. The calculated puncture site (x- and y-axes) is marked with an external marker (e.g., oil-containing), and a MRI check is performed without additional contrast administration.
- If the marker position is incorrect, then a new calculation is performed and the marker position corrected. If the marker position is correct, then the skin is disinfected and local anesthesia may be administered. The puncture cannula is inserted 5–10 mm deeper than the calculated depth (z-axis).
- The position of the needle is checked by performing an MRI T1-weighted series without contrast. If the position is incorrect, then the needle is repositioned and rechecked. If the position is correct, then the marker is advanced and released into the breast tissue (wire, coil/clip).
- Perform a postlocalization MRI check (when indicated with contrast administration) as a final confirmation of the correct wire or coil/clip marking. If the position is incorrect (>10 mm from lesion) and the localization marker used is a repositionable wire, then the wire may be relocated. Alternatively, a second marker can be placed opposing the first, placing the localized lesion between the two markers. The position of oil/clips markers usually cannot be corrected.
- Conclude the localization procedure and carry out postlocalization mammograms in CC and ML projections for the surgeon

Special case: For nonmass lesions, a localization marker may not necessarily be placed within the finding. It is often better for the surgeon's orientation to place markers at relevant lesion borders (e.g., margins for segmental resection). In this situation, it is not necessary to correct the marker when it is more than 10 mm from the lesion.

Before neoadjuvant chemotherapy, the tumor is marked at its original borders.

Report: Was the target finding reproducible? (yes/no)
- Position of target finding (quadrant, clock-time position, distance from the skin)
- What marker was used? (single-/double-hook wire, J-wire, clip/coil)
- Marker position relative to lesion (in cm)
- Associated findings (e.g., hematoma after biopsy)

Specimen radiography: Recommended, especially after coil/clip or wire localization to confirm their removal

Documentation:
- MRI-image of target finding (subtraction image)
- MRI-image documentation of marker's position
- Mammography in CC and ML projection

Quality criteria:
- Distance of marker to lesion < 10 mm in 90 % of cases (not applicable for diffusely enhancing lesions with marking of surgically relevant borders)
- Complete surgical excision in > 95 % of cases (final assessment made in interdisciplinary conference)
- Correlation of histopathology with MRI findings (final assessment made in interdisciplinary conference)

* German Radiology Association's Breast Diagnostics Working Group 2007

Checklist: MRI-guided Vacuum-assisted Biopsy

1. Establish indication.
2. Confirm that there is no correlating finding on mammography and/or US.
3. Obtain informed consent (in advance).
4. Position patient comfortably in open breast surface coil with biopsy option.
5. Choose appropriate puncture equipment (grid, post and pillar).
6. Position external marker at estimated target position (arbitrary zero-point).
7. Perform dynamic MR mammography examination with image subtraction.
8. Identify target.
9. Calculate appropriate x-, y-, and z-coordinates.
10. Move external marker to appropriate puncture site and perform MRI check.
11. Disinfect breast skin and optional administration of local anesthesia.
12. Choose appropriate marker material (wire, coil, clip).
13. Percutaneous introduction of localization cannula.
14. Perform MRI check of needle position in relation to target lesion and correct position, if necessary.
15. Advance wire or release coil/clip marker.
16. Perform MRI check of marker position in relation to target lesion (possibly with additional contrast administration).
17. If necessary, position second marker.
18. Remove needle cannula, apply compression.
19. Release breast from localization device. Move patient.
20. Perform final mammograms in two orthogonal planes.
21. Optional: create photomontage showing individual lesions and marker positions.

6

Clinical Cases (MRI-guided Localization)

Clinical Case 1: MRI-guided Localization Wire Placement (Fig. 6.54)

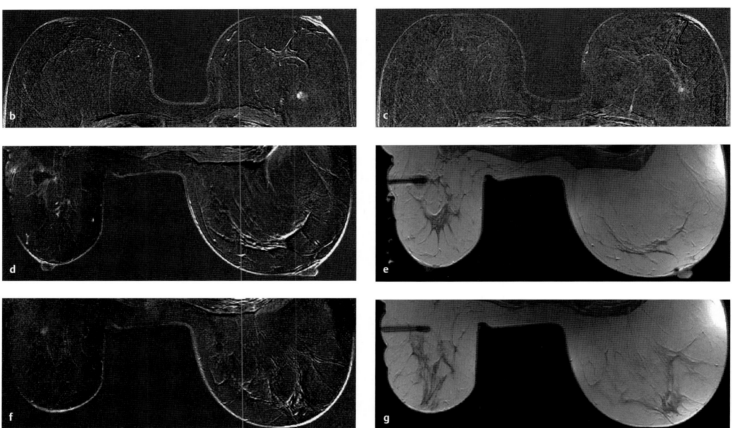

Tips and Tricks

When a diagnostic surgical excision of a focal MRI-lesion is performed, one should strive to place the localization wire tip in the center of the lesion.

Fig. 6.54a–h Preoperative MRI-guided localization of ipsilateral bifocal findings. The diagnostic MR mammography shows two hypervascularized findings in the lateral aspect of the left breast (subtraction MIP) (**a**). Subtraction slice image of larger lesion in the upper outer quadrant of the left breast (**b**). Subtraction slice image of smaller lesion in the lower outer quadrant of the left breast (**c**). MRI-guided VAB of the larger lesion revealed an ILC (B5b). Documentation of the preoperative MRI-guided localization of the biopsy cavity in the upper outer quadrant (**d, e**), and the smaller lesion in the lower outer quadrant of the left breast (**f, g**) shows exact placement of both hook wires. Annotated photo (**h**). *Final histology*: ILC, pT1b pN0 G2 (lesion 01), and CLIS (lesion 02).

Clinical Case 2: MRI-guided Coil/Clip Placement (Fig. 6.55)

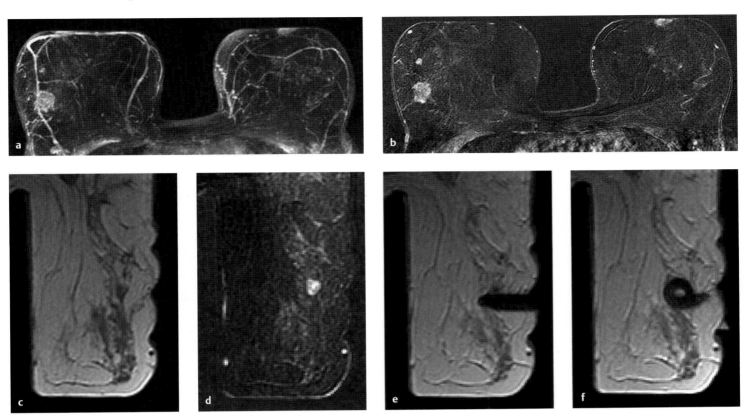

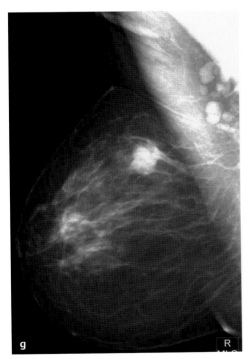

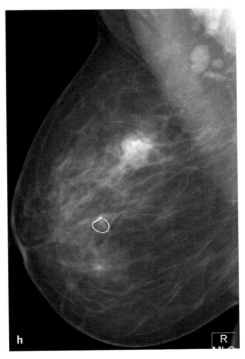

Fig. 6.55a–h Preoperative MRI-guided placement of a coil marker in an ipsilateral secondary finding in a patient with a BI-RADS 6 lesion. Highly suspicious lesion on palpation, mammography, and US in the upper outer quadrant of the right breast. The preoperative staging MR mammography shows the index tumor with typical morphology and a second ventrally located, hypervascularized, round finding of 5-mm diameter (subtraction MIP) (**a**). Subtraction slice image (**b**). US-guided CNB of the index tumor revealed an IDC (BI-RADS 6). Because surgery was to be performed in an external medical facility, the secondary finding was marked using an Ariadne thread hook wire (coil). T1-weighted precontrast image (**c**). Subtraction image of secondary finding (**d**). MRI check with needle cannula in place (**e**). MRI check after releasing coil (**f**). Mammography in MLO projection showing index tumor and suspicious axillary lymph node (**g**). Final mammographic documentation in MLO projection showing coil (**h**). *Final histology*: IDC, pT1c pN1 G2 (index tumor), and a papilloma (secondary lesion).

Tips and Tricks

Lesions that are to be surgically removed at an external medical facility or at a later date should preferably be marked with a coil or clip. Placing a localization wire in these situations increases the risk of dislocation and infection.

Clinical Case 3: Trifocal Findings—MRI-guided Marking of the Relevant Target Volume (Fig. 6.56)

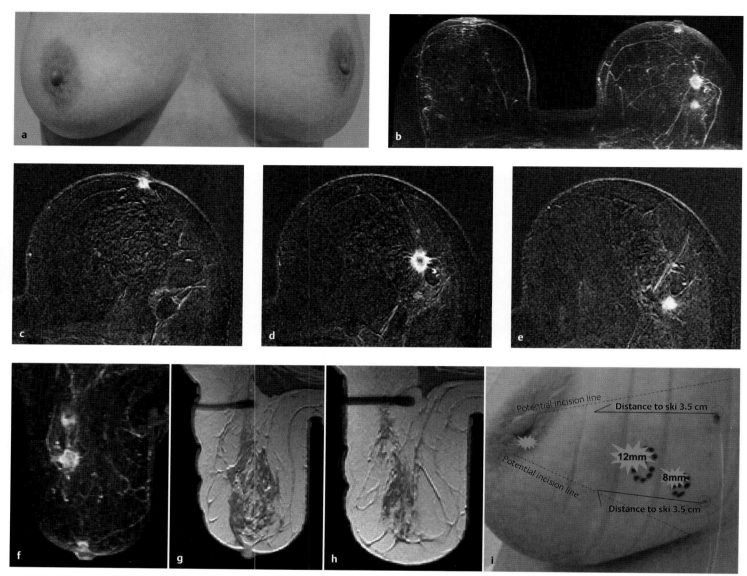

Fig. 6.56a–i MRI-guided marking of the target volume in a patient with trifocal findings. Recent development of a discrete retraction of the left nipple (**a**). No palpable findings. Mammography and US revealed a suspicious lesion in the lateral aspect of the left breast (no images). US-guided CNB revealed an IDC (B5b, BI-RADS 6). The preoperative staging MR mammography shows the index tumor with typical morphology (**d**). In addition, a second hypervascularized finding of 5-mm diameter is shown in the left retromamillary region (**c**), and a third hypervascularized finding of 7-mm diameter in the lower outer quadrant (**e**). All lesions are seen on the subtraction MIP (**b**). In the interdisciplinary conference, it was decided to perform a quadrantectomy after preoperative localization of the relevant target volume borders. Documentation images during MRI-guided localization show all three tumor manifestations in the subtraction MIP (**f**). T1-weighted documentation of two localization wires near the chest wall marking the cranial (**g**) and caudal (**h**) borders of the quadrant to be excised. Annotated photo shows the positions of the lesions, localization wires, and the target volume (**i**). *Final histology*: trifocal breast cancer: pT1c pN0 G2 R0.

Tips and Tricks

When a segmental resection or quadrantectomy is planned, it often makes more sense to place markers at the relevant borders of the target volume than to place one marker within the lesion.

Clinical Case 4: MRI-guided Localization of a Target Volume (Fig. 6.57)

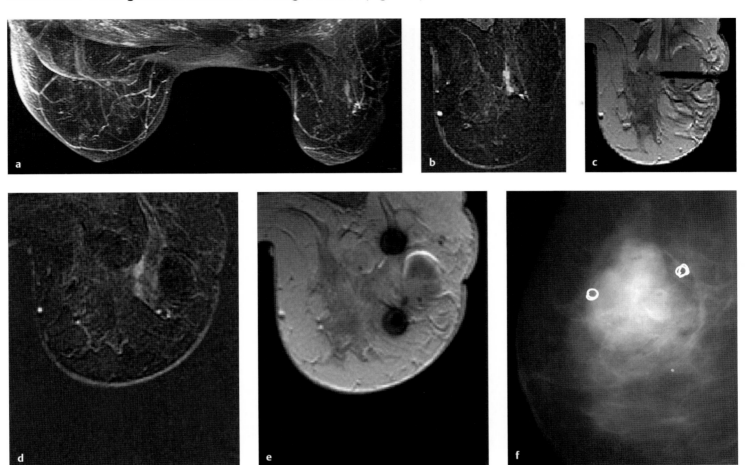

6

Fig. 6.57a–f MRI-guided VAB of a linear enhancement in the right breast with placement of two coil markers at the relevant borders with respect to onco-logic aspects. MR mammography was performed as a supplemental diagnostic procedure in a patient with extremely dense breast tissue (ACR density type IV) and revealed a linear enhancement in the right breast (no image). Imaging before MRI-guided VAB clearly reproduced the target linear enhancement in the right breast (subtraction MIP) (**a**). Subtraction slice image (**b**). T1-weighted documenta-tion after harvesting 12 tissue samples (9-gauge) (**c**). *Histology*: IDC (DCIS) (patho-logic classification: B5a). Preoperative localization was performed a few days later for surgery in an external medical facility. Subtraction image shows the linear enhancement after biopsy without interfering enhancement around the biopsy cavity (**d**). T1-weighted documentation after placement of an MRI-compatible coil marker at the dorsal and ventral ends of the enhancement (**e**). (Note: mastectomy is usually recommended for a DCIS larger than 4 cm. In this case, the coil markers were deliberately placed 4 cm apart. A tumor reaching both coils would provide the indication for mastectomy). Final mammographic documentation shows the post-biopsy hematoma and both coil markers (**f**). The suspicious lesion and both coils were completely excised in the following open surgery. The hematoma was aspi-rated percutaneously before surgery. *Final histology*: DCIS (28-mm diameter): pTis pN0 G2 R0 (tumor-free safety margin >10 mm). Breast conserving therapy was per-formed.

Tips and Tricks

Before performing a preoperative localization, the planned surgical pro-cedure should be discussed in the interdisciplinary conference to decide whether the tumor center or the relevant target volume borders should be localized.

Clinical Case 5: MRI-guided Localization of Residual Tumor—BI-RADS 6 (Figs. 6.58 and 6.59)

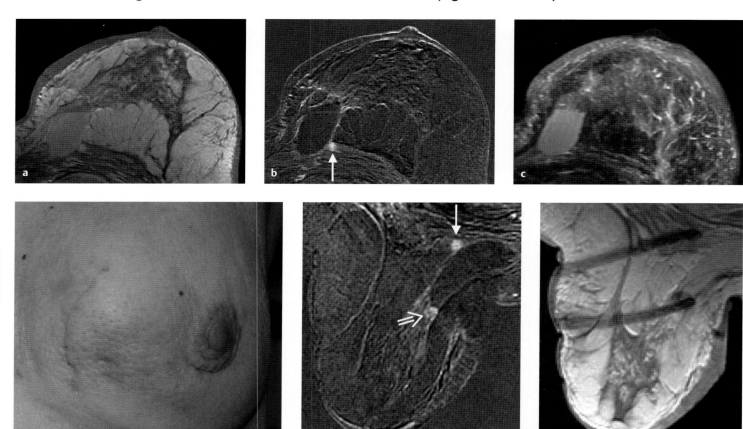

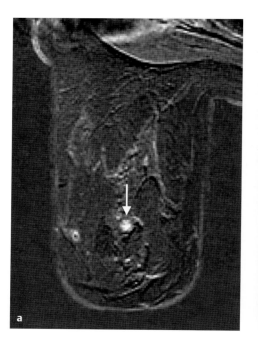

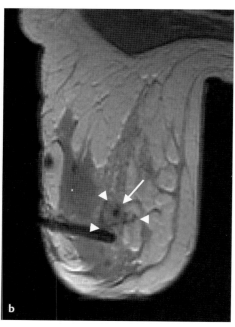

Fig. 6.58a–f MRI-guided localization of residual tumor after open biopsy of a breast carcinoma. MR mammography was performed 5 days after surgery for breast cancer because of pathologic evidence of tumor at the resection margins (R1). The T1-weighted GE postcontrast image shows the oval hemorrhagic resection cavity with sedimentation (**a**). The corresponding subtraction slice image shows a hypervascularized lesion near the chest wall (arrow) (**b**). The corresponding water-sensitive IR-sequence image provides no additional information (**c**). Clinical photograph of the breast postoperatively shows swelling due to hemorrhagic resection cavity (**d**). Imaging before MRI-guided localization clearly reproduces the suspicious hypervascularization near the chest wall (arrow), as well as a second ambiguous hypervascularization at the ventral resection cavity border (double arrow) (**e**). T1-weighted documentation after placement of two localization wires (**f**). *Histology*: Resection cavity with two areas of residual tumor at the ventral and dorsal borders.

Fig. 6.59a, b MRI-guided localization of residual tumor after VAB of a breast carcinoma. MRI-guided VAB revealed IDC in the left breast (B5b). Imaging before MRI-guided localization of the resection cavity shows residual tumor at the resection cavity border (arrow) (**a**). Wire localization with tip in the residual tumor, next to an US-visible clip marker placed in the biopsy cavity after VAB (**b**). Arrowheads designate the clip marker dimensions. The single arrow designates the central metal clip. *Histology*: residual tumor.

Tips and Tricks

After MRI-guided VAB, it is preferable to preoperatively localize the potential residual tumor than to localize the center of the biopsy cavity.

Further Reading

AG Mammadiagnostik der Deutschen Röntgengesellschaft. Empfehlungen zur MR-mammografie. RöFo 2005;177:474–475

AG Mammadiagnostik der Deutschen Röntgengesellschaft. Empfehlungen zur MR-gestützten Interventionen der Mamma. RöFo 2007;179:429–430

Daniel BL, Freeman LJ, Pyzoha JM, et al. An MRI-compatible semiautomated vacuum-assisted breast biopsy system: initial feasibility study. J Magn Reson Imaging 2005;21(5):637–644

Gebauer B, Bostanjoglo M, Moesta KT, Schneider W, Schlag PM, Felix R. Magnetic resonance-guided biopsy of suspicious breast lesions with a handheld vacuum biopsy device. Acta Radiol 2006;47(9):907–913

Fischer U, Vosshenrich R, Döler W, Hamadeh A, Oestmann JW, Grabbe E. MR imaging-guided breast intervention: experience with two systems. Radiology 1995;195(2):533–538

Fischer U, Rodenwaldt J, Hundertmark C, Döler W, Grabbe E. MRI-assisted biopsy and localization of the breast. [Article in German] Radiologe 1997;37(9):692–701

Fischer U, Kopka L, Grabbe E. Magnetic resonance guided localization and biopsy of suspicious breast lesions. Top Magn Reson Imaging 1998;9(1):44–59

Helbich TH. Localization and biopsy of breast lesions by magnetic resonance imaging guidance. J Magn Reson Imaging 2001;13(6):903–911

Heywang-Köbrunner SH, Heinig A, Pickuth D, Alberich T, Spielmann RP. Interventional MRI of the breast: lesion localisation and biopsy. Eur Radiol 2000;10(1):36–45

Kuhl CK, Morakkabati N, Leutner CC, Schmiedel A, Wardelmann E, Schild HH. MR imaging—guided large-core (14-gauge) needle biopsy of small lesions visible at breast MR imaging alone. Radiology 2001;220(1):31–39

Kuhl CK, Elevelt A, Leutner CC, Gieseke J, Pakos E, Schild HH. Interventional breast MR imaging: clinical use of a stereotactic localization and biopsy device. Radiology 1997;204(3):667–675

Lehman CD, Deperi ER, Peacock S, McDonough MD, Demartini WB, Shook J. Clinical experience with MRI-guided vacuum-assisted breast biopsy. AJR Am J Roentgenol 2005;184(6):1782–1787

Liberman L, Bracero N, Morris E, Thornton C, Dershaw DD. MRI-guided 9-gauge vacuum-assisted breast biopsy: initial clinical experience. AJR Am J Roentgenol 2005;185(1):183–193

Orel SG, Rosen M, Mies C, Schnall MD. MR imaging-guided 9-gauge vacuum-assisted core-needle breast biopsy: initial experience. Radiology 2006;238(1):54–61

Perlet C, Heywang-Kobrunner SH, Heinig A, et al. Magnetic resonance-guided, vacuum-assisted breast biopsy: results from a European multicenter study of 538 lesions. Cancer 2006;106(5):982–990

Schrading S, Simon B, Wardelmann E, Schild HH, Kuhl CK. MR gesteuerte Vakuumbiopsie der Mamma. RöFo 2007;179:45

Viehweg P, Bernerth T, Kiechle M, et al. MR-guided intervention in women with a family history of breast cancer. Eur J Radiol 2006;57(1):81–89

Viehweg P, Heinig A, Buchmann J, et al. MRT-gestützte Intervention der Brust bei Patientinnen mit einem histologisch gesicherten Mammakarzinom. Senologie 2007;4:28–34

6

7 Instrumentation

F. Baum

The instrumentation used in breast diagnosis includes devices for tissue sample collection and tools for marking lesions to be examined. Special examination equipment and positioning aids facilitate optimal access to the breast. However, some conventional biopsy devices can affect certain key imaging procedures. For example, some biopsy devices produce considerable artifacts in magnetic resonance imaging (MRI); those that do not carry the label "MRI-compatible."

Various techniques are available for specimen collection. Fine needle aspiration biopsy (FNAB) is used for collecting single cells (cytology). Core needle biopsy (CNB) and vacuum-assisted biopsy (VAB) facilitate the collection of tissue samples (histology).

Fine Needle Aspiration Biopsy

Fine needle aspiration (**Figs. 7.1, 7.2, 7.3, 7.4, 7.5, 7.6, 7.7, 7.8**) uses biopsy needles with outer diameters of 19–26 gauge. Needle tips are available in different point styles. The Chiba needle (**Figs. 7.4** and **7.5**) has a beveled tip that permits easy puncture of the tissue. As the needle advances, asymmetric tissue displacement at the needle tip causes a shift away from the beveled side.

The crown-point tip of the Franseen needle (**Fig. 7.6**) facilitates the extraction of cells during puncture. When the stylet is introduced, the needle has a symmetric point.

Fine needle aspiration is almost exclusively performed under ultrasound (US) guidance. For this reason, it is essential that the examiner be able to guide the syringe and advance the plunger with one hand, while holding the ultrasonic transducer with the other. This is possible with special puncture aids (**Figs. 7.1** and **7.2**).

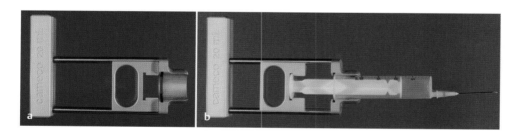

Fig. 7.1 Cameco handle. Cameco handle without syringe (**a**), and with cylinder and plunger resting in the corresponding nuts of syringe holder and movable plunger guide (**b**). The design enables the examiner to determine the needle direction by angulation of the entire holder and, at the same time, to create negative pressure by operating the plunger with the same hand.

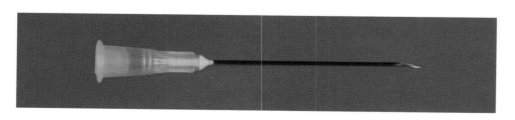

Fig. 7.2 Binder valve. The Binder valve is used with commonly available syringes. It consists of a valve and a spacer (**a**). The valve is attached to the Luer nose between puncture needle and syringe cylinder (**b**). With the valve closed, the syringe plunger is completely pulled back and fixed by the spacer, thus maintaining negative pressure. Once the needle tip has reached the lesion to be examined, suction is produced by pressing the Binder valve.

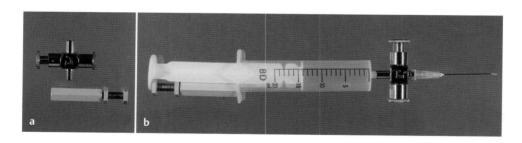

Fig. 7.3 Beveled puncture needle. Puncture needles that are commonly used for collecting blood may also be used for puncturing tissues or cysts. Because these needles do not have a stylet, negative pressure should be created only after penetrating the target lesion. Needle sizes: 19, 20, 21, 22, 23, 24, 25, 26 gauge; lengths: 25, 30, 40, 50, 60, 70, 80, 120 mm.

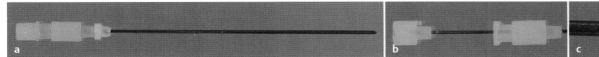

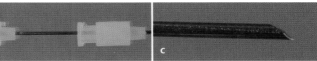

Fig. 7.4 Chiba biopsy needle (Cook Medical, Bloomington, IN). Chiba needle with stylet (**a**), partially withdrawn stylet (**b**), beveled needle point (**c**). Needle sizes: 18, 20, 2-, 22, 23 gauge; lengths: 10, 15, 20 cm.

Available also as EchoTip needle designed to enhance needle visibility during ultrasonic imaging. Needle sizes: 18, 20, 21, 22 gauge; lengths: 10, 15, 20, 25 cm.

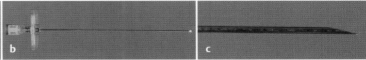

Fig. 7.5 Chiba needle (Bard Biopsy Systems, Tempe, AZ). Chiba needle with stylet (**a**), Chiba needle with mountable plastic wing and stylet clip for optimal handling (**b**), beveled needle point (**c**). Needle sizes: 18, 20, 22, 23 gauge; lengths: 9, 12, 15, 22, 28 cm.

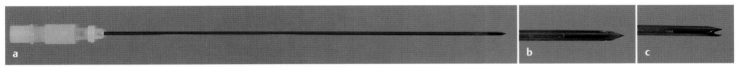

Fig. 7.6 Franseen needle (Cook Medical, Bloomington, IN). Franseen needle with stylet (**a**), needle point with stylet (**b**), needle point without stylet, showing crown-point tip (**c**). Needle size: 18 gauge; length: 15 cm.

Available also as EchoTip needle designed to enhance needle visibility during ultrasonic imaging. Needle size: 22 gauge; length: 15 cm.

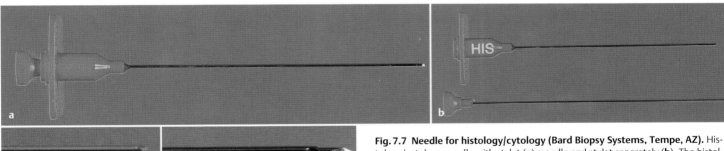

Fig. 7.7 Needle for histology/cytology (Bard Biopsy Systems, Tempe, AZ). Histology/cytology needle with stylet (**a**), needle and stylet separately (**b**). The histology/cytology needle has no point but a sharpened edge (**c**). The stylet has a lancet point and extends beyond the needle opening (**d**). After penetrating the target lesion with the needle point, the stylet is used to create negative pressure for aspiration in the needle by pulling it back. Needle sizes: 18, 20, 21 gauge; lengths: 10, 15, 20 cm.

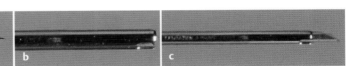

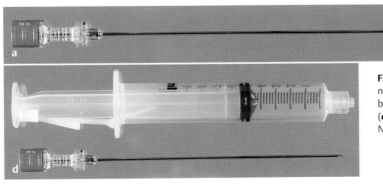

Fig. 7.8 Core biopsy needle (Bard Biopsy Systems, Tempe, AZ). The core biopsy needle (**a**) has no point but a sharpened edge (**b**). The stylet is beveled and extends beyond the needle opening (**c**). The set includes a syringe with a plunger stopper (**d**) for maintaining the negative pressure in the needle while directing the needle. Needle sizes: 16, 17, 18, 20, 21 gauge; lengths: 5, 10, 15, 20, 28, 40 cm.

Core Needle Biopsy

The aim of performing a CNB is to collect cohesive cell clusters. A typical biopsy needle (**Fig. 7.9**) is composed of a hollow cannula (x) with a puncture needle inside (y); the puncture needle has at its end a tissue reservoir (notch) (z). First, the puncture needle penetrates the target lesion; then the cannula cuts off the tissue inside the notch, and a specimen of the glandular tissue is recovered with the needle.

Characteristic features of a biopsy needle are needle size and needle advance (stroke). There are semi-automatic (**Figs. 7.10, 7.11, 7.12, 7.13, 7.14, 7.15, 7.16**) and automatic biopsy devices (**Figs. 7.17, 7.18, 7.19, 7.20, 7.21, 7.22**).

Semi-automatic Biopsy

The cannula of a semi-automatic biopsy device has a spring mechanism that is tensioned using a plunger on the handle. The puncture needle is advanced into the target lesion by hand, and the cannula then cuts off the tissue by means of spring action. Semi-automatic devices are offered as single-use only.

Fig. 7.9 Diagram of a biopsy needle. Biopsy needle before and after biopsy (**a**), and with the puncture needle advanced (**b**).

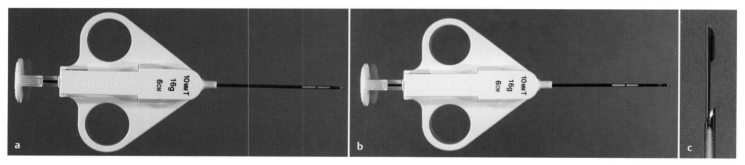

Fig. 7.10 Quick-Core biopsy needle (Cook Medical, Bloomington, IN). Quick-Core biopsy needle (**a**), in the cocked position (**b**), advanced specimen notch (**c**). Needle sizes: 16, 18, 20 gauge; lengths: 6, 9, 15 cm; stroke: 10 mm. Needle sizes: 14, 16, 18, 20 gauge; lengths: 6, 9, 15, 20 cm; stroke: 20 mm.

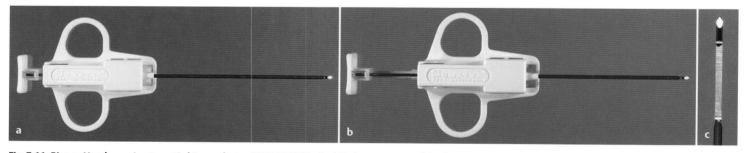

Fig. 7.11 Biopsy-Handy semi-automatic biopsy device (SOMATEX Medical Technologies GmbH, Teltow, Germany). Biopsy-Handy biopsy device (**a**), in the cocked position (**b**), advanced specimen notch (**c**). MRI-compatible; needle sizes: 14, 16, 18, 20 gauge; lengths: 10, 15, 20 cm; stroke: 20 mm.

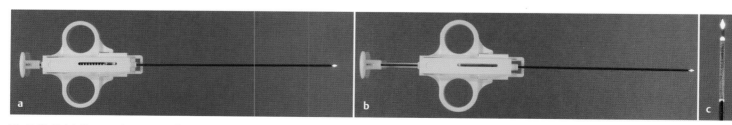

Fig. 7.12 Quick-Shot semi-automatic biopsy system (SOMATEX Medical Technologies GmbH, Teltow, Germany). Quick-Shot biopsy device (**a**), in the cocked position (**b**), advanced specimen notch (**c**). Needle sizes: 14, 16, 18, 20 gauge; length: 10 cm; stroke: 15 or 22 mm, optional.

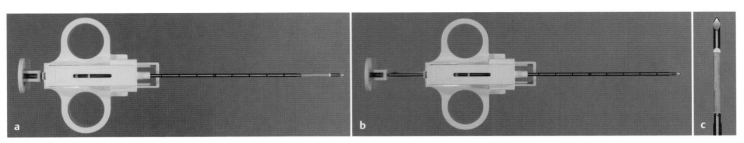

Fig. 7.13 Semi-automatic biopsy gun (Invivo Corp., Orlando, FL). Invivo semi-automatic biopsy device (**a**), in the cocked position (**b**), advanced specimen notch (**c**). MRI-compatible; needle size: 14, 16, 18 gauge; lengths: 10, 15 cm; stroke: 20 mm.

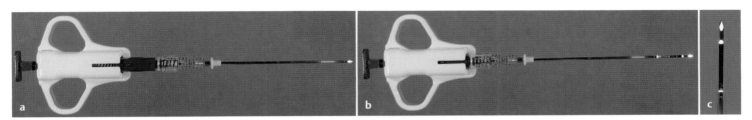

Fig. 7.14 LUX 2 semi-automatic biopsy device (OptiMed, Ettlingen, Germany). LUX 2 semi-automatic biopsy device (**a**), with advanced puncture needle (**b**), notch (**c**). Needle sizes: 14, 16, 18 gauge; lengths: 10, 16, 20 cm; stroke: 12 or 25 mm, optional.

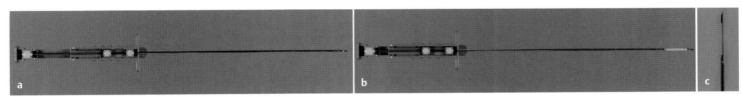

Fig. 7.15 Unicut needle biopsy device (Bard Biopsy Systems, Tempe, AZ). Unicut needle biopsy device (**a**), with advanced puncture needle (**b**), notch (**c**). The system is without a spring mechanism and is shown here only for the sake of completeness. To obtain a tissue specimen, the notch of the puncture needle is first advanced into the target tissue, then the cutting cylinder is manually advanced beyond the notch. Needle sizes: 14, 16, 17, 18 gauge; lengths: 7.5, 11.5, 15, 20 cm; stroke: 20 mm.

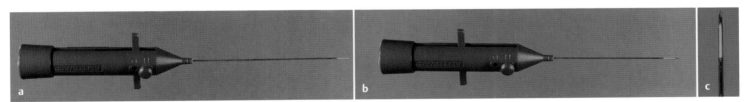

Fig. 7.16 Autovac disposable full cut biopsy instrument (Bard Biopsy Systems, Tempe, AZ). Autovac single-use biopsy needle (**a**), in the cocked position (**b**), needle point (**c**). This jet needle does not have a notch. The cannula itself acts as the cutting cylinder for obtaining the specimen. Recovering the specimen is occasionally problematic if the tissue is firm, since the tissue sample is not mechanically cut off at the needle point but remains connected with the breast tissue. Detachment is facilitated by rotating the needle after the jet advance or by gentle gyrating movements of the needle tip. Needle sizes: 17, 18, 20, 21 gauge; lengths 10, 15, 20 cm; stroke: 20, 30, or 40 mm, optional.

Automatic Biopsy

The cannula and puncture needle of an automatic biopsy device are operated with spring mechanisms that need to be tensioned prior to using the device. Here, the needle is placed in front of the target lesion; the sudden advance of the puncture needle and the advance of the cannula occur automatically after pulling the trigger.

Reusable automatic devices (**Figs. 7.17** and **7.18**) are available in addition to single-use devices (**Figs. 7.19** and **7.22**). A reusable biopsy needle is inserted into a sterilizable needle holder. Different needle sizes and lengths are available. Automatic biopsy devices have a variable stroke.

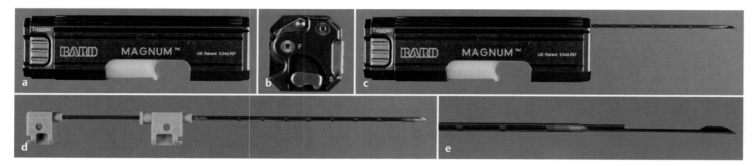

Fig. 7.17 Magnum reusable biopsy system (Bard Biopsy Systems, Tempe, AZ). Magnum automatic hand-held device (**a**), mechanism for setting needle advance and unlocking the system (**b**), device with biopsy needle (**c**), disposable biopsy needle (**d**), advanced specimen notch (**e**). Needle sizes: 12, 14, 16, 18, 20 gauge; lengths: 10, 13, 16, 20 cm; stroke: 15 or 22 mm, optional.

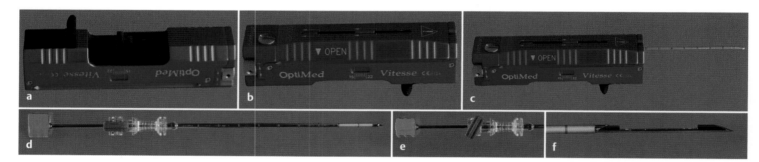

Fig. 7.18 Vitesse reusable biopsy system (OptiMed, Ettlingen, Germany). Vitesse automatic hand-held device (**a, b**), device with biopsy needle (**c**), biopsy needle (**d**), turning knob for arresting biopsy needle (**e**), advanced specimen notch (**f**). If necessary, shipping of a tissue specimen inside the needle is possible by arresting the puncture needle using the turning knob. Needle sizes: 19.5, 18, 16, 14 gauge; lengths: 10, 15, 20, 28 cm; stroke: optional from 10 to 22 mm.

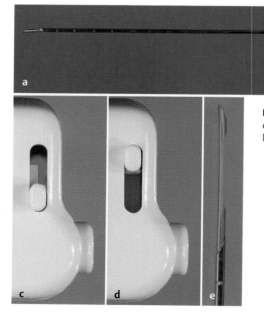

Fig. 7.19 TSK disposable automatic biopsy gun (Invivo Corp., Orlando, FL). TSK automatic biopsy device (**a**), cocking mechanism (**b**), locked (**c**), unlocked (**d**), needle point with notch (**e**). Needle sizes: 14, 16, 18 gauge; lengths: 10, 15 cm; stroke: 20 mm.

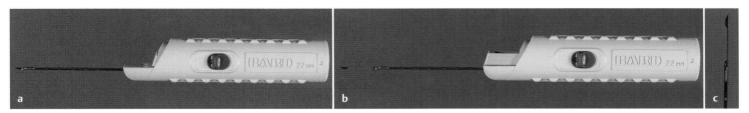

Fig.7.20 Max-Core disposable core biopsy instrument (Bard Biopsy Systems, Tempe, AZ). Max-Core automatic biopsy device (**a**), in the cocked position (**b**), specimen notch (**c**). Needle sizes: 14, 16, 18, 20 gauge; lengths: 10, 16, 20 cm; stroke: 20 cm.

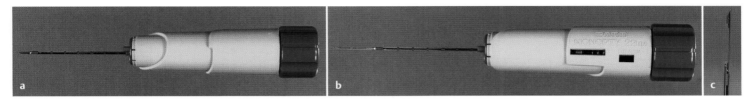

Fig. 7.21 Monopty disposable core biopsy instrument (Bard Biopsy Systems, Tempe, AZ). Monopty automatic biopsy device (**a**), in the cocked position (**b**), specimen notch (**c**). Needle sizes: 14, 16, 18, 20 gauge; lengths: 10, 16, 20 cm; stroke: 22 or 11 mm.

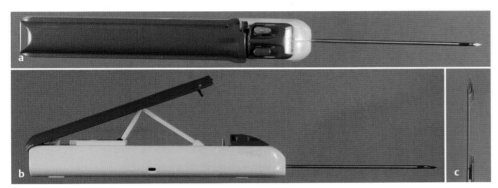

Fig. 7.22 Celero vacuum-assisted core biopsy device (Suros Surgical Systems, Inc., Indianapolis, IN). Suros Celero spring-loaded, disposable biopsy device (**a**), lever mechanism for cocking the needle and creating negative pressure (**b**), needle point with notch (**c**). This instrument is a hybrid between a CNB needle and a VAB device. By using a vacuum during jet biopsy, the quality of the biopsy specimen is improved. Prior to triggering the needle advance, negative pressure is created at the needle point. This is done to prevent displacement of tissue during jet biopsy and to achieve better filling of the notch. A hinged lever on the handle operates the mechanism of this biopsy device. Two knobs are moved during tissue sampling: first, the spring mechanism is cocked and a vacuum created, then the needle is advanced. Needle size: 12 gauge; length: 12.25 cm; stroke: 25 mm.

7

Vacuum-assisted Biopsy Systems (Figs. 7.23, 7.24, 7.25, 7.26)

Unlike other biopsy methods, VAB systems use needles with a lateral aperture into which the tissue is pulled by negative pressure. A cutting cylinder extracts a sample from the tissue. By rotating the aperture, several cubic centimeters of tissue can be removed from around the center of the needle position. Needle sizes vary from 8 to 11 gauge.

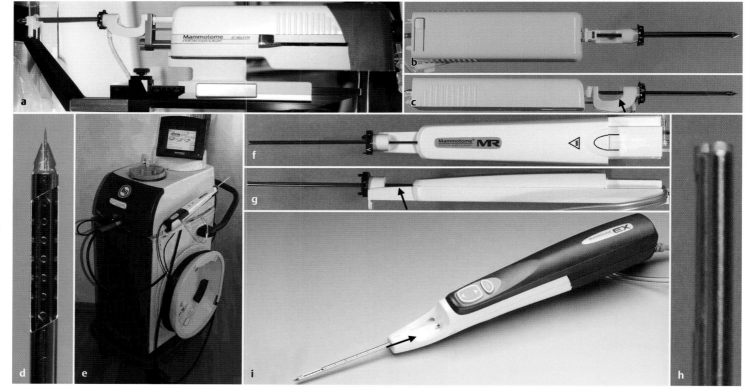

Fig. 7.23 Mammotome biopsy system (Ethicon Endo-Surgery, Cincinnati, OH). Stereotactic Mammotome (**a–e**). Mammotome for stereotactic breast biopsy (**a**), biopsy needle viewed from above (**b**) and from the side (**c**), coaxial needle point with tissue acquisition aperture and vacuum holes (**d**), vacuum pump (**e**). The Stereotactic Mammotome encloses a spring mechanism to trigger the jet advance. A free-standing vacuum pump is connected to the needle holder by a tubing system. The pump creates negative pressure for pulling tissue through the aperture into the biopsy needle, and also for aspirating blood from the biopsy cavity. The tissue specimen is cut out by a rotating cutter inside the needle. By withdrawing the hollow cutter within the needle, the specimen is moved backward and can be collected at the specimen collection chamber (arrows), while the biopsy needle itself remains in the lesion under examination. This step is repeated with every rotation of the aperture. Needle sizes: 14, 11 , 8 gauge; lengths: 8.2 or 9.2 cm. Mammotome magnetic resonance (MR) biopsy system (**f–h**). For magnetic resonance imaging (MRI-) guided tissue collection, a special hand-held device without jet advance and a special coaxial needle are available. View from above (**f**), view from the side (**g**), MRI-compatible coaxial needle with blunt point (**h**). The vacuum pump remains outside the magnetic field. MRI-compatible; needle sizes: 11 and 8 gauge; lengths: 11.5 and 14.5 cm.
Mammotome for ultrasound(US)-guided biopsy (**i**).

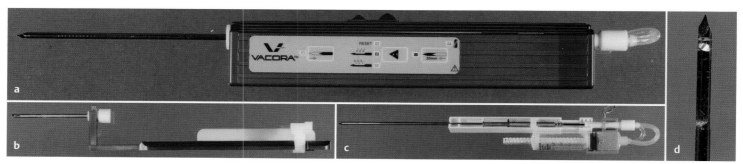

Fig. 7.24 Vacora VAB system (Bard Biopsy Systems, Tempe, AZ). Vacora needle holder with the needle inserted (**a**), sliding carriage for stereotactic biopsy, with fixed coaxial needle (**b**), single-use needle (**c**), needle point with notch (**d**). The Vacora system has a syringe cylinder (**c**) for creating the necessary negative pressure. Prior to biopsy, a coaxial needle is first placed in front of the lesion to be examined. Then, the biopsy needle is placed into the lesion using an integrated jet advance. After aspiration, the tissue specimen is cut out by a hollow cutter rotating outside. When the biopsy needle is withdrawn, the specimen is removed from the notch. After turning the notch and placing the needle again into the lesion, the process is repeated. The mechanism is operated by an electromotor located in the needle holder. A lithium-ion battery serves as power supply. The device is not MRI-compatible, but may be used in the vicinity of the magnetic field. Needle size: 10 gauge; lengths: 11.8 and 14 cm; stroke: 20 mm.

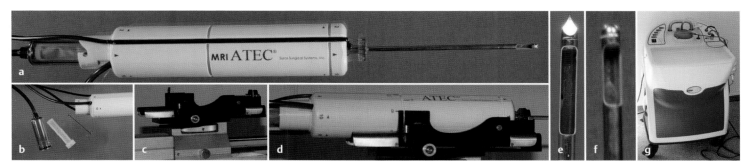

Fig. 7.25 ATEC breast biopsy system (Suros Surgical Systems, Inc., Indianapolis, IN). ATEC disposable handpiece (**a**), specimen reservoir with insert (**b**), jet biopsy needle holder without (**c**) and with the biopsy needle in place (**d**), needle with lancet point (**e**), needle with blunt point (**f**), vacuum pump (**g**). This system has a freestanding vacuum pump. Permanent negative pressure aspirates the tissue into the notch of the needle and the blood from the biopsy cavity. For stereotactic VAB, the biopsy needle has a special holding device (**c**) to facilitate the jet advance. For MRI-guided biopsy, the system is used with a coaxial needle. The tissue specimen is cut out by a rotary cutter inside the needle and is automatically aspirated into a receptacle (**b**) from which specimens are collected once the examination is complete. During the rotation of the notch, the biopsy needle remains in the lesion under examination. Biopsy needles are available with lancet points and blunt points. The device operates on compressed air;. Furthermore, it is possible to flush the biopsy cavity. MRI-compatible; needle sizes: 12 and 9 gauge; lengths: 9 and 11 cm; stroke: 20 mm.

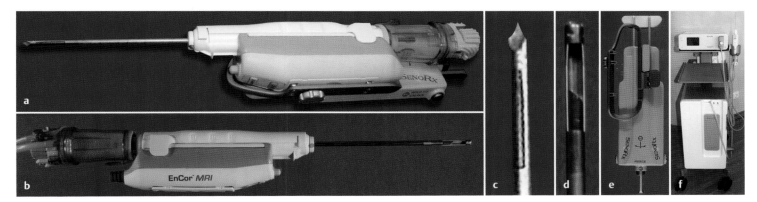

Fig. 7.26 EnCor biopsy system (SenoRx, Inc., Irvine, CA). EnCor hand-held device with biopsy needle for stereotactic procedure (**a**), MRI-compatible EnCor device (**b**). Stereotactic needle point (**c**), MRI-compatible blunt needle point (**d**). Holding device for jet advance during stereotactic biopsy (**e**). The EnCor system has only recently been introduced. It has a free-standing vacuum pump (**f**) to which the needle holder is connected with a tubing system. The tissue specimen is cut out by a rotary cutter inside the needle and is automatically aspirated into a receptacle at the end of the needle holder; the biopsy needle itself remains in the lesion under examination. This step is repeated with every rotation of the notch—which the device does automatically. The tissue specimens are collected from the receptacle once the examination is complete. MRI-compatible; needle sizes: 10 and 7 gauge; length: 11 cm; stroke: 20 mm.

7

Large Core Excision Biopsy
(Figs. 7.27, 7.28, 7.29)

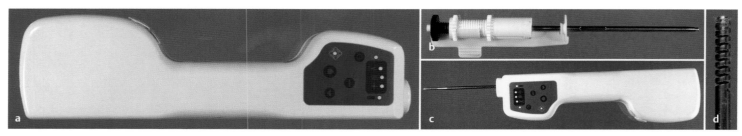

Fig. 7.27 MEDINVENTS Coramate automated large core biopsy system (Siemens, Berlin/Munich, Germany). Coramate hand-held device (**a**), biopsy needle (**b**), Coramate hand-held device with needle (**c**), cutting helix (**d**). Excision biopsy allows the collection of tissue specimens without a jet advance. A hollow metal spiral cuts in a screw-like fashion into the target tissue. The biopsy specimen is secured inside the spiral. Prior to tissue removal, a coaxial needle is advanced to the lesion to be examined, and the tissue specimen is cut out from the focal lesion. After withdrawal of the needle, the specimen is released from the needle using a comb-like tool that reaches into the cavities of the cutting helix. Needle sizes: 12 and 8 gauge; length: 11 cm.

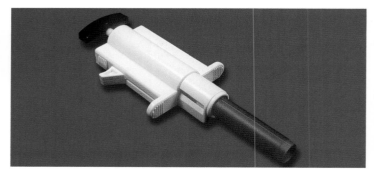

Fig. 7.28 Advanced Breast Biopsy Instrument (ABBI; United States Surgical Corporation, Norwalk, CT). The ABBI system has been designed as a diagnostic as well as a therapeutic tool. After the introduction of VAB, its use is now rather limited. The objective has been to completely remove palpable small carcinomas in an image-guided procedure called buttonhole surgery. After locating the lesion and determining its depth using a mammographic stereotactic unit, the lesion is first kept in place with a hook wire. Subsequently, a tissue sample is removed from the breast containing both lesion and hook wire. In this procedure, however, the tissue in the entire access path—from the skin level to the lesion—is also resected. Once the desired depth of the biopsy is reached and the tumor is inside the cutting cylinder, the tissue is cut out with a built-in cautery wire loop snare and then recovered from the breast. The cutaneous incision is closed with dermal stitches. Because of the high rate of follow-up resections due to incomplete tumor resection (>50% follow-up resections for tumors of <10 mm in diameter), the ABBI system has not proved successful as a therapeutic tool. Diameters of the cutting cylinder: 5, 10, 15, 20, and 30 mm.

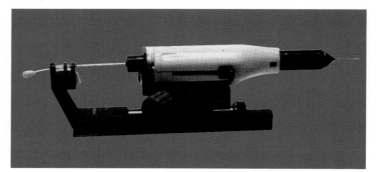

Fig. 7.29 SiteSelect breast biopsy system (SiteSelect Medical Technologies, Pharr, TX). The SiteSelect system is used for a minimally invasive approach (CNB) together with a stereotactic unit. After locating the lesion, a needle is advanced and the lesion is kept in place with a hook wire. The target tissue is then encircled and cut out with a cautery wire. The biopsy specimen is passed through the widened puncture channel in the breast. Dermal stitches are required to close the cutaneous incision. Diameters of cutting cylinders: 5, 10, 15, and 20 mm.

Coaxial Needles (Figs. 7.30, 7.31, 7.32, 7.33, 7.34, 7.35, 7.36, 7.37, 7.38, 7.39, 7.40)

Coaxial needles matching the biopsy needles are available. They consist of a stylet and a cannula; the cannula serves as an "introducer" sheath once the stylet has been removed. The use of coaxial needles is recommended to prevent unnecessary trauma by repeatedly puncturing the breast. Furthermore, coaxial needles are easier to place in the glandular tissue because of their sharper bevel points. In an MRI-guided biopsy, documentation of the needle position is only possible when using a coaxial needle.

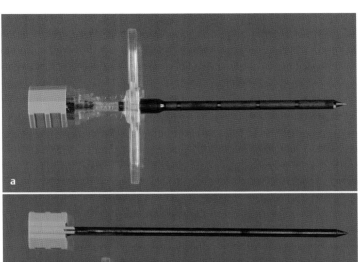

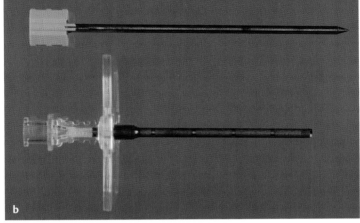

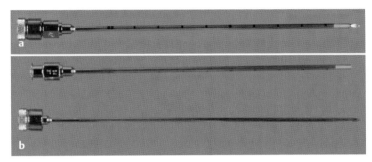

Fig. 7.30 Quick-Core coaxial biopsy needle (Cook Medical, Bloomington, IN). Cook coaxial needle (**a**), introducer sheath and stylet (**b**). Needle sizes: 14, 16, 19 gauge; lengths: 7, 13, 18 cm.

Fig. 7.31 Coaxial needle (SOMATEX Medical Technologies GmbH, Teltow, Germany). SOMATEX coaxial needle (**a**), stylet and introducer sheath (**b**). MRI-compatible; needle sizes: 16, 15, 13 gauge; lengths: 5, 10, 15 cm.

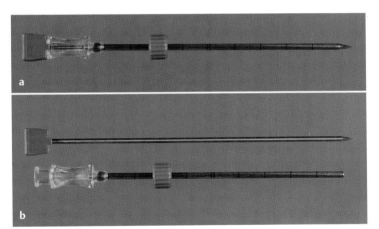

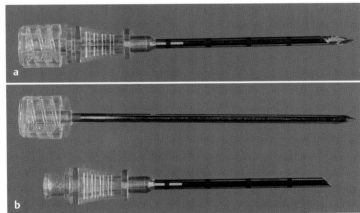

Fig. 7.32 Coaxial needle (Invivo Corp., Orlando, FL). Invivo coaxial needle (**a**), stylet and introducer sheath (**b**). MRI-compatible; needle sizes: 12, 14, 16 gauge; length: 6, 9, 11 cm; stroke: 20 mm.

Fig. 7.33 Coaxial needle (Bard Biopsy Systems, Tempe, AZ). Coaxial needle for the Magnum reusable biopsy system (**a**), stylet and introducer sheath (**b**). May be used with the following BARD biopsy systems: Magnum, Max-Core, Monopty, and Unicut. Needle sizes: 11, 13, 14, 15, 16, 17, 19 gauge; length: 7, 10, 13, 17 cm.

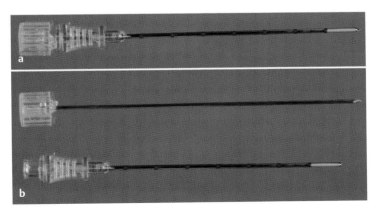

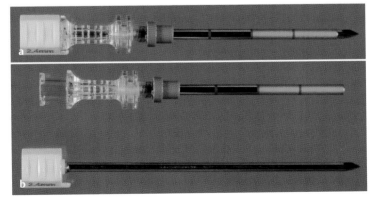

Fig. 7.34 Autovac coaxial needle (Bard Biopsy Systems, Tempe, AZ). Autovac coaxial needle (**a**), stylet and introducer sheath (**b**). Needle sizes: 17, 18, 20, 21 gauge; lengths: 7.5, 12.5, 17.5 cm.

Fig. 7.35 Coaxial needle for Vitesse automatic device (OptiMed, Ettlingen, Germany). OptiMed coaxial needle (**a**), introducer sheath and stylet (**b**). Needle sizes: 13, 14, 17, 18 gauge; lengths: 10, 15, 20 cm.

7

7

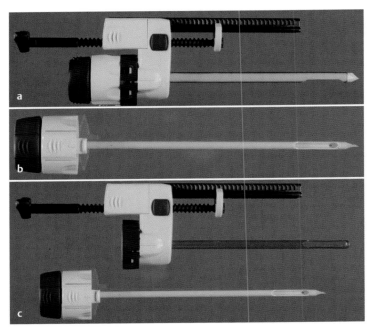

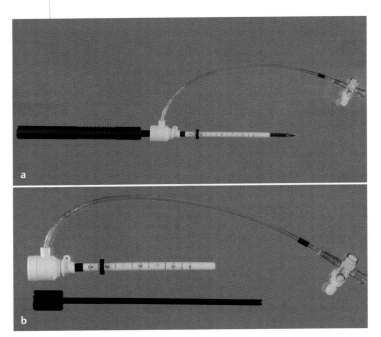

Fig. 7.36 Coaxial needle for the Mammotome MR biopsy system (Ethicon Endo-Surgery, Cincinnati, OH). Complete coaxial needle (**a**), stylet with notch (**b**), introducer sheath and stylet (**c**). Unlike other coaxial needles, this one has a notch. The system is equipped with a catch to limit the needle's advance. MRI-compatible; needle sizes: 7, 19 gauge; length: 8 or 9 cm.

Fig. 7.38 Coaxial needle for the ATEC VAB device (Suros Surgical Systems, Inc., Indianapolis, IN). Suros ATEC MRI introducer set: introducer sheath with stylet (**a**), introducer sheath and obturator (**b**). MRI-compatible; needle sizes: 8 and 11 gauge; length: 9 cm.

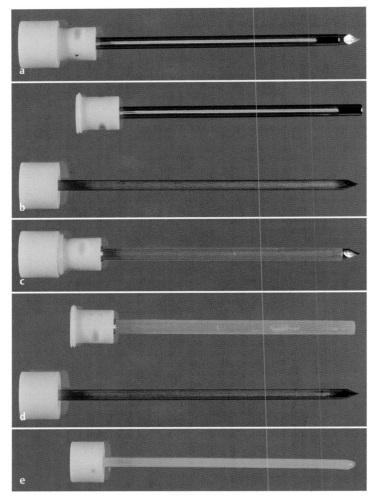

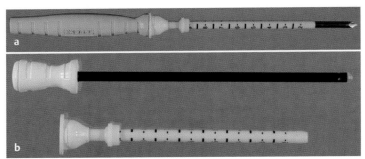

Fig. 7.39 Coaxial needle for the EnCor MRI VAB device (SenoRx, Inc., Irvine, CA). EnCor MRI coaxial needle: introducer sheath with stylet (**a**), obturator and introducer sheath (**b**). MRI-compatible; needle sizes: 6.5 and 9.5 gauge; length: 9 cm.

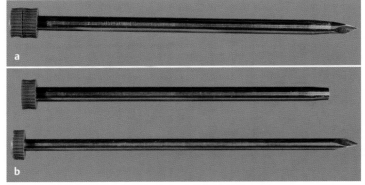

Fig. 7.40 Coaxial needle for the Coramate biopsy device (Siemens, Berlin/Munich, Germany). Coramate coaxial needle (**a**), introducer sheath and stylet (**b**). Needle sizes: 7 and 11 gauge; length: 9 cm.

Fig. 7.37 Coaxial needles for the Vacora VAB device (Bard Biopsy Systems, Tempe, AZ). Vacora coaxial needle for stereotactic biopsy (**a**), introducer sheath (metal) and stylet (**b**). Needle size: 9 gauge; lengths: 8.5 and 10.7 cm.
Vacora coaxial needle for MRI (**c**), introducer sheath (plastic) and stylet (**d**), obturator (**e**). MRI-compatible; needle size: 8 gauge; lengths: 8.5 and 10.7 cm.

Preoperative Localization

Prior to the treatment of nonpalpable lesions, preoperative markings are required. Here, we distinguish between one-stage and two-stage procedures. In case of one-stage marking, which is commonly performed with hook wires, surgery follows immediately. In the case of two-stage marking, the therapeutic procedure is independent of it in space and time; both clips and coils are used for this purpose.

Hook Wires (Figs. 7.41, 7.42, 7.43, 7.44, 7.45, 7.46, 7.47, 7.48, 7.49)

We distinguish between retractable and nonretractable hook wires. After release, retractable wires can be withdrawn into the localization needle so that their position may be corrected. The wires are anchored by means of the hook at the wire end; single-hook and double-hook wires are available.

> **Tips and Tricks**
>
> If the glandular tissue is very lipomatous, the use of double hooks is recommended. If the tissue structures are firm, good anchoring is achieved with single hooks.

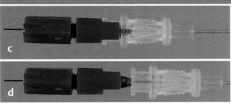
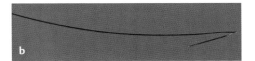
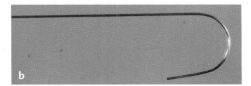

Fig. 7.41 Homer Mammalok (Mitek, Westwood, MA). Homer Mammalok localization needle with hook wire (**a**), Homer Mammalok hook wire (**b**). Nut locked (**c**) and withdrawn (**d**). The direction in which the hook wire leaves the puncture needle can be controlled; it is indicated to the examiner by a protrusion on the wire stabilizer, which fits into a notch in the needle hub. Needle size: 20 gauge; needle length: 10 cm.

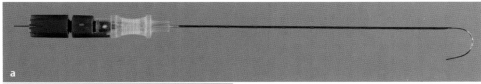

Fig. 7.42 Kopans localization hook wires (Cook Medical, Bloomington, IN). Kopans localization hook wire, nonretractable (**a, b**). Localization needle with hook wire (**a**), tip of Kopans hook wire (**b**). Needle sizes: 20, 21 gauge; needle lengths: 5, 9, 15 cm. MRI-compatible: needle sizes: 20, 21 gauge; lengths: 9, 15 cm.

Kopans localization hook wire with reinforcement, nonretractable (**c, d**). Localization needle with hook wire (**c**), tip of Kopans hook wire (**d**). The wire is reinforced 2 cm in front the hook to prevent damage during surgery. Needle sizes: 20, 21 gauge; needle lengths: 5, 9, 15 cm. MRI-compatible: needle sizes: 20, 21 gauge; needle lengths: 9, 15 cm.

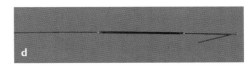
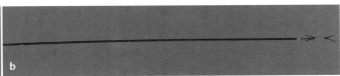

Fig. 7.43 X-Reidy breast localization needle (William Cook, Europe A/S, Bjaeverskov, Denmark). Reidy localization needle with a nonretractable X-shaped hook wire (**a**), tip of hook wire (**b**). Needle sizes: 18 and 19.5 gauge; needle lengths: 5, 9, 15 cm.

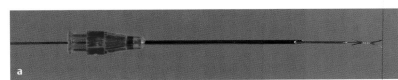
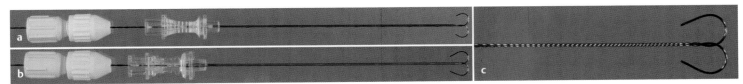

Fig. 7.44 Duo System (SOMATEX Medical Technologies GmbH, Teltow, Germany). Duo System correctable localization needle (**a**), MRI Duo System localization needle (**b**), tip of hook wire (**c**). Relatively rigid hook wire made of two twisted wires. Not MRI-compatible: bare metal, black calibration. Needle size: 19.5 gauge; needle lengths: 5, 9, 12 cm.

MRI-compatible: black metal, light calibration. Needle sizes: 18 and 19.5 gauge; needle lengths: 5, 9, 12 cm.

7

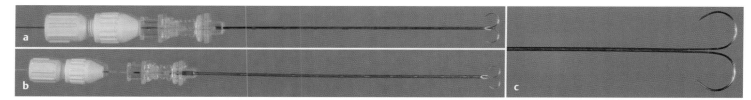

Fig. 7.45 Tuloc localization system (SOMATEX Medical Technologies GmbH, Teltow, Germany). Tuloc retractable localization needle (**a**), Tuloc MRI-compatible localization needle (**b**), tip of hook wire (**c**). Relatively rigid hook wire split by laser technique. Not MRI-compatible: bare metal, black calibration. Needle size: 19.5 gauge; needle lengths: 5, 9, 12 cm. MRI-compatible: black metal, light calibration. Needle size: 18 and 19.5 gauge; needle lengths: 5, 9, 12 cm.

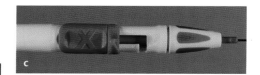

Fig. 7.46 Duo System PREMIUM localization system (SOMATEX Medical Technologies GmbH, Teltow, Germany). Retractable Duo System localization needle with a handle (**a**), tip of hook wire (**b**), slide with bayonet mechanism (**c**). The handle permits single-handed use of the marker wire especially during US. The wire is advanced and released by the bayonet mechanism. Needle size: 19.5 gauge; needle lengths: 5, 9, 12 cm.

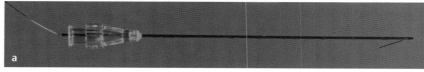

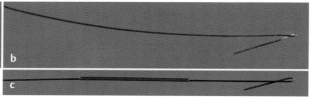

Fig. 7.47 Single-hook wire localization needle (Invivo Corp., Orlando, FL). Invivo localization needle with nonretractable-hook wire (**a**), tip of hook wire (**b**). MRI-compatible: needle sizes: 18 and 20 gauge; needle lengths: 8, 10, 15 cm. Tip of hook wire with reinforcement (**c**).

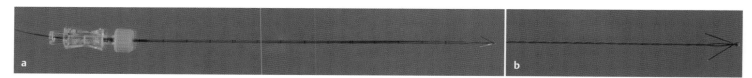

Fig. 7.48 Double hook wire localization needle (Invivo Corp., Orlando, FL). Nonretractable localization needle with hook wire (**a**), tip of hook wire (**b**). MRI-compatible: needle size: 18 and 20 gauge; needle lengths: 8, 10, 15 cm.

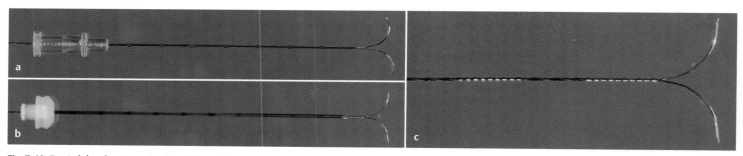

Fig. 7.49 DuaLok localization wire (Bard Biopsy Systems, Tempe, AZ). Retractable DuaLok localization needle (**a**), MRI-compatible DuaLok localization needle (**b**), tip of hook wire (**c**). Needle size: 20 gauge; needle lengths: 57, 77, 107, 137 mm. MRI-compatible: needle size: 20 gauge; needle lengths: 77, 107 mm.

Clips and Coils (Figs. 7.50, 7.51, 7.52, 7.53, 7.54, 7.55, 7.56, 7.57, 7.58, 7.59, 7.60)

Provided it was possible to completely remove suspicious lesions by vacuum-assisted biopsy, the site is marked with clips or coils. The same applies to marking tumor outlines prior to neoadjuvant chemotherapy. In a two-stage procedure, clip and coil markings permit mammographic localization of lesions visible only in MRI scans. Coils are metal spirals; clips are mainly bent metal wires. Puncture needles with handles for single-handed operation facilitate their application under ultrasound guidance; during MR mammography, handles occasionally strike the equipment casing.

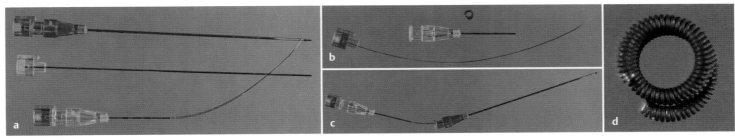

Fig. 7.50 EchoTip localization needle with Müller-Schimpfle coil (Cook Medical, Bloomington, IN). Puncture needle, pusher, and introducer sheath with guide wire (**a**), coil, introducer sheath, and guide wire (**b**), guide wire with the coil inside the puncture needle (**c**), coil (**d**). The coil is introduced into the needle by means of the guide wire, and it is released at the needle tip by the pusher. MRI-compatible; needle size: 19.5 gauge; length: 9 cm; coil winding: 4 mm.

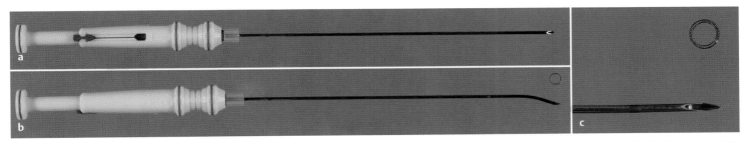

Fig. 7.51 O-Twist Marker (BARD GmbH, Karlsruhe, Germany). Loaded puncture needle (**a**), needle with bent tip for anchoring the coil in the wall of the biopsy cavity (**b**), coil (**c**). MRI-compatible; needle size: 20 gauge; length: 13.7 cm; coil winding: 3 mm.

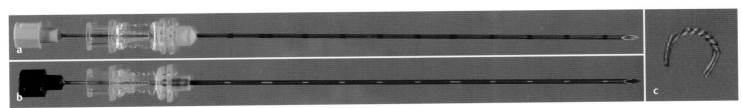

Fig. 7.52 Tumark (SOMATEX Medical Technologies GmbH, Teltow, Germany). Loaded puncture needle with pusher (**a**), loaded MRI-compatible puncture needle (black metal with light calibration) with pusher (**b**), clip (**c**). MRI-compatible; needle size: 18 gauge; length: 12 cm.

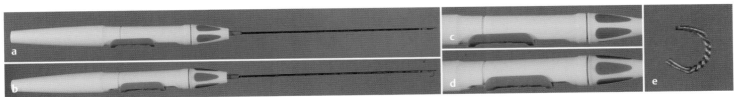

Fig. 7.53 Tumark Professional (SOMATEX Medical Technologies GmbH, Teltow, Germany). Puncture needle with handle (**a**), the same with a clip at the needle tip (**b**), slider for clip release, in backward position (**c**) and in forward position (**d**), clip (**e**). The tool facilitates precise clip marking, particularly during US examination. MRI-compatible; needle size: 18 gauge; length: 12 cm.

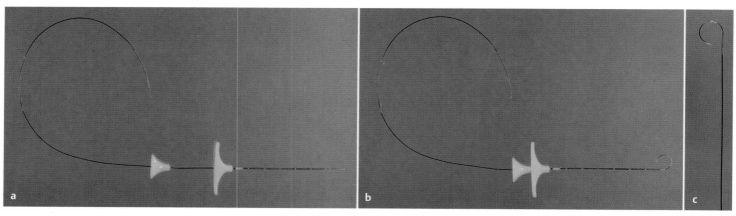

Fig. 7.54 RepoLoc (Ariadne localization coil; Bard Biopsy Systems, Tempe, AZ). Localization needle with pusher, loaded with coil (**a**), coil pushed forward (**b**), Ariadne localization coil with thread (**c**). Because of the thread, there is little hindrance if the coil travels a large distance and is retained for a long time. The risk of damaging the thread during surgery is high. MRI-compatible; needle size: 18 gauge; length: 10 cm.

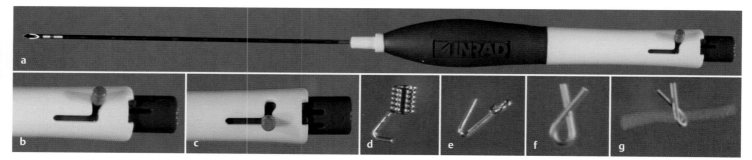

Fig. 7.55 UltraCLIP breast tissue markers (Bard Biopsy Systems, Tempe, AZ). Puncture needle with handle (**a**), sliding knob for releasing the clip (**b, c**). Various clip styles (**d–f**), clip with sponge for detection by US (**g**). Various clip styles allow for spatial correlations when using several clips. MRI-compatible; needle size: 20 gauge; lengths: 9 and 12 cm.

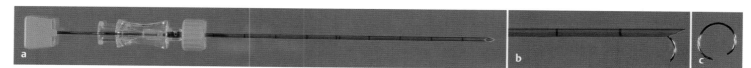

Fig. 7.56 ClipLoc soft tissue marker (Invivo Corp., Orlando, FL). Loaded puncture needle with pusher (**a**), clip in needle tip (**b**) and clip (**c**). MRI-compatible; Needle size: 18 gauge; lengths: 10, 13, and 15 cm.

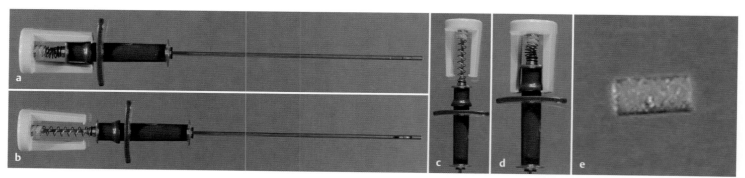

Fig. 7.57 ATEC clip marker (Suros Surgical Systems, Inc., Indianapolis, IN). Puncture needle with handle (**a**) and loaded with clip (**b**), sliding clamp in unlocked position (**c**) and in locked position (**d**), marker clip (**e**). Marker clip for use in ATEC VAB system. MRI-compatible; Needle size: 15 gauge; length: 10 cm.

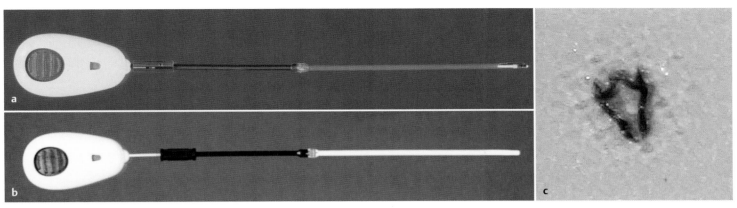

Fig. 7.58 Marker clip (Ethicon Endo-Surgery, Cincinnati, OH). Clip applicator with clip carrier loaded (**a**) and unloaded (**b**), clip (**c**). Marker clip for use in Mammotome VAB system. MRI-compatible; Needle size: 14 gauge; length: 20 cm.

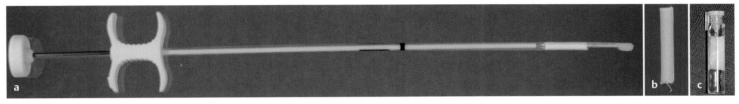

Fig. 7.59 MammoMark (Ethicon Endo-Surgery, Cincinnati, OH). Clip applicator (**a**), collagen marker, dry (**b**), collagen marker with water, swollen (**c**). Bioabsorbable marker made of collagen. Caveat: protein allergy. MRI-compatible; Needle size: 14 gauge; length: 20 cm; marker length: 11 mm.

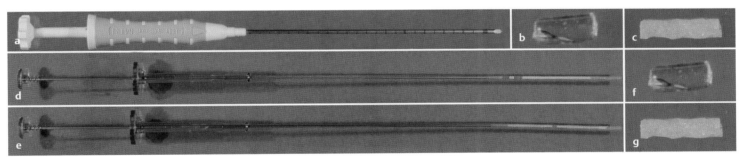

Fig. 7.60 GelMark UltraCor, SenoMark UltraCor MRI, GelMark, GelMark Ultra, and SenoMark (SenoRx, Inc., Irvine, CA). GelMark UltraCor puncture needle with handle (**a**), metal clip (**b**), polyglycolic acid pellet (**c**). MRI-compatible; Needle size: 14 gauge; lengths: 10 and 13 cm.
GelMark, GelMark Ultra, and SenoMark (**d–g**). Applicators (**d, e**), metal clip (**f**), pellet (**g**). MRI-compatible; needle sizes: 8, 9, 10, 11 gauge; varied lengths.
These applicators are for commonly used VAB devices. Pellets made of polyglycolic/polylactic acid or collagen are visible during US examination (caveat: protein allergy). Steel or titanium clips are visible during mammography or MRI. Metal clips are available in various styles to allow for spatial correlations, e. g., when marking a tumor.

7

Specimen Radiography

Post- or perioperative specimen radiography is performed to document the complete resection of a lesion. In addition, it documents the precise position of the lesion for both the surgeon and the pathologist to facilitate necessary follow-up resections and/or specific processing of the preparation. Appropriate agreement is required for orientation. It is customary to identify the cut edges of the specimens with thread markings, both close and distant to the mammilla and close and distant to the skin. Special containers are available to facilitate the mammographic examination of specimens (**Figs. 7.61, 7.62, 7.63**). Radiography should be performed in two orthogonal planes.

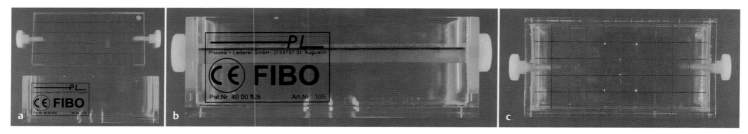

Fig. 7.61 FiboBox (Plieske + Lederer, Sankt Augustin, Germany). FiboBox and lid with radiopaque grid (**a**), closed FiboBox viewed from the side (**b**) and viewed from above (**c**).

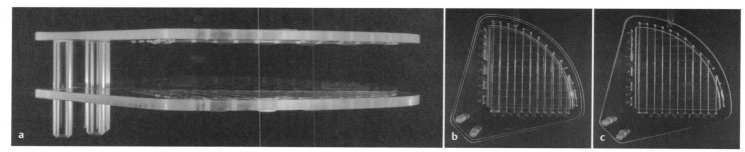

Fig. 7.62 Symadi: Specimen holder (Symadi, Krefeld, Germany). Specimen holder viewed from the side (**a**), from above (**b**), and from above with radiographic grid inserted (**c**). The holder is made of two acrylic glass paddles with a nylon cover and a mountable radiopaque grid. Specimen radiography in the second plane is not possible without repositioning.

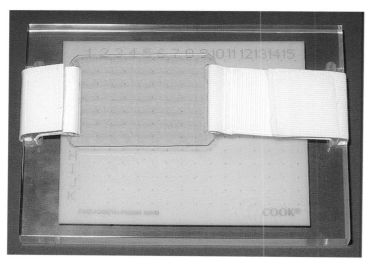

Fig. 7.63 Specimen holder (Cook Medical, Bloomington, IN). Acrylic plate with stippled grid and pressure plate with rubber band fixtures. Specimen radiography in the second plane is not possible without repositioning.

Galactography

Galactography needles are used for injecting contrast medium into the mammary ducts (**Figs. 7.64, 7.65, 7.66, 7.67, 7.68, 7.69**). Very fine, blunt needles are used for this purpose; they may be straight or with a 90° angle. Sialography needles are also used for fine needle aspiration of mammary duct tissue. In addition to individual needles, sets are available consisting of a needle, tubing, and syringe.

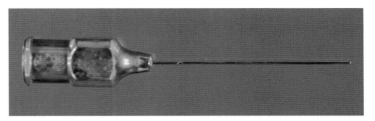

Fig. 7.64 Galactography needle with Luer-Lock hub. Needle size: 30-gauge; length: 30 mm.

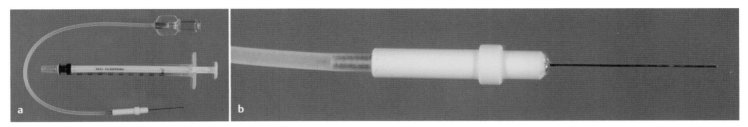

Fig. 7.65 Sialography / galactography needle (Peter Pflugbeil GmbH, Zorneding, Germany). Sialography set with needle, connecting tube, and microliter syringe (**a**), sialography needle (**b**). Needle size: 30 gauge; length: 25 mm; tube length: 15 cm.

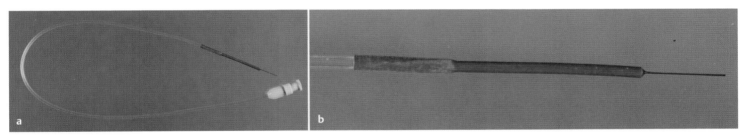

Fig. 7.66 Rabinov sialography catheter (Cook Medical, Bloomington, IN). Sialography needle with connecting tube (**a**), cannula (**b**). Needle size: 30-gauge; length: 25 mm; tube length: 32 cm.

Fig. 7.67 Jabczenski ductogram needle (Cook Medical, Bloomington, IN). Jabczenski ductogram needle with connecting tube (**a**) and angled needle tip (**b**). Needle size: 30 gauge; length: 25 mm; angled tip: 5 mm; tube length: 15 cm.

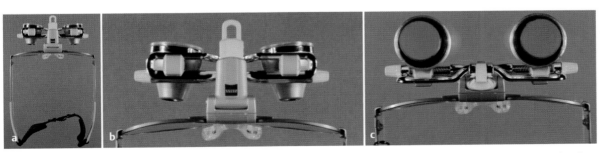

Fig. 7.68 EyeMag Smart loupe (Carl Zeiss, Oberkochen, Germany). Binocular loupe with 2.5 × magnification (**a**) and hinged oculars (**b, c**). The system can be supplemented with a head light.

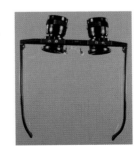

Fig. 7.69 Binocular spectacle magnifier (Eschenbach Optik, Nurnberg, Germany). Binocular loupe with 4 × magnification.

Stereotactic Mammography

Stereotactic biopsy systems are used to calculate the exact location of the lesion to be examined by mammography. We distinguish between dedicated systems (**Fig. 7.70**) and diagnostic devices that can be retrofitted (**Figs. 7.71** and **7.72**). Examination using a dedicated system is performed in the prone position, whereas examination using retrofitted diagnostic devices is mostly performed in the sitting position, but with some devices also in the prone or lateral position. When using old stereotactic systems with conventional imaging, the examination is also performed in the sitting position. However, these devices are rarely used today because of the delay in image processing.

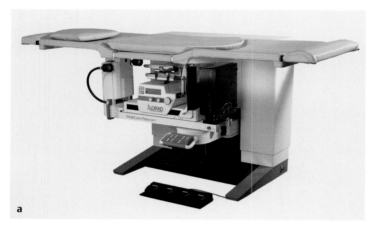

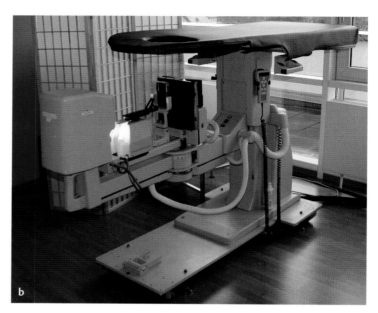

Fig. 7.70 Dedicated stereotactic biopsy systems (Lorad Medical Systems, Danbury, CT). Premium stereotactic table (**a**), **Siemens (Berlin/Munich, Germany)** Fischer stereotactic table (**b**). Positioning of the patient on the Lorad table is optional (feet to the left or right) and permits 360° of access to the breast. Needle guidance is parallel to the table-top. Positioning of the patient on the Fischer table is preset and prevents caudal access to the breast; lateral access must be selected as an alternative. Needle guidance is diagonal to the table axis.

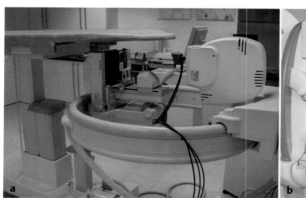
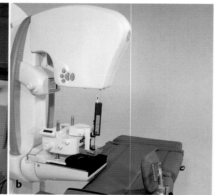

Fig. 7.71 Diagnostic mammography systems with intervention possible in the prone position. Giotto Image (I.M.S., Bologna, Italy) (**a**): The ring-shaped gantry of the Giotto diagnostic system makes it possible to use this device in the horizontal optical path. Needle guidance is parallel to the table-top. **GE Senographe DS (GE Healthcare, Chalfont St., Giles, UK)** (**b**): Craniocaudal access is performed in the sitting position. For lateral access, examination may be performed in the prone position. Needle guidance is parallel to the optical path.

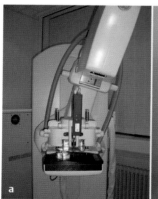
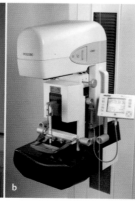
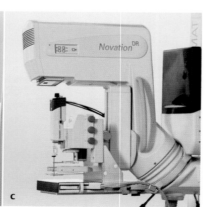

Fig. 7.72 Diagnostic mammography systems with optional intervention in the sitting position. GE Senographe DS (GE Healthcare, Chalfont St., Giles, UK) (**a**), **Lorad Selenia (Lorad Medical Systems, Danbury, CT).** (**b**), **Siemens Novation (Berlin/Munich, Germany)** (**c**): all procedures are performed in the sitting position. Needle guidance is parallel to the optical path.

MRI-guided Breast Biopsy

Coils

For MRI-guided breast biopsy, open diagnostic coils are used. They permit optimal breast positioning as well as access for interventions in the prone position (**Figs. 7.73, 7.74, 7.75, 7.76, 7.77**). Alternatively, shoulder coils with breast positioning aids are also used (**Fig. 7.78**). Interventions in the supine position are obsolete today.

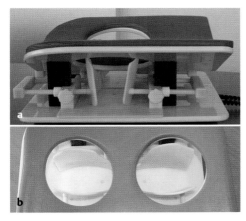
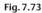

Fig. 7.73

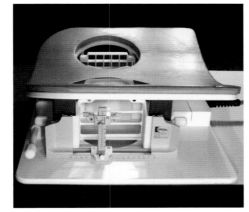

Fig. 7.74

Fig. 7.73 Four-channel breast coil (Invivo Corp., Orlando, FL) (a). View from above (**b**).

Fig. 7.74 Four-channel breast coil (Philips Healthcare, Amsterdam, the Netherlands).

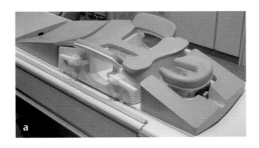

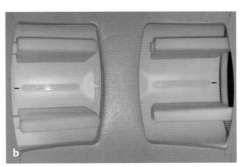

Fig. 7.75 Eight-channel breast coil (GE Healthcare, Chalfont St., Giles, UK) (a). View from above (**b**).

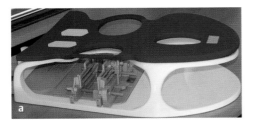

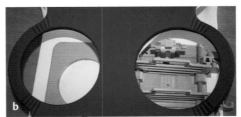

Fig. 7.76 Eight-channel breast coil (Noras MRI Products, Hochberg, Germany). Breast coil with Flex Coil cover (**a**), view from above (**b**). Open coil design with 360° access.

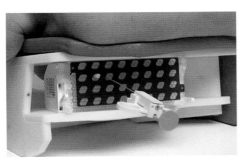

Fig. 7.77

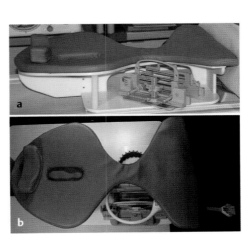

Fig. 7.78

Fig. 7.77 Four-channel breast coil (Machnet BV, Eelde, the Netherlands).

Fig. 7.78 Shoulder coil (Noras MRI Products, Hochberg, Germany). Positioning aid (**a**), shoulder coil inserted (**b**).

Positioning Aids

For positioning the breast during MRI-guided biopsy, perforated plastic plates, grids, and post and pillar systems are used (**Figs. 7.79, 7.80, 7.81, 7.82, 7.83, 7.84, 7.85, 7.86**).

7

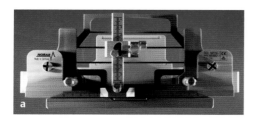
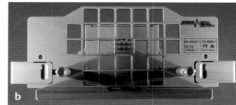

Fig. 7.79   MRI positioning aids for open breast coils, first generation (Noras MRI Products, Hochberg, Germany). Noras positioning aid with post and pillar (**a**) and grid (**b**). Noras positioning aid for Siemens (Berlin/Munich, Germany) coil with post and pillar (**c**) and grid (**d**).

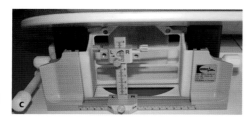
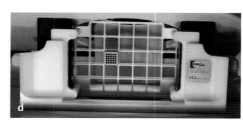

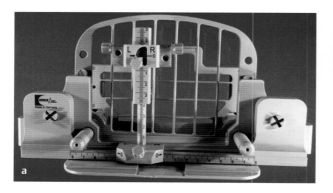
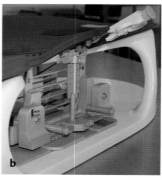

Fig. 7.80 Positioning aid for open breast coils, second generation (Noras MRI Products, Hochberg, Germany). Positioning aid with grid (**a**) and post and pillar system (**b**). Option of 360° rotation and maximum post and pillar amplitude.

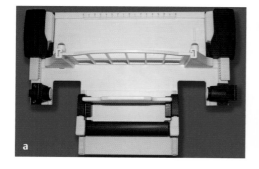
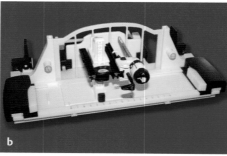

Fig. 7.81 Positioning aid for open breast coils (Invivo Corp., Orlando, FL). Positioning aid with grid (**a**) and post and pillar, here shown with Mammotome coaxial needle (**b**).

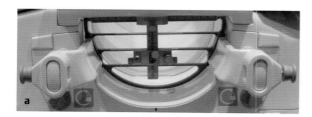
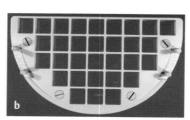

Fig. 7.82 Positioning aid (Noras MRI Products, Hochberg, Germany) for General Electric eight-channel coil. Positioning aid with post and pillar system (**a**) and grid (**b**).

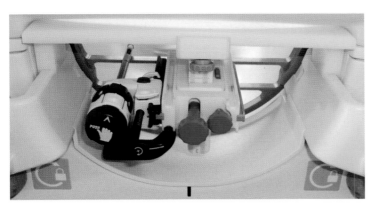

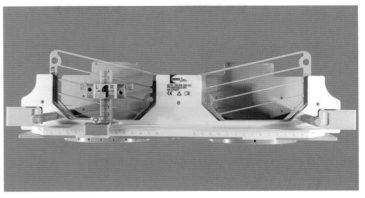

Fig. 7.83 Positioning aid (Invivo Corp., Orlando, FL) for General Electric eight-channel coil. Positioning aid, here shown with Mammotome coaxial needle. Grids are available for this system as well.

Fig. 7.84 Double positioning aid for frontal intervention (Noras MRI Products, Hochberg, Germany). Bilateral, frontal positioning aid.

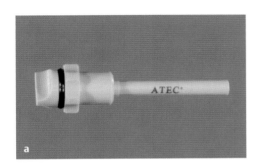

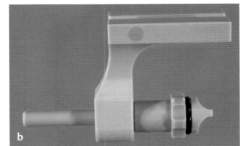

Fig. 7.85 Marking pins. Marker pin for insertion into the guide rail (**a**), with guide rail (**b**). For grid and post and pillar system. Clearly visible in T1-weighted MRI.

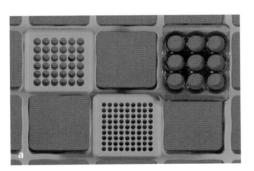

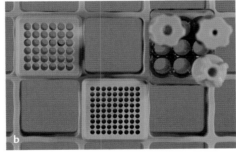

Fig. 7.86 Needle guide blocks (for needles of 23, 19, 14, 12, 11 gauge). Needle guide blocks for grid (**a, b**), sleeves for grid and post and pillar system (**c**).

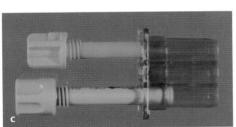

Additional Instrumentation
(Figs. 7.87 and 7.88)

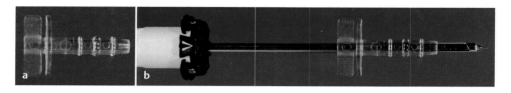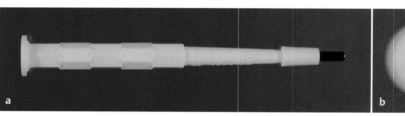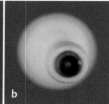

Fig. 7.87 Mammotome cover sleeve. Cover sleeve (**a**), mounted cover sleeve (**b**). The sleeve allows a biopsy specimen to be obtained at skin level by covering the exposed tissue acquisition opening.

Fig. 7.88 BIOPSY PUNCH skin punch (Stiefel Laboratories GmbH, Offenbach am Main, Germany). Extremely sharp stainless-steel blade, with ergonomic plastic handle, viewed from the side (**a**) and from above (**b**).

8 Specimen Processing for Pathologic Diagnosis

F. Baum

Cytologic Smears

In the diagnosis of breast anomalies, cytologic smear examinations are usually performed when a bloody nipple discharge is present. Despite the fact that a bloody nipple discharge is caused by intraductal papillomas and other benign changes in approx. 95% of cases, exfoliative cytology is performed to exclude the presence of malignant cells in the nipple discharge. A negative cytologic result, however, does not reliably exclude malignancy.

To attain secretion for a cytologic smear, the breast should be gently massaged from the periphery toward the nipple. By slightly squeezing behind the nipple, the subareolar secretion accumulation can then be expressed and collected on one end of a glass slide. A second specimen slide is then used to smear the secretion drop across the greater length of the first slide for cytologic examination (**Fig. 8.1**). The smear is most commonly air-dried and then labeled and prepared for transportation to the cytopathologist.

Aspiration Cytology

The indication for the performance of a fine needle aspiration biopsy (FNAB) is limited to the aspiration of symptomatic or complicated cysts, the diagnostic work-up of palpable lumps without correlating imaging abnormalities, and the diagnostic work-up of suspicious axillary lymph nodes.

Fluids. The syringe in which aspirated fluids (e.g., from a cyst) are collected is closed with a stopper and labeled with the patient data before being sent to cytopathology. The fluid is then centri-

fuged and the precipitate smeared onto a specimen slide, air-dried, and stained (Giemsa stain) for microscopic examination.

Solid lesions. FNAB of a solid lesion (e.g., lymph node) is performed by rapidly passing the needle back and forth in various directions, 1 to 2 cm through the lesion, while applying a vacuum (negative pressure) to obtain cellular material. After the pressure in the syringe has been allowed to equalize, the needle is removed from the breast. The contents of the syringe and needle are then carefully expressed onto a glass slide. For this, the syringe is first disconnected from the needle and filled with air by drawing back the plunger. The Luer-slip is then held closely over the glass slide and the material expressed by applying positive pressure (**Fig. 8.2**). This procedure is repeated after reconnecting the needle to the syringe after the plunger has been drawn back (**Fig. 8.3**).

> ### Tips and Tricks
>
> Occasionally, the aspirated material can be scanty and located in the syringe, making it difficult to retrieve. In such cases, it is sometimes possible to use a long needle to salvage the sample for the cytologic smear. Alternatively, saline solution can be aspirated into the syringe through the puncture needle, retrieving the cellular material herein. The syringe is closed with a stopper and then centrifuged at the laboratory. The precipitate is then used to prepare the cytologic smear.

Viscous aspirate. Cytologic specimens of viscous aspirate are best obtained by applying flat pressure with the spreading slide on the slide with the sample drop and then distributing it by moving the slide sideways (**Fig. 8.4**).

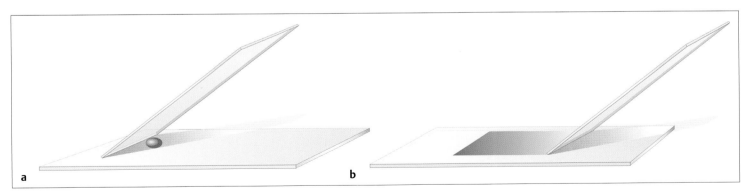

Fig. 8.1 a, b Smearing fluid aspirate.

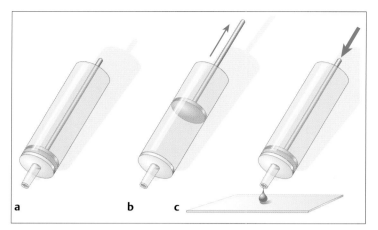

Fig. 8.2a–c Removing aspirate from a syringe.
a Syringe with aspirate.
b The plunger is drawn back slowly.
c The Luer-slip is held closely over the glass slide and the material expressed by rapidly applying positive pressure.

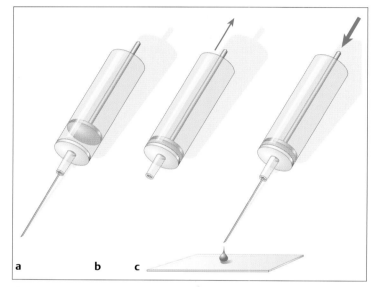

Fig. 8.3a–c Removing aspirate from the puncture needle.
a Syringe and puncture needle with aspirate.
b After removing the needle, the plunger of the syringe is drawn back slowly.
c After replacing the needle, it is held closely over the glass slide and the material expressed by rapidly applying positive pressure.

Core Needle Biopsy and Vacuum-assisted Biopsy Specimens

Optimal operational and organizational structures as well as good communication between the pathologist and the diagnostic physician are essential prerequisites for effective cooperation. Reliable transportation and handling of the samples, as well as the prompt and correct technical processing of tissue specimens are part of these structures and ensure a prompt histologic diagnosis to the benefit of the patient involved.

Tissue containers for specimen processing. Tissue samples obtained by minimally invasive interventions usually have a cylindrical shape. The sample structure reflects the corresponding anatomic structures of the sampled organ. The appropriate handling and processing of these specimens preserves these anatomic structures and facilitates the pathologist's orientation and

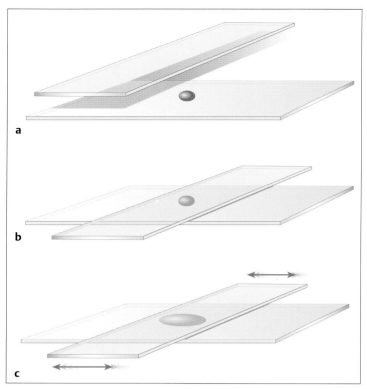

Fig. 8.4a–c Preparing a smear of viscous aspirate.
a Viscous aspirate.
b Flat pressure is applied with the spreading slide.
c By displacing the slide sideways, a smear is produced.

the pathologic evaluation. This is especially important when tissue specimens are long and thin. For this purpose, specimens are placed directly in labeled tissue capsules for the pathology laboratory. Lining the capsules with filter paper maintains a stable specimen position within the container. In general, three to five biopsy specimens are placed in one capsule and arranged in parallel arrays (**Fig. 8.5**).

Clustered microcalcifications. Because microcalcifications often correspond to areas of necrosis in intraductal tumors, it is especially important that these be histologically identified in the biopsy specimens of abnormalities containing microcalcifications. To facilitate this for the pathologist, arrange the biopsy specimens in parallel arrays on filter paper (e.g., coffee filters) during harvesting for specimen radiography. These can then be separated according to whether they contain calcifications or not, and placed into separate capsules (three tissue samples per capsule). Final specimen radiography of the capsules facilitates the correlation of the macroscopic appearance of the tissue samples with the location of the microcalcifications because the specimens normally retain their shape and position during processing (**Fig. 8.6**).

Another way to optimize the histologic detection of microcalcifications in the tissue specimens is to mark the areas containing microcalcifications with ink after specimen radiography. The pathologist then sees the ink marking and can begin with the examination of these sections.

Fixation, embedding, and sectioning. Optimal fixation of biopsy specimens is a prerequisite for further specimen processing. Sectioning with a microtome requires that the biopsy speci-

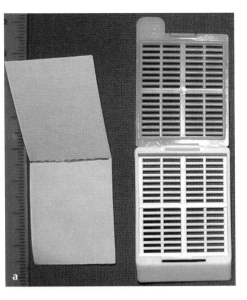

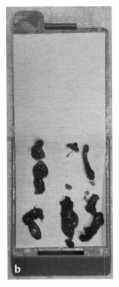

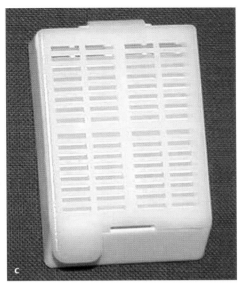

Fig. 8.5a–c Specimen capsules for pathologic processing.
a Specimen capsule and filter paper.
b Specimen capsule with inserted filter paper and three tissue samples.
c Closed specimen capsule ready for transport.

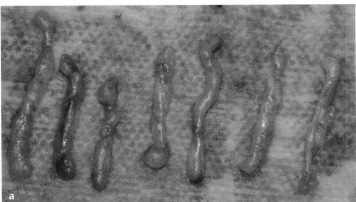

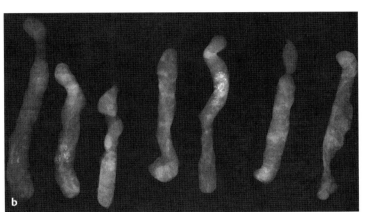

8

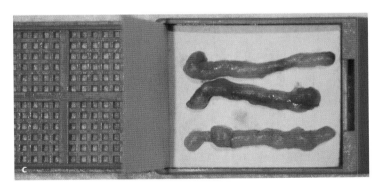

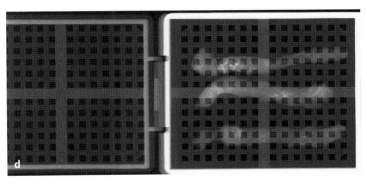

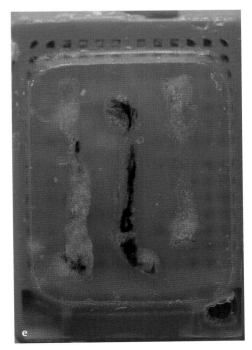

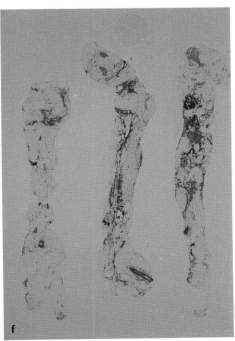

Fig. 8.6a–f Specimen handling of tissue samples obtained from a finding containing microcalcifications.
a Specimens arranged on filter paper.
b Specimen radiograph.
c Specimen capsule holding samples with microcalcifications.
d Specimen radiograph of this capsule.
e Same specimens in paraffin block.
f Stained histologic section.

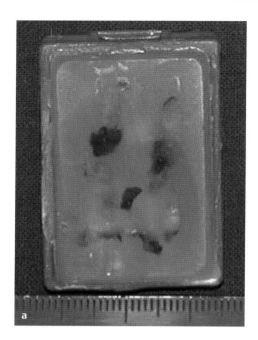

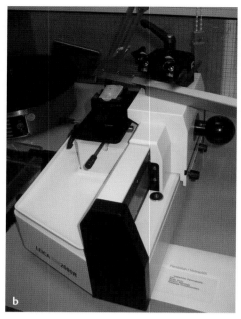

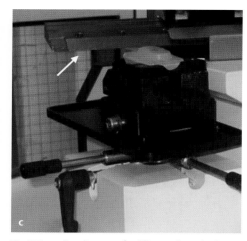

Fig. 8.7a–c Specimen embedding and sectioning.
a Specimens in paraffin block.
b Microtome.
c Microtome sled with cutting blade.

mens be of homogeneous consistency. The first step required to achieve this is to solubilize the fatty tissue fraction out of the specimens by immersing them in formalin. This process begins with the immersion of the tissue capsules in formalin-filled containers before they are sent to the pathology laboratory, and should be continued overnight before further processing. After the fat fraction has been removed, the specimens are embedded in paraffin blocks (**Fig. 8.7a**). Because the mechanical resistance of paraffin is similar to that of the prepared tissue samples, it is well suited to obtain a uniform cutting. A microtome is the mechanical instrument used to cut the paraffin blocks containing the specimen tissue to attain high-quality histologic sections of approx. 5 µm thickness (**Figs. 8.7b, Fig. 8.7c**), thin enough to be transparent for microscopic examination. These are then mounted on a microscope slide.

Staining. Before staining the histologic sections with hematoxylin and eosin, the paraffin is melted away at 80 °C and residual paraffin removed with a xylol solution. The razor-thin specimen section remaining on the slide is then placed in a dye bath (**Fig. 8.8**). Finally, microscopic examination can be performed after retreatment with a xylol solution and drying.

Specimen radiography of paraffin blocks. Special cooperation between the diagnostic physician and the pathologist is required when despite the detection of microcalcifications on specimen radiography, the pathologist cannot find microcalcifications in the initial histologic sections. To perform additional sectioning selectively, the paraffin blocks can be x-rayed to identify areas of microcalcifications (**Fig. 8.9**).

Frozen section. Although the pathologic examination of histologic sections after processing in formalin is more reliable, frozen sectioning may occasionally be more expedient. For this, the specimens are transported in a saline solution, then quick-frozen using liquid nitrogen for microtome slicing. Due to the mechanical resistance encountered with microcalcifications, these may be lost or cause damage to the histologic sections during microtome

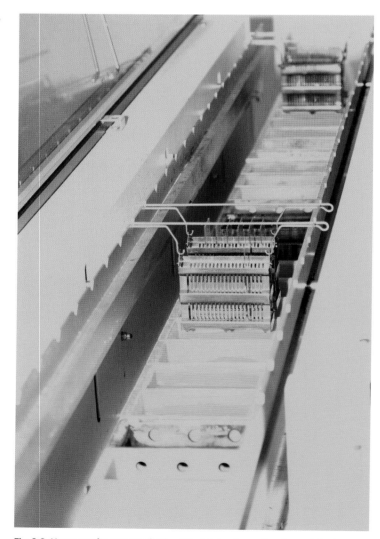

Fig. 8.8 Hematoxylin staining bath with staining trays. Specimen slides in staining trays are immersed for approx. 2 minutes in the appropriate staining solutions.

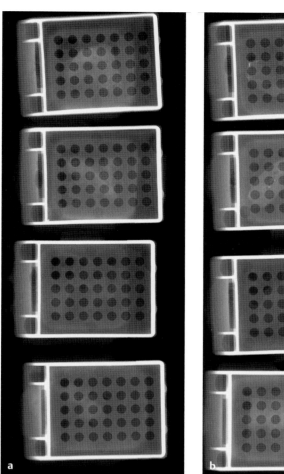
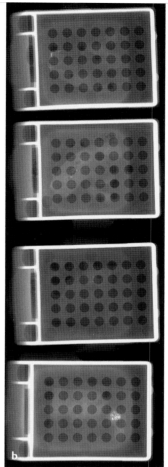
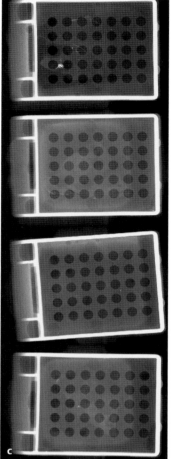
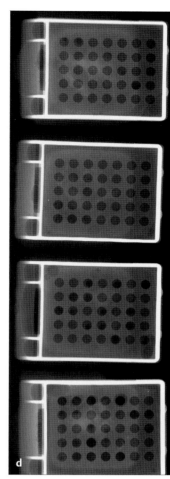

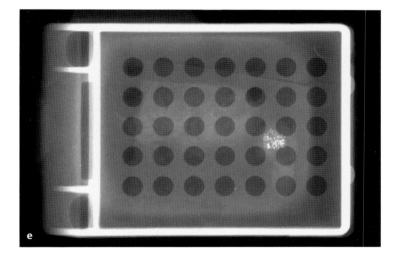

Fig. 8.9a–e Specimen radiography of paraffin blocks. Pathologic examination of a surgical specimen failed to detect the expected microcalcifications. Specimen radiography of specimen capsules (**a–d**) identified those containing samples with microcalcifications in series **b** and **c**. One enlarged view (**e**).

8

slicing, rendering the frozen section preparations impossible to interpret. For this reason, frozen sections of nonpalpable lesion biopsies with microcalcifications are strongly discouraged.

Correlation of specimen to patient. If there is uncertainty as to whether a specimen has been obtained from a specific patient, genetic testing can resolve this problem.

Tips and Tricks

To reduce time it takes to transport a specimen to the pathology laboratory, especially when performing a frozen section preparation, consider using a bike courier or taxi company.

9 Perioperative Specimen Imaging

U. Fischer

When an excisional biopsy is performed for a nonpalpable breast lesion, imaging must verify that the suspicious lesion has been removed and biopsy is representative. This is not usually necessary for palpable findings because it can be assumed that the surgeon is able to reliably excise these.

Which imaging technique to perform for this perioperative check is dependent upon whether the biopsied lesion is most reliably identified on mammography (specimen radiography), or ultrasound (US) (specimen US). Specimen magnetic resonance imaging (MRI) has not been established as a reliable method to verify correct excision.

> **Good Practice Recommendation**[*]
>
> Preoperative localization and postoperative specimen imaging should always be performed when a nonpalpable breast lesion is excised (Grade of Recommendation A, Level of Evidence 3b).
> [*] European S3 guidelines

Specimen Radiography

Mammography of surgically excised tissue—a specimen radiograph—is essential after open surgery of mammographic abnormalities associated with microcalcifications. Pertinent information derived from the specimen radiograph is whether any microcalcifications are detected at all, whether the biopsy is representative and/or the microcalcifications completely excised, and whether the microcalcifications are centrally or marginally located in the specimen.

A specimen radiograph is also obligatory after surgical removal of nonpalpable breast lesions. The target abnormality can often be radiographically detected within the specimen, especially when the surrounding tissue is lipomatous. In such cases, the specimen radiograph is a reliable documentation of the representative lesion excision.

Examination in two planes. Specimen radiography should be performed in two orthogonal planes (craniocaudal [CC] and mediolateral [ML]) (**Fig. 9.1**). This can be done by placing the specimen in a commercially available container (e.g., a Bollmann specimen chamber) or in any other suitable, x-ray transparent container (**Fig. 9.2**). Some containers, however, require that the specimen be repositioned for radiography, occasionally making topographic orientation more difficult. Others take anatomic relationships with regard to the axilla and other defined landmarks into consideration.

Fixation. The assignment of the specimen configuration to the anatomic topography is facilitated when the surgical specimen is fixed or mounted on a carrier medium, and can be x-rayed on this medium without further manipulation. To facilitate this, the materials used must allow the specimen to be firmly fastened, as well as be easily x-rayed without producing disturbing artifacts. One material possessing these qualities is Styrofoam. Other materials, such as cork, often possess interfering, radiopaque inclusions (**Fig. 9.3**). As an aid to the pathologist, it is also possible to place markers on relevant areas of the tissue specimen as seen on the specimen radiograph and then take another radiograph for documentation (**Fig. 9.4**).

> **Good Practice Recommendation**[*]
>
> Specimen radiography of tissue samples obtained from abnormalities associated with microcalcifications should be performed in magnification technique.
> [*] European S3 guidelines

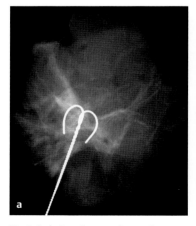
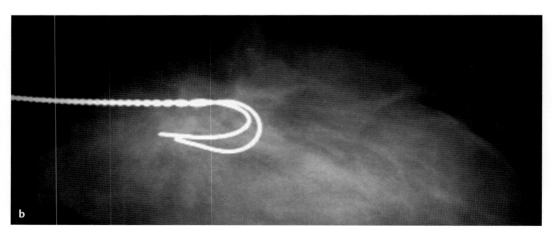

Fig. 9.1a,b Specimen radiographs in two planes. Surgical specimen with localization wire in place in the craniocaudal (CC) projection (**a**) and lateral projection (**b**).

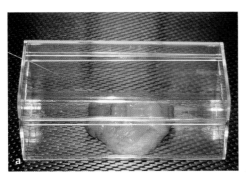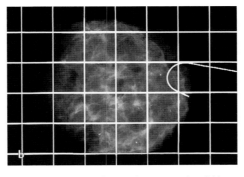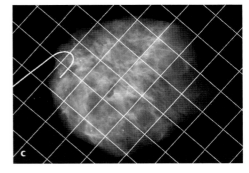

Fig. 9.2a–c Containers used in specimen radiography. Simple Plexiglas box without marker aids (**a**). Bollmann specimen chamber with integrated wire grid scale (**b**). SYMADI (Krefeld, Germany) specimen holder allowing anatomically oriented specimen fastening (**c**).

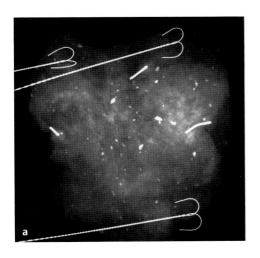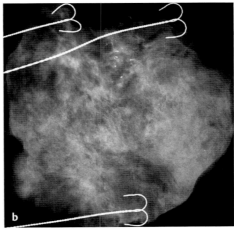

Fig. 9.3a,b Mounting specimens for radiography. Specimen radiograph of a specimen mounted on a cork slab showing multiple radiopaque artifacts (**a**). Repeat specimen radiograph after repositioning specimen onto Plexiglas plate is artifact-free (**b**).

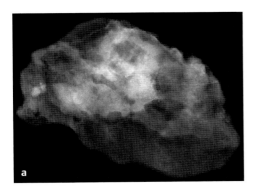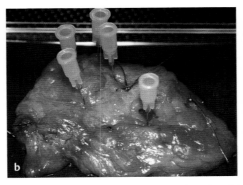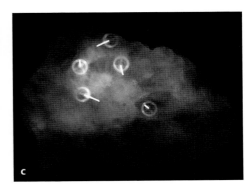

Fig. 9.4a–c Specimen marker placement. Surgical specimen showing microcalcifications in central and marginal areas of the tissue specimen (**a**). Appropriate placement of markers (**b**). Repeat specimen radiograph shows markers placed to facilitate the pathologist's orientation (**c**).

Reporting. The following information and remarks pertaining to a specimen radiograph should be included in the written report:

- A statement about the presence or absence of microcalcifications.
- A statement about whether the target microcalcifications have been completely or incompletely removed (in comparison to the diagnostic mammogram) (**Figs. 9.5, 9.6, 9.7**).
- A statement about the location (central or marginal) of the excised microcalcifications within the specimen (as deduced from the specimen radiograph in two orthogonal planes).
- A statement about whether or not a re-excision is recommended, and in which direction (cranial / caudal / medial / lateral / ventral / dorsal).

Specimen Ultrasound

Perioperative specimen US can be helpful for the evaluation and documentation of the representative and/or complete excision of nonpalpable, noncalcified lesions that are sonographically visible (**Fig. 9.8**).

Good Practice Recommendation*

Specimen US can be performed on tissue samples obtained from abnormalities that have been preoperatively localized under US-guidance.

*European S3 guidelines

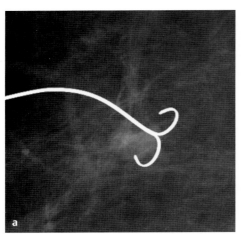
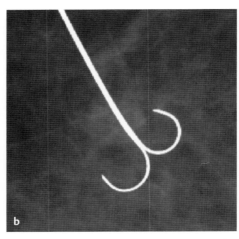
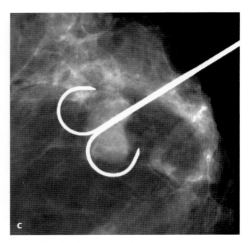

Fig. 9.5a–c Verification of complete lesion excision. Enlarged partial view of the preoperative mammography after needle localization of an ambiguous lesion in two planes (**a, b**). Specimen radiograph documents complete excision (**c**).

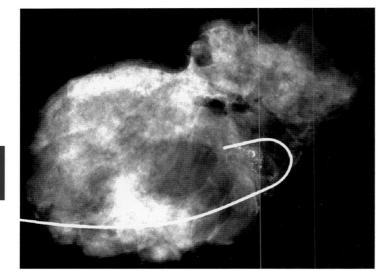

Fig. 9.6 Verification of the complete excision of target microcalcifications. Specimen radiograph shows localization wire and completely excised microcalcification cluster.

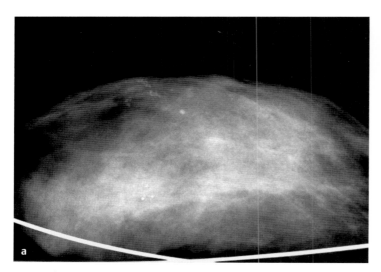
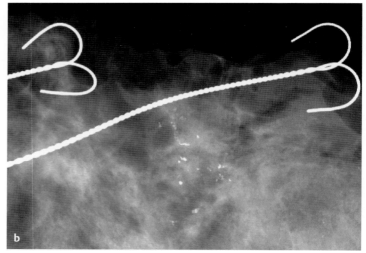

Fig. 9.7a,b Specimen radiographs showing the incomplete excision of target microcalcifications. Specimen radiograph in lateral x-ray beam projection shows that the excised microcalcifications reach the specimen margins (**a**). Specimen radiograph in orthogonal x-ray beam projection (**b**).

9

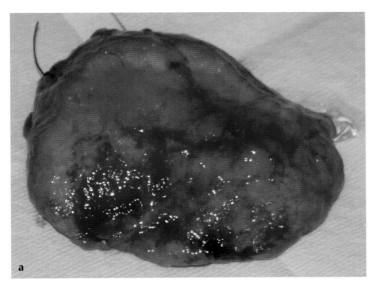

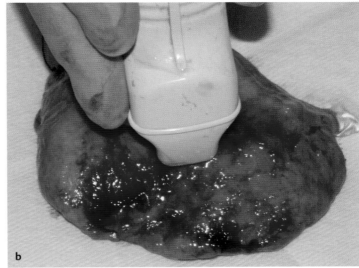

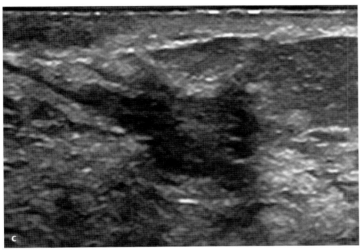

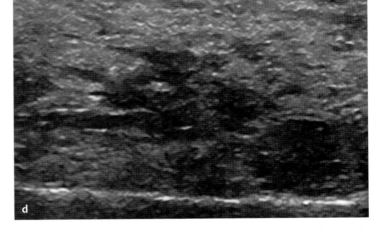

Fig. 9.8a–d Specimen US. Surgical specimen of a nonmass lesion (**a**). Transducer is placed on the specimen for US (**b**). Preoperative b-scan US image shows hypo-echoic lesion with radial structures (**c**). Specimen US with definite reproduction of echo alterations corresponding to the preoperative US image (**d**).

Specimen Magnetic Resonance Imaging

Presently there is no effective perioperative method of verifying the correct excision of a breast lesion seen only on MR mammography because there is no technique with which to simulate the in vivo perfusion conditions in such a specimen. Attempts to perform a specimen magnetic resonance imaging (MRI) in a T1-weighted, fat-saturation technique after intraoperative administration of a bolus injection of contrast material immediately before lesion excision have only shown reliable results in a few individual cases involving large lesions (**Fig. 9.9**). This approach cannot be recommended as a routine approach, however, considering the great logistic efforts involved, and the limited reliability of the method's results.

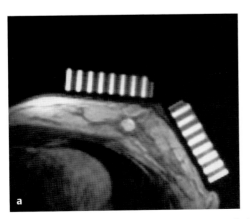

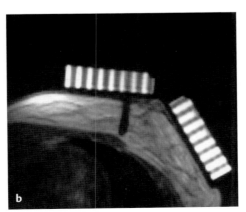

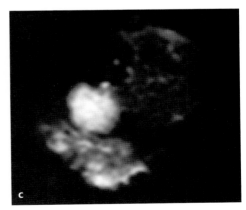

Fig. 9.9a–c Specimen MRI. Image documentation of a hypervascularized retro-mammillary target lesion during preoperative localization in the supine position (**a**). Verification of correct wire position protruding through lesion (**b**). Specimen MRI (T1-weighted fat saturation) performed after intraoperative administration of gadolinium immediately before excision. Verification of the target lesion within the specimen (**c**).

10 Galactography, MR Galactography, Ductoscopy

U. Fischer

Galactography

Galactography, or ductography, is a mammographic technique for visualization of a mammary duct and its segmental branches by injecting a water-soluble contrast agent into the milk duct. Galactography is usually performed as part of the evaluation of a unilateral spontaneous bloody nipple discharge to determine the size, extent, and localization of an intraductal proliferation. It is not usually possible, however, to differentiate between malignant and benign galactographic findings. The sensitivity of galactography is approx. 70 to 85%, the specificity however, is only 40 to 60%.

Technique

Preparation and materials. Before galactography is performed, at least one recent mammographic image of the ipsilateral breast should be made available to ensure that if intraductal microcalcifications are present, these are not overlooked because of superimposition by the contrast material (**Fig. 10.1**). It is also recommended that secretion be obtained for cytologic analysis before performing the procedure.

Galactography is usually performed with the patient in the supine position. Special blunt-tipped galactography needles may be used to cannulate the appropriate duct orifice. Alternatively, lymphography or sialography (30-gauge) needles may be used (**Fig. 10.2**). Some work groups prefer using a right-angle bent cannula (e.g., Jabczenski end-port, right-angle cannula).

> **Tips and Tricks**
>
> Before inserting the cannula into the milk duct, the needle system must be flushed with contrast material to avoid the introduction of air bubbles, which could be mistaken for filling defects caused by proliferative lesions on galactography (**Fig. 10.3**).

Cannulation. After disinfection of the nipple, the secreting milk duct must be identified and is best visualized using a bright light and magnifying glasses (magnification factor 3×–5×). Possible incrustations on the papillary surface of the nipple should be carefully removed using a moist pad or disinfection swab. To locate the correct duct, only a minimal amount of fluid must be discharged from the nipple. The cannula is then inserted into the duct using mild pressure. Once the needle has passed beyond the sphincter of the orifice, it will normally advance easily without further resistance unless the duct's course has a sharp retromammillary deflection, or a retromammillary tumor is present. Contrary to some reports in the literature, dilation of the duct opening before galactography is definitely superfluous. Rash probing and/or antegrade cannulation using strong pressure is painful and can quickly lead to traumatization of the nipple surface or to injury and paraductal administration of contrast material.

Contrast administration. After correct cannulation of the appropriate milk duct, water-soluble contrast material is injected using mild pressure. Normally, only 0.5–1 mL is administered. Reports in the literature of administration of 3 mL and more pertain to cases with pronounced duct ectasia. Oil-containing contrast agents are generally no longer used. When the patient reports of a mild feeling of pressure in the breast, contrast injection is terminated and the needle removed from the duct while slightly pulling the nipple ventrally. The duct orifice is then closed using a liquid bandage spray. Any contrast material that has been expelled from the duct should be carefully removed from the skin surface before performing the galactography images. Some work groups prefer to tape the cannula in place before the image is taken.

While moving from the examination table to the mammography unit, the patient should support the underside of the examined breast with the contralateral hand to avoid expression of the contrast material.

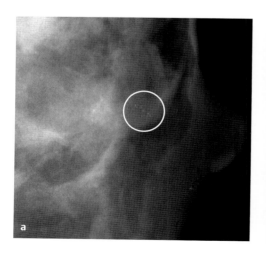

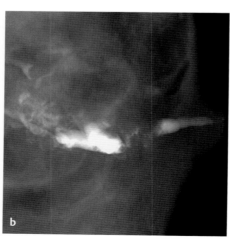

Fig. 10.1a,b Masking of microcalcifications by intraductal contrast material in galactography. Mammography performed before galactography shows a retromammillary cluster of microcalcifications (circle) (**a**). Microcalcifications are masked by intraductal contrast material injected for galactography (**b**).

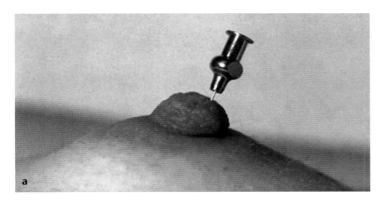

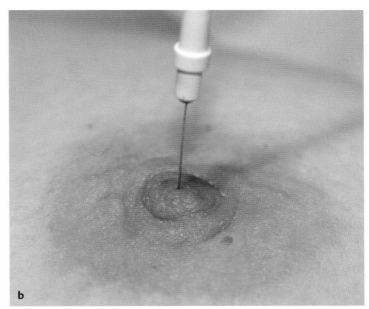

Fig. 10.2a,b **Insertion of a needle into a secreting duct for galactography.** Lymphography needle (**a**). Sialography needle (**b**).

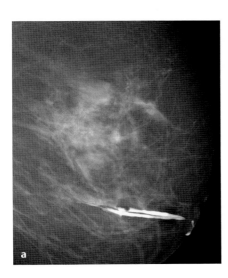

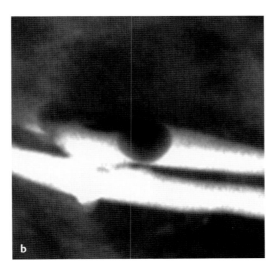

Fig. 10.3a,b **Air bubble artifact in galactogram.** Two straight, communicating ducts of normal caliber in galactogram. Round, well-defined filling defect in one duct correlates with an air bubble introduced when contrast was injected (**a, b**). Magnified partial view (**b**).

10

X-ray images. Galactography is a mammography examination in two orthogonal planes (craniocaudal [CC] and mediolateral [ML]) performed after injection of contrast material into the secreting milk duct. Breast compression should not be too firm to avoid expression of contrast material before the images have been completed. Once the images have been acquired, however, the nipple can be wiped clean of the spray bandage with a moist pad, and most of the contrast material is expressed by gently massaging the appropriate breast segment from the periphery toward the nipple.

Indications

Pathologic secretion. Statements in the literature pertaining to the appropriate indications for performing galactography are inconsistent. Some work groups consider the secretion from a single milk duct to be an indication. Others perform a galactography only when the discharge is bloody (**Fig. 10.4**). Nevertheless, most agree that galactography is indicated in a patient with a spontaneous, pathologic secretion from one milk duct. In general, a pathologic secretion is considered to be bloody. A bloody secre-

tion can be verified either by cytologic examination, or more quickly by gently touching a urine test strip to the expressed discharge. A secretion is always considered pathologic, however, when cytology reveals cells with atypia or carcinoma.

A milky secretion, which is usually bilateral and discharged from multiple ducts, is not a pathologic secretion. Outside of the lactational period, however, one should consider hyperprolactemia as a possible cause. Note that the manual provocation of breast secretion is no longer part of the routine clinical breast examination. By squeezing the nipple, it is often possible to obtain a secretion from many women's breasts.

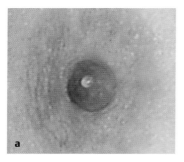
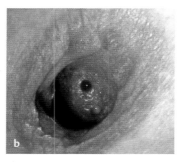
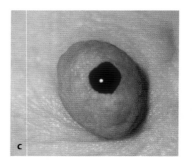
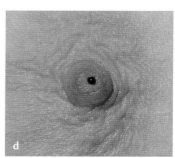

Fig. 10.4a–d Clinical appearance of breast secretions. Watery discharge from one duct (**a**). Green and yellowish discharge from several ducts (**b**). Pathologic secretions from one milk duct: fresh bloody discharge (**c**), older, brownish bloody discharge (**d**).

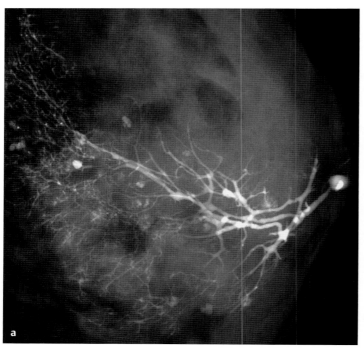
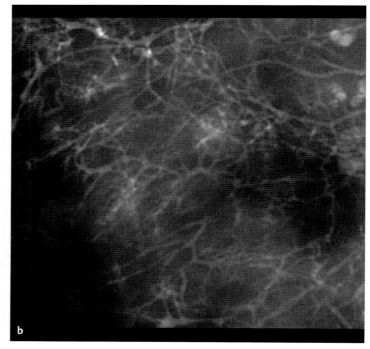

Fig. 10.5a, b Normal galactography findings. Normal galactogram showing a milk duct and it's branches from the nipple to the chest wall (**a**). Contrast material is also seen in paraductal cysts. Magnified partial view (**b**).

The Written Report and Evaluation Criteria

The written galactography report should include information on the number of cannulated milk ducts, the amount of injected contrast material, and whether complications (description) occurred. Galactographic findings include

- a normal duct system
- duct ectasia (found in approx. 50% of cases, usually without clinical significance)
- a filling defect
- duct truncation

Consequences. When galactography reveals a normal duct system, a short-term clinical examination can be recommended to evaluate whether the discharge is persistent or not. A diagnostic excision is usually unnecessary (**Figs. 10.5** and **10.6**).

Duct ectasia is found in over 50% of cases and has no clinical significance. The duct widening is commonly believed to be a result of fibrocystic changes, subacute or chronic inflammatory changes, or secretory disease (**Figs. 10.7** and **10.8**).

Filling defects and duct truncations are pathologic findings that usually require surgical or interventional therapy. The most frequent causes of such findings are solitary intraductal papillomas, papillomatosis, or intraductal carcinomas (DCIS) (**Figs. 10.9, 10.10, 10.11, 10.12, 10.13, 10.14, 10.15**). Stagnant, thickened secretions and detritus within a milk duct can also cause intraductal filling defects and duct truncations, resulting in false-positive findings (**Fig. 10.16**).

Failure rate. In approximately 5% of cases, it will be impossible even for the experienced examiner to perform a galactography. In the literature, failure rates of up to 50% have been reported.

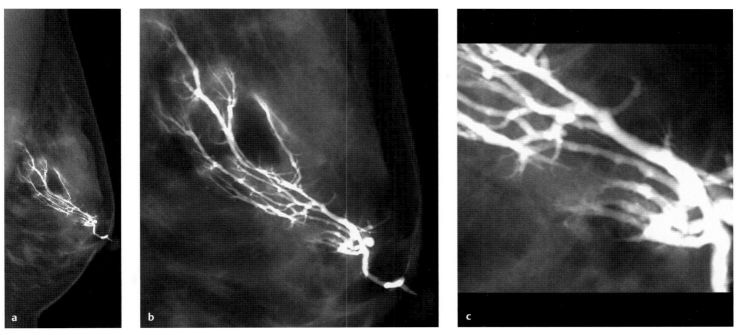

Fig. 10.6a–c Normal galactography findings with displacement of ductal structures. Normal galactogram shows a localized displacement of ductal branches caused by a simple cyst. Galactogram (**a**). Partial view (**b**). Magnified partial view (**c**).

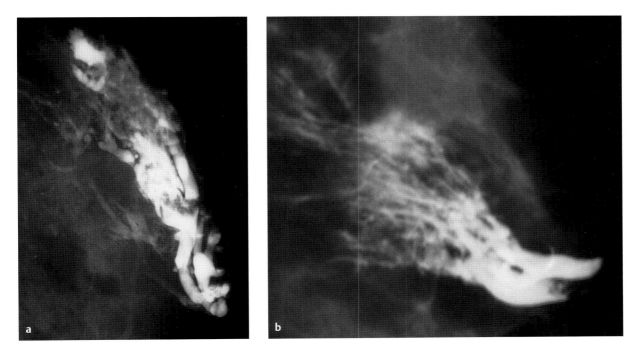

Fig. 10.7a, b Duct ectasia. Several milk ducts with pronounced duct ectasia and a duct diameter up to 10 mm. Limited evaluation of the galactography due to superimposition of several ducts in both planes (**a, b**).

10

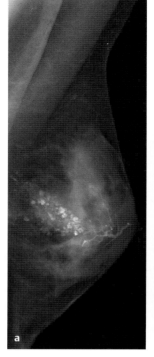

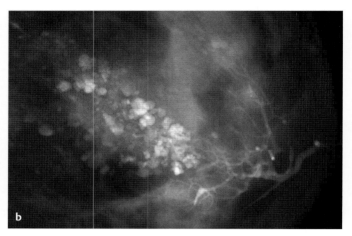

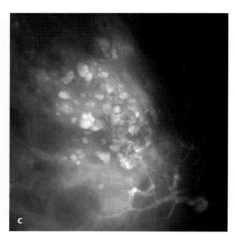

Fig. 10.8a–c Cystic alteration of a duct segment. Normal galactogram findings in the retromammillary region. Pronounced cystic alteration of a duct segment showing numerous paraductal cysts (**a**). Partial view (**b**). Magnified partial view (**c**). No therapeutic consequences.

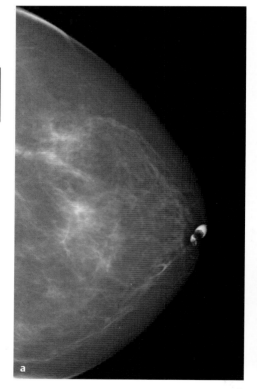

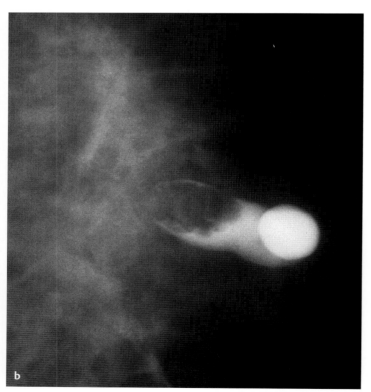

Fig. 10.9a, b Retromammillary papilloma. Galactography shows short duct ectasia with localized filling defect and normal caliber of distal duct segment (**a**). Partial view (**b**). *Histology*: papilloma.

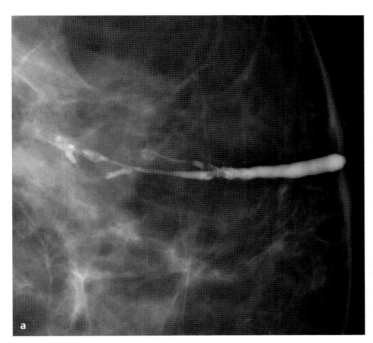
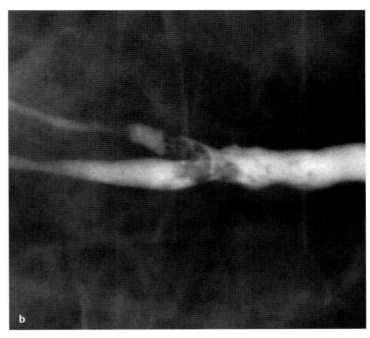

Fig. 10.10a, b Papilloma. Galactography shows a long duct of normal caliber with localized, irregular filling defect at a bifurcation (**a**). Partial view (**b**). *Histology*: papilloma.

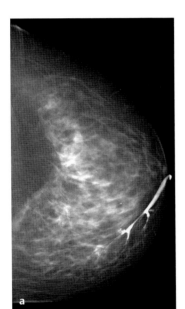
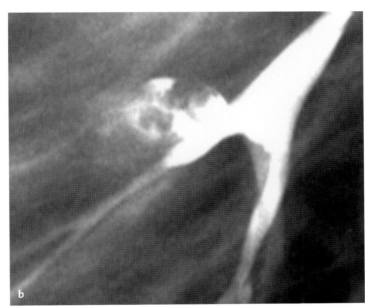

Fig. 10.11a, b Papilloma. Patient with bloody discharge from the left nipple. Two milliliters of contrast material were injected into the appropriate duct. The galactography shows a filling defect caused by a proliferative lesion within a paraductal cyst and a focal duct ectasia and truncation. Mammography in CC projection (**a**). Partial view (**b**). Complete removal by MRI-guided VAB. *Histology*: papilloma.

10

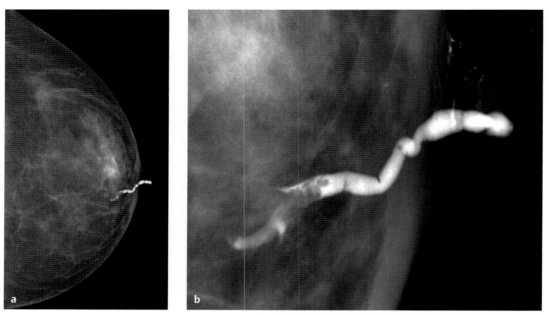

Fig. 10.12a,b Papillomatosis. Galactography shows a winding duct of normal caliber with long, irregular filling defect and duct truncation (**a**). Partial view (**b**). *Histology*: papillomatosis.

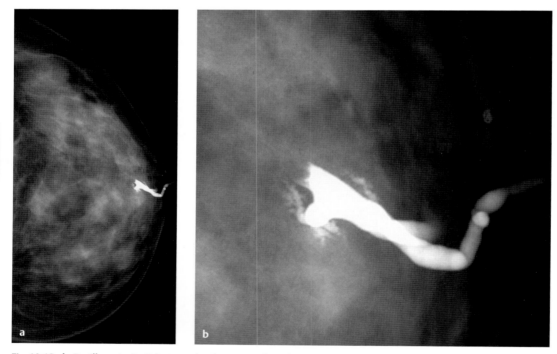

Fig. 10.13a,b Papillomatosis. Galactography shows a winding, slightly ectatic duct with complete duct truncation 3 cm from the nipple (**a**). Partial view (**b**). *Histology*: papillomatosis.

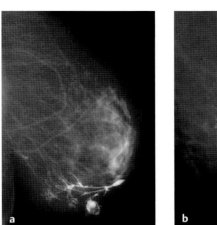
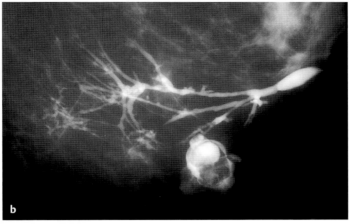

Fig. 10.14a,b Invasive papillary carcinoma. Galactography shows a duct of normal caliber with a filling defect within a paraductal cyst (**a**). Magnified view (**b**). *Histology*: invasive papillary carcinoma, pT1a (4 mm).

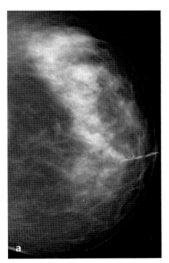
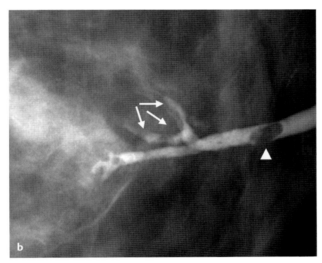

Fig. 10.15a,b Invasive ductal carcinoma (IDC). Galactography shows a long duct of normal caliber with a localized spreading of the ductal branches at a bifurcation (**a**). The magnified view shows marginal filling defects (arrows) and an air bubble artifact (arrow tip) (**b**). Removal of lesion by MRI-guided VAB (see **Fig. 6.49**, p. 116). Surgical reresection showed no residual lesion. *Histology*: IDC. Pathologic classification: vbT1b.

10

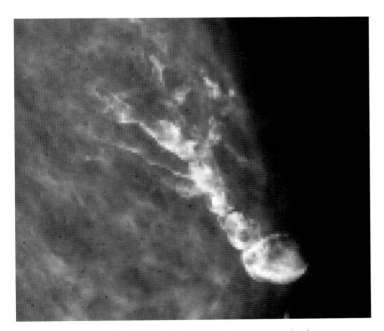

Fig. 10.16 Duct ectasia with intraductal detritus. Galactography shows pronounced duct ectasia with heterogeneous filling defects throughout the contrasted duct segments. *Histology*: Duct ectasia with a substantial amount of thickened secretions. No evidence of papilloma or carcinoma.

Contraindications and Complications

Contraindications. Galactography should not be performed in patients with mastitis or a breast abscess so as not to aggravate the condition. According to the literature, a known allergy against an iodine-containing contrast material is considered a relative contraindication. In such cases, the use of a gadolinium-containing contrast material is recommended.

Complications. The most relevant complication of galactography is the development of an infection, which can begin with an iatrogenic galactophoritis and lead to mastitis and/or abscess formation. This possible complication must be specifically discussed with the patient when obtaining the informed consent.

Another possible complication of galactography is the occurrence of a vasovagal reaction during manipulation of the nipple.

Less significant complications are the injury of a milk duct during cannulation and the subsequent extravasation of contrast material, which can be seen on galactography (**Fig. 10.17**). This contrast material outside the breast duct system is normally reabsorbed within a few days, making a repeat examination possible. Should the patient experience pain, mild analgesics can be prescribed. If an excessive volume of contrast material is injected into the milk duct, an extravasation can occur in the smaller, distal duct branches or lobuli (**Fig. 10.18**). This normally does not impair the examination. However, the extraductal contrast material is transported by, and is often visualized in the lymph vessels.

There are no reports of intolerance to the intraductal administration of water-soluble contrast materials.

10

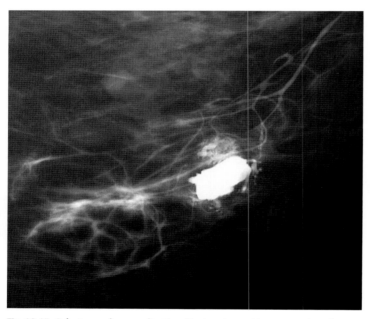

Fig. 10.17 Galactography complication. Duct rupture with extravasation of contrast.

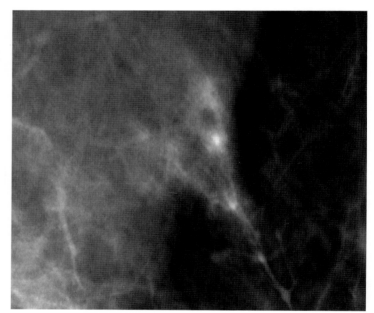

Fig. 10.18 Extravasation of contrast during galactography. Injection of too large a volume of contrast material. Contrast extravasation at the distal end of the milk duct near the chest wall.

MR Galactography

Procedure

The visualization of a secreting duct is also possible using magnetic resonance imaging (MRI), e.g., after cannulation of the appropriate milk duct and intraductal injection of a highly diluted MRI contrast material (contrast-enhanced MR galactography). High-resolution, T1-weighted fat-saturated sequences are used in the imaging process. In general, however, the spatial resolution of contrast-enhanced MR galactography is significantly lower than that of conventional (x-ray) galactography. Other work groups have reported the use of water-sensitive T2-weighted sequences to visualize the milk ducts on MRI without prior intraductal administration of contrast material (T2-MR gal-

actography). Both techniques are under investigation; presently they are of no significant value in the clinical routine (**Figs. 10.19, 10.20**).

Of considerably higher relevance is the performance of high-resolution contrast-enhanced MR mammography using the routine examination protocol. In this technique, even very small proliferating lesions within a milk duct can be directly visualized due to their hypervascularization. In addition, considering that the most common cause of pathologic secretion is of papillary origin, finding a lesion on MR mammography opens up the therapeutic possibility of removing such a lesion, provided that it is small (< 10 mm), by vacuum-assisted biopsy. Multiple lesions, if few, may also be removed by vacuum-assisted biopsy. Thus, open surgery can be avoided in many cases (see Chapter 6).

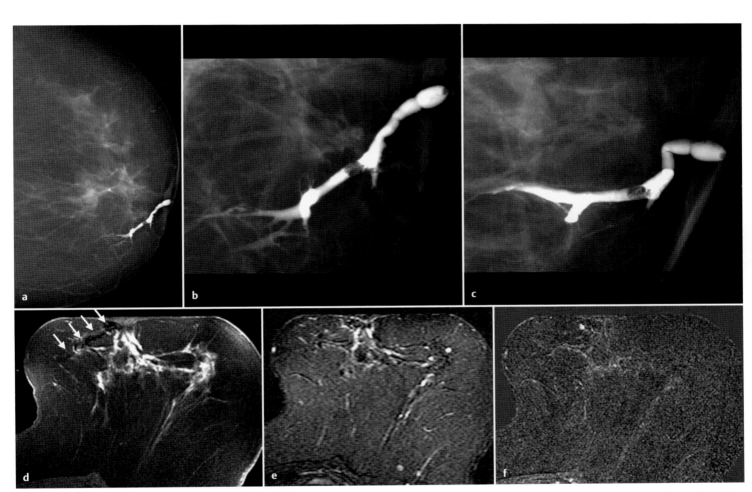

Fig. 10.19a–f Galactography, contrast-enhanced MR galactography, T2-weighted MR galactography, and diagnostic MR mammography. Imaging performed in the diagnostic work-up of a patient with a bloody discharge from the left breast. Visualization of the secreting milk duct on conventional galactography using a mixture of a radiocontrast- and paramagnetic contrast material for duct injection. Galactography shows localized filling defect approx. 2 cm from the nipple. Galactography in CC projection (**a**). Magnified partial view in CC (**b**) and medio-lateral oblique (MLO) projection (**c**). High-resolution T1-weighted fat-saturation image of the left breast (contrast-enhanced MR galactography) shows undesirable signal loss within the contrast-filled duct due to an overly high concentration of contrast material (aliasing effect, arrows) (**d**). No signal is seen in the contrast filled milk duct on T2-MR galactography (**e**). The subtraction image of the diagnostic examination shows a hypervascularized lesion of 3-mm diameter in the retromammillary region of the left breast (**f**). This lesion was completely removed by MRI-guided VAB. *Histology*: papilloma.

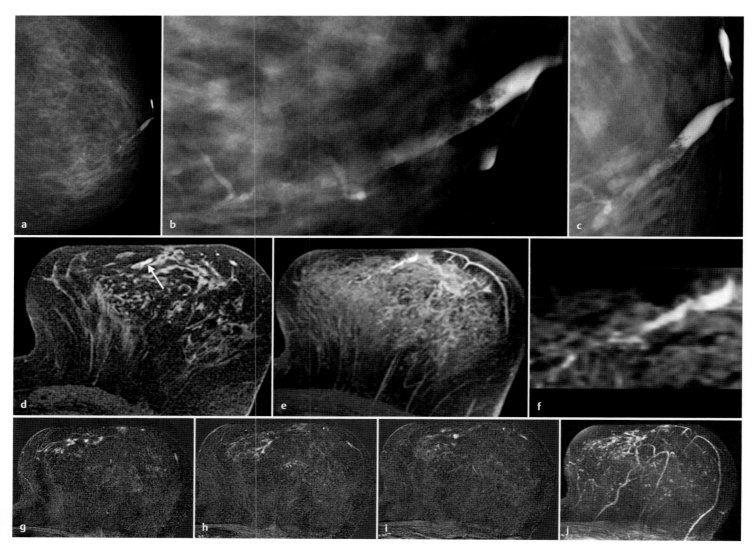

10

Fig. 10.20a–j Galactography, contrast-enhanced MR-galactography, T2-MR-galactography and diagnostic MR-mammography. Imaging performed in the diagnostic work-up of a patient with a bloody discharge from the left breast. Visualization of the secreting milk duct on conventional galactography using a mixture of a radiocontrast and paramagnetic contrast material for duct injection. Galactography shows a long filling defect and duct truncation. Galactography in CC projection (**a**). Magnified partial view in CC (**b**) and MLO projection (**c**). High-resolution T1-fat saturation (fat-sat) image of the left breast (contrast-enhanced MR-galactography) visualizes the signal intense, contrast-filled milk duct showing a filling defect (arrow) (**d**). T1-fat-sat maximum intensity projection (MIP) shows the entire milk duct (**e**). Partial view of the MIP using selected slice images (**f**). Subtraction slice images of the high-resolution MR mammography show numerous nodular, linear, and linear-branching enhancing lesions in correlation with an extensive papillomatosis (**g–i**). The subtraction MIP shows the segmental distribution of the papillomas (**j**). Because the papillomas are distributed over several centimeters, there is no option of removing the lesions by VAB. *Histology after surgical excision*: papillomatosis.

Ductoscopy

Methods and Materials

Diagnostic ductoscopy. Mammary ductoscopy is an endoscopic procedure, which has been available for several years and allows the direct visualization of the ductal lining and intraductal changes in patients with pathologic nipple discharge (**Fig. 10.21**). The procedure can be performed using local anesthesia or under full anesthesia. Dilators in various diameters up to 1.3 mm are used to widen the ductal orifice. Modern microendoscopes used for ductoscopy have an outer diameter of 1.1 mm or less.

Interventional ductoscopy. New developments aim to improve the interventional capabilities of modern microendoscopes, including the development of an additional working chamber for the introduction of biopsy brushes, forceps, microbiopsy instruments, and the aspiration of lavage fluid for cytologic analysis. Current investigations are focused on fluorescence or spectography-based techniques, which can facilitate the detection of intraductal lesions and direct tissue sampling during ductoscopy. Subjects for future investigation are the use of laser ductoscopes able to excise intraductal papillomas, and the development of 3D tracking systems.

Surgical milk duct excision. At present, milk ducts in which an intraductal finding has been detected on ductoscopy (when performed in an operating room) are excised along a guiding shaft. Depending upon the location of the finding, the breast incision is performed as a longitudinal splitting of the nipple, or along the perimeter of the areola. Both operative procedures have the advantage of being less traumatic and more anatomically suited than a nonselective ductectomy.

Significance. In summary, the performance of mammary ductoscopy is possible. Its final significance as a diagnostic and therapeutic procedure performed when pathologic nipple discharge is present must be further evaluated. The use of this method, therefore, cannot be generally recommended now.

Further Reading

Funovics MA, Philipp MO, Lackner B, Fuchsjaeger M, Funovics PT, Metz V. Galactography: method of choice in pathologic nipple discharge? Eur Radiol 2003;13(1):94–99

Gregl A. Color Atlas of Galactography. Stuttgart: Schattauer; 1980

Grunwald, S, Ohlinger R, Euler U, et al. Minimalinvasive Diagnostik sezernierender Brusterkrankungen durch Milchgangsendoskopie. Endosk heute. 2005;18(4):186–189

Grunwald S, Heyer H, Paepke S, et al. Diagnostic value of ductoscopy in the diagnosis of nipple discharge and intraductal proliferations in comparison to standard methods. Onkologie 2007;30(5):243–248

Hou MF, Huang TJ, Liu GC. The diagnostic value of galactography in patients with nipple discharge. Clin Imaging 2001;25(2):75–81

Jacobs VR, Kiechle M, Plattner B, Fischer T, Paepke S. Breast ductoscopy with a 0.55-mm mini-endoscope for direct visualization of intraductal lesions. J Minim Invasive Gynecol 2005;12(4):359–364

Jacobs VR, Paepke S, Ohlinger R, Grunwald S, Kiechle-Bahat M. Breast ductoscopy: technical development from a diagnostic to an interventional procedure and its future perspective. Onkologie 2007;30(11):545–549

Krämer SC, Rieber A, Görich J, et al. Diagnosis of papillomas of the breast: value of magnetic resonance mammography in comparison with galactography. Eur Radiol 2000;10(11):1733–1736

Ohlinger R, Paepke S, Jacobs VR, et al. Stellenwert der Duktoskopie in der Mammadiagnostik. Gynakologe 2006;39:538–544

Orel SG, Dougherty CS, Reynolds C, Czerniecki BJ, Siegelman ES, Schnall MD. MR imaging in patients with nipple discharge: initial experience. Radiology 2000;216(1):248–254

Schulz-Wendtland R, Aichinger U, Krämer S, Schaaf H, Tartsch M, Bautz W. [Galactoscopy—is it a new interventional method for breast diagnosis?]. Rofo 2002;174(8):1015–1017

Woods ER, Helvie MA, Ikeda DM, Mandell SH, Chapel KL, Adler DD. Solitary breast papilloma: comparison of mammographic, galactographic, and pathologic findings. AJR Am J Roentgenol 1992;159(3):487–491

10

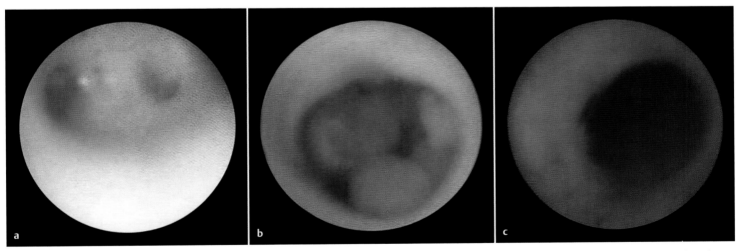

Fig. 10.21a–c Ductoscopy. Ductoscopic images. Normal bifurcation (**a**). Conglomerate of several papillomas (**b**). Intraductal carcinoma (**c**). (Images kindly provided by VR Jacobs and S Paepke from the Gynecology Department of the Technical University of Munich, Germany).

11 Sentinel Lymph Node Mapping and Dissection

T. Kuehn

The prognosis of mammary carcinoma depends on both local tumor control and adequate adjuvant systemic therapy. Chemotherapy, hormone therapy, and antibody therapy are used individually and in a targeted way. Selection of the systemic treatment approach depends on the likely effectiveness of different substances (predictive factors, such as estrogen and progesterone receptor status, HER2 status) and on the urgency of therapy (prognostic factors). In clinical practice, the nodal status is the most important prognostic factor, substantially influencing the adjuvant treatment decision.

Axillary lymphadenectomy. For many decades, axillary lymph node dissection (ALND) has been an integral component of primary surgical therapy of mammary carcinoma. The objective has been to determine the pathologic nodal (pN) status for designing the adjuvant therapy plan and to secure local tumor control if lymph nodes are positive. ALND therefore represented both a diagnostic and a preventative therapeutic measure.

Numerous studies, however, have demonstrated that ALND is associated with high morbidity in the shoulder–arm region and considerably affects the patient's quality of life (Kuehn et al, 2000; Keramopoulos et al, 1993). Research has therefore focused on how to identify patients with negative nodal status to save them from radical axillary dissection.

Evaluating the Nodal Status

Imaging procedures. The imaging procedures available for evaluating the nodal status are ultrasound (US), magnetic resonance imaging (MRI), and positron emission tomography (PET). It has not been possible to obtain acceptable diagnostic accuracy for any of these procedures (Fehr et al, 2004; Rajesh et al, 2002; Rieber et al, 2002; Schirrmeister et al, 2001; Yoshimura et al, 1999).

Alternative surgical procedures. As an alternative to open axillary dissection, an endoscopic method for ALND was developed some years ago. Lymph nodes were removed through the endoscopic access following liposuction and dilatation of the axilla with CO_2 gas. Because of high equipment costs, long surgery times, and comparatively low reduction in morbidity, this procedure did not find its way into routine clinical practice (Kuehn et al, 2001).

Lymphatic mapping and sentinel lymph node dissection. Sentinel lymph node dissection (SLND) is based on the orderly lymph drainage of solid tumors (**Table 11.1**). Accordingly, lymphogenic metastasis first occurs through one or more defined and reproducibly located lymph nodes called sentinel lymph nodes (SLNs) (**Fig. 11.1**). The pathway of tumor metastasis can be mapped by lymphography. Here, a dye or radioactive substance is injected near the tumor for visualization of lymph drainage. The tracers used are phagocytized by cells in the SLNs, and the SLNs are then detected either visually (dyes), by imaging (lymphoscintigraphy), and/or with a gamma probe (radioactive tracer).

If no tumor cells are detected in the SLNs, it may be assumed that the other lymph nodes (nonsentinel lymph nodes [NSLNs]) are tumor-free as well, thus making their removal unnecessary. If the SLNs are histologically positive, it cannot be ruled out that subsequent lymph nodes are also affected; complete axillary lymph node dissection with the removal of 10 lymph nodes from levels I and II is therefore required.

Table 11.1 Definitions of terms: sentinel lymph node, sentinel lymph node excision, lymphatic mapping, and nonsentinel lymph node.

Term	Definition
Sentinel lymph node (SLN)	SLNs are the first lymph nodes found in the lymphatic drainage of mammary carcinoma and thus have the highest probability of containing metastases. SLNs are mapped using radioactive tracers and/or dyes (lymphography). All lymph nodes identified by an afferent lymphatic pathway or the uptake of dye, radionuclide, or both tracers are called SLNs.
Sentinel lymph node dissection (SLND)	SLND is the removal of all lymph nodes that meet the definition of a SLN. Only marked lymph nodes are removed.
Lymphatic mapping	Lymphatic mapping is the functional imaging of lymphatic drainage from the breast or from a tumor area.
Nonsentinel lymph node (NSLN)	NSLNs are axillary lymph nodes that do not take up any tracer.

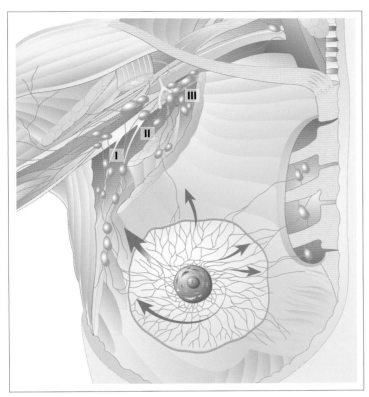

Fig. 11.1 Axillary and mediastinal lymph nodes. Diagram of axillary and mediastinal lymph nodes showing sentinel nodes and levels I–III.

siderable advantage of SLND as compared with standard axillary dissection (Fleissig et al, 2006; Veronesi et al, 2003).

SLN biopsy has therefore become the standard of care to determine the pN-status in patients with early breast cancer.

Anatomy and Physiology of Lymphatic Drainage of the Breast

The introduction of lymphatic mapping has led to renewed interest in the network of lymph vessels and the functional anatomy of the lymphatic drainage from various regions of the breast. An understanding of the lymphatic system is of utmost importance for choosing the tracer and the injection techniques to be used. Although not all aspects of physiology and pathophysiology of the lymphatic drainage from the breast are fully understood, the current view may be summarized as follows (Romrell and Bland, 1998):

Blind-ended lymph capillaries transport the lymph from the parenchymal tissue of the breast through a system of communicating vessels. There are three main directions of drainage:

- lymph vessels draining directly through the parenchymal tissue to the lymph nodes
- lymph vessels draining along the mammary ducts through the subareolar plexus to the axillary lymph nodes
- lymph nodes draining a deep plexus at the base of the breast and through the transpectoral pathway into the axillary and internal lymph nodes

Clinical Value of Sentinel Lymph Node Dissection

SLND is a targeted means of staging to establish the nodal status in patients with mammary carcinoma. The aim is to reduce the morbidity of the standard procedure (complete ALND), without loss of staging accuracy (Kuehn et al, 2005).

False-negative rate. Numerous validation studies have shown that SLND has a false-negative rate (FNR) of 5 to 29% (Kim et al, 2006; Kuehn et al, 2004). In a meta-analysis by Kim and co-workers covering 69 studies and involving over 8000 patients, a mean sensitivity of 92.6% was found (FNR of 7.4%). When calculating the FNR, the number of false-negative cases does not refer to the entire collective, but only to the number of patients with positive nodal status; hence, the rate of women with incorrectly classified nodal status and thus receiving systemic undertreatment is very low.

Due to considerable interinstitutional variability of the FNR (an FNR of up to 60% was found in individual studies), it is essential to pay close attention to clear and standardized procedural instructions to achieve widely reproducible results at a high level (see below).

Relapse rate. Data on the local relapse rate following SLND are now available from numerous studies on several thousand patients (Palesty et al, 2006; Smidt et al, 2005). They all show that the rate lies far below 1% in patients who develop clinically apparent axillary lymph node (ALN) metastasis after SLND.

Postoperative morbidity. Several randomized studies on postoperative morbidity are available; they clearly document the con-

Mapping and imaging of the lymphatic flow by means of tracers has greatly extended our knowledge on the lymphatic drainage of the breast. Currently, the following ideas greatly influence the tracer injection techniques used for SLND.

The entire breast and the overlying skin drain into one or more axillary SLNs. Only regions near the thoracic wall may have additional drainage through the mediastinal lymph node chain. Dermal, subdermal, and periareolar injection can only map the axillary SLNs; deep injection near the tumor or into the tumor also maps the mediastinal SLNs in up to 29% of cases (Borgstein et al, 2000; Nathanson et al, 2001; Roumen et al, 1999; Tanis et al, 2001). Hence, the question of mediastinal lymph drainage depends less on the quadrant than on the proximity of a tumor to the thoracic wall.

Sentinel Lymph Node Mapping

SLNs are mapped by using either dyes or radioactive tracers. The use of radionuclides has been established in clinical practice as a standard procedure because of higher detection rates, better reproducibility, and less tissue trauma. The dye method is considered as an optional supplement to make it easier for the surgeon to find the SLN under image guidance.

Dye Method

In Germany, patent blue V (Guerbet Laboratories, Birmingham, UK) is usually used for SLN dye mapping. Immediately before surgery (following skin disinfection and sterile coverage), approx. 3 mL of a diluted solution (1:1 with physiological saline) are injected near the tumor (**Fig. 11.2a**). It is important to ensure that skin tattooing is avoided (no injection near the skin, avoidance of

11

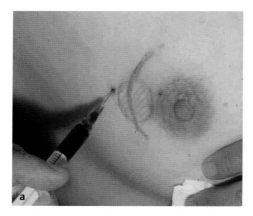
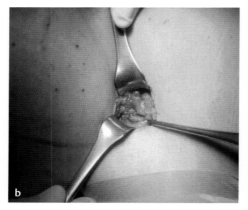
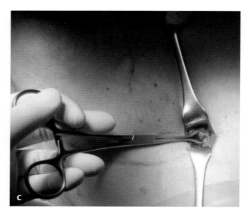

Fig. 11.2a–c **Dye method.** Injection of dye in the periphery of the tumor (**a**). Exposed sentinel lymph node, dye-stained (**b, c**).

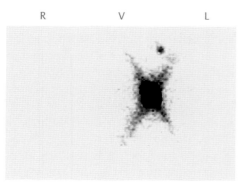
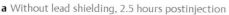
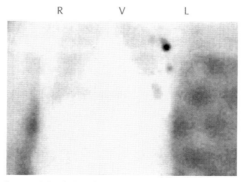

Fig. 11.3a,b **Lymphoscintigraphy.** Tracer injected in the periphery of the tumor, nuclear medicine imaging of axillary tumor site; (**a**) without lead shielding, 2.5 hours postinjection, (**b**) with lead shielding, 2.5 hours postinjection.

a Without lead shielding, 2.5 hours postinjection   **b** With lead shielding, 2.5 hours postinjection

multiple injections, withdrawal of the syringe plunger when retracting the needle). The axillary incision should be performed 5 minutes after injection of the dye and not before. However, this time interval should not exceed 15 minutes because if the intervals are too long the rate of detection is reduced (Kuehn et al, 1999) (**Fig. 11.2b,c**).

Lymphoscintigraphy

Lymphoscintigraphic mapping still is the standard procedure for imaging the SLNs (**Fig. 11.3**). The mapping may be performed using a 1-day or 2-day protocol.

Radiotracer and activity. The radiopharmaceuticals used are ^{99m}Tc-labeled colloids with a particle size of 20–100 nm. Based on the current understanding of lymphatic drainage from the breast (see above), the injection is performed in such a way that SLN removal is as little hampered by blooming artifacts as possible. Periareolar intradermal injection of small volumes (0.1–0.2 mL) of radiotracer is therefore increasingly used.

The activity should be chosen such that a sufficient target signal is achieved at the time of surgery despite the radioactive decay. When surgery is scheduled to take place 24 hours after the injection, the activity should be 150–250 MBq. With the half-life of ^{99m}Tc being 6 hours, the activity may be cut by half if surgery takes place 6 hours earlier. One-day protocols use a total activity between 10 and 50 MBq.

Radiographs. When performing lymphoscintigraphy, static images should be taken at two levels. Preoperative marking of the SLN on the skin is not required. The nuclear medicine report should indicate the localization of SLNs and also the assumed number of tracer-accumulating lymph nodes.

Combined Radionuclide and Dye Method

Lymphography using a combination of blue dye and radionuclide is advised.

Advantages. The combination of both mapping techniques offers visual guidance for the surgeon and may save time in many cases. SLNs that are completely infiltrated by a tumor and no longer take up radiotracer because of the tumor burden may be detected by the blue staining of the afferent lymphatic pathway. In these cases, this may prevent a false-negative result.

Disadvantages. The disadvantages of dye mapping include additional costs, the waiting period required between the injection and the incision into the skin, and the possibility of transient (and in rare cases, permanent) skin tattoos.

Indications for Sentinel Lymph Node Dissection

Tumor size. The indications for SLND were limited initially to small, unifocal primary tumors of up to 2 cm in diameter and with a clinically negative nodal status. However, the range of indications for SLND is widening. The aim is to reduce the proportion of women with negative nodal status who receive complete axillary lymph node dissection. As shown by numerous studies, SLND allows making a statement about the nodal status even with larger tumors (Bedrosian et al, 2000; Chung et al, 2001). Hence, the size of the tumor is no longer a criterion restricting the indication for SLND.

Biopsies and previous surgery. SLND is also possible after minor excision biopsies. In case of major previous surgery (e.g., quadrantectomy), the results are not reproducible with certainty, particularly not regarding detection.

Multifocal carcinomas. According to today's understanding of the functional lymphatic anatomy of the breast, SLND makes it possible to predict reliably the nodal status even in multifocal carcinomas. The clinical studies available confirm the concept (Ferrari et al, 2006; Knauer et al, 2006). According to recommendations of the American Society of Clinical Oncology (ASCO), the indication for SLND in case of limited evidence is classified as acceptable (Lyman et al, 2005).

Clinically suspicious lymph nodes. Clinically suspicious lymph nodes have been viewed, so far, as an exclusion criterion for SLND. As the term "clinically suspect" is not clearly defined, primary ALND was performed in numerous women with palpable axillary lymph nodes (particularly following core needle biopsy), although it was shown in the end that the histologic lymph node status was negative. The new S3 guidelines therefore stipulate that clinical suspicion of advanced lymph node involvement or tumor-infiltrated lymph nodes are the only contraindications for SLND. In case of questionable axillary lymph node involvement (palpation, US), numerous surgeons now indicate primary axillary dissection exclusively based on targeted tissue biopsy. Fine needle aspiration (FNA), core needle biopsy (CNB), and targeted lymph node removal after preoperative wire localization may be used here.

Neoadjuvant chemotherapy. SLND is not recommended after neoadjuvant chemotherapy (NCT) (Kuehn et al, 2005; Lyman et al, 2005). This applies particularly to patients with clinically sus-picious lymph nodes at the time of first diagnosis. Critical evaluation of SLND after NCT is based on theoretical considerations and unfavorable rates of success as compared with primary surgery patients (detection rate 96 versus 90%, FNR 7.3 versus 12.1%; Xing et al, 2006). As no prospective studies are available on the value of SLND in the context of neoadjuvant treatment protocols, SLND is currently not indicated after primarily systemic treatment. The German SENTINA study is internationally the first targeted, prospective study in which SLND has been examined in different subgroups (Bauerfeind and Kuehn, 2007).

Advanced lymph node involvement. Currently, SLND is strongly contraindicated only when advanced axillary lymph node involvement is suspected.

Surgical Methods

Sentinel lymph node mapping. SLND may be performed following a 1-day or 2-day protocol. For organizational reasons (reliable planning of the surgical procedure), most hospitals use the 2-day protocol. SLN mapping by radiocolloid injection and subsequent scintigraphy are preformed on the day before the surgery; blue dye mapping may follow during surgery on the next day, if necessary.

SLND is usually performed before resection of the primary tumor. This time sequence makes optimal use of the waiting period for intraoperative histologic examination; if dye mapping is to be used as well, SLND should be performed within a time frame of 5–15 minutes after injection of the dye.

Sentinel lymph node identification. The surgical procedure begins with careful exploration of the breast and thoracic wall, and of the axilla (if necessary, also the extra-axillary lymphatic drainage areas). The radiation fields of the primary tracer injected and the tracer-accumulating lymph nodes must be found and visualized individually. Scattered radiation from the injection site may lead to problems with SLN visualization (**Fig. 11.4**). An SLN can only be identified as such when there is decreased signal intensity between the injection site and the axilla.

Preoperative mapping of the SLN by the nuclear medicine physician has proven to be impractical because changes in positioning may cause considerable shift in the preoperative mapping. With the gamma probe, the surgeon has a reliable instrument available for certain identification of the SLN.

11

R V L R V L

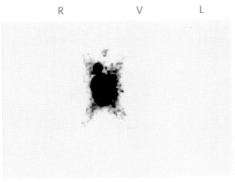 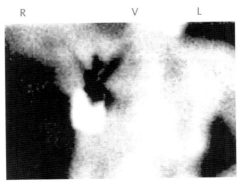

Fig. 11.4a,b Potential errors in mapping sentinel lymph nodes. Nuclear medicine imaging of axillary tumor site; (**a**) without lead shielding, 2.5 hours postinjection: highly scattered radiation; (**b**) with lead shielding, 2.5 hours postinjection: without signal reduction between tumor and lymph nodes.

a Without lead shielding, 2.5 hours postinjection   **b** With lead shielding, 2.5 hours postinjection

Sentinel lymph node removal. The point of maximum signal intensity in the axilla is located transcutaneously with the hand-held gamma detection probe; it helps to pinpoint the site of incision. After cutting into the skin, the axillary cavity should first be palpated as not to overlook lymph nodes completely infiltrated by tumor, which may lead to false-negative results in rare cases. During further preparation, care should be taken to use only non-traumatic and bloodless surgical techniques while repeatedly using the gamma probe to minimize tissue trauma. Lymph nodes with accumulated radionuclide should be isolated and selectively removed. Removal of NSLNs or larger portions of fat should be avoided. After removal, the SLN must be examined away from the surgical area for its actual radionuclide accumulation. The SLN should be safely stored and the number of counts documented. When the lymph node shows no accumulation after removal, it is labeled a NSLN and sent separately for pathologic examination. When the combined tracer method has been used, all lymph nodes with blue staining and/or radionuclide accumulation, or those clearly showing an identifiable lymphatic pathway, are labeled SLNs. The number of counts measured, the method of detection, and the localization of all SLNs (levels I, II, or others) should be documented, as well as the maximum residual activity in the axilla after termination of the SLND procedure. Finally, it should be checked whether there is agreement between the number of SLNs detected by lymphography and those actually removed.

More than three sentinel lymph nodes. In approx. 15% of cases, more than three lymph nodes are mapped as SLN. So far, it has not been clarified whether the removal of all mapped lymph nodes will bring any benefit for the patient. Some studies have shown that removal of the first three SLNs achieves 98% accuracy for establishing a positive nodal status (Kennedy et al, 2003). The optimal approach in case of multiple lymph nodes with accumulated tracer has not been established yet. The German Society of Senology recommends that, initially, up to three tracer-accumulating lymph nodes should be removed. When more SLNs are identified, the procedure may be limited by using a count ratio. Here, accumulating lymph nodes that show in vivo only one-third of the activity of the lymph node with the highest accumulation (or ex vivo one-tenth of this activity) should not be called SLNs and, hence, not be removed.

Pathology

The SLN is examined both intraoperatively and postoperatively (**Fig. 11.5**).

Intraoperative examination. Intraoperative examination allows for same-day surgery when complete axillary lymph node dissection is indicated by a positive SLN. Intraoperative examination involves cutting the SLN into 3-mm thick slices. When malignancy is suspected macroscopically, either rapid section diagnosis or touch imprint cytology is performed.

Postoperative examination. Postoperative examination of the SLN provides the basis for local or systemic treatment. The extent of the examination depends on the clinical importance of the results. The minimum objective of the examination is the detection of macrometastases (>2 mm). Desirable but not obligatory is the identification of micrometastases as well (<2 mm, but >0.2 mm) because the involvement of further lymph nodes must be expected in approx. 20% of these patients. Histologic examination of the SLN does not aim for the detection of isolated tumor cells (ITCs). Macrometastases, micrometastases, and ITCs are defined by the TNM classification system of the International Union Against Cancer (UICC).

For final processing, the SLN slices are embedded in paraffin, and serial sections are prepared at 500-µm intervals. This ensures that macrometastases are detected in 100% of cases. Emphasis should be placed on homogeneous and complete serial sectioning of the SLN preparations because macrometastases may be overlooked in unevenly distributed serial sections cut only from the surface of tissue blocks.

Importance of Local and Systemic Treatment Decisions

SLND is used for axillary staging and provides important information for planning local and systemic treatment. Whereas primary ALND has been used as a preventive treatment, SLND now facilitates the targeted selection of patients who require axillary dissection.

Negative and positive nodal status. It is uncontested that, in patients with negative nodal status (pN0[sn]), the removal of other lymph nodes can be omitted. No further treatment of axillary lymph nodes is required, and systemic treatment is based on the guideline for treating patients with negative nodal status.

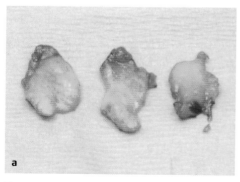
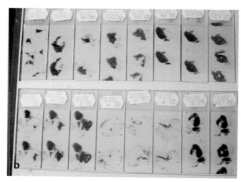
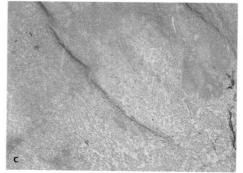

Fig. 11.5a–c Histologic processing of sentinel lymph nodes. Dissected nodes (**a**), serial sections, 500 µm in thickness (**b**), microscopy showing metastasis (**c**).

With a positive SLN, axillary dissection with removal of at least 10 lymph nodes from levels I and II is indicated, and systemic treatment is based on the guideline for treating patients with positive nodal status.

Other situations. Introduction of lymphatic mapping also brings with it new situations that require well-founded and standardized recommendations regarding further treatment planning. The following issues are central:

- the importance of micrometastases and ITCs for local and systemic treatment planning
- the value of extra-axillary lymph nodes

Micrometastases and occult tumor cells. According to the TNM classification system currently in use, metastases in SLNs of >0.2 mm and <2 mm in diameter are classified as micrometastases pN1(mic) (sn). Metastases of <0.2 mm without tissue response are called occult tumor cells pN0(i+) (sn). There is consensus that micrometastases and occult tumor cells are of no prognostic significance. Therefore, low-volume metastases cannot be used as the deciding factor for a systemic therapeutic approach (e. g., chemotherapy). The data are unclear with respect to the clinical importance of minor lymph node involvement for local tumor control and the necessity of ALND. Most authors recommend axillary dissection at stage pN1(mic) (sn). At stage pN0 (i+), axillary dissection is largely avoided (Kuehn et al, 2005; Lyman et al, 2005).

Extra-axillary lymph nodes. Lymphatic mapping has made it possible also to include the nonaxillary regions of lymphatic drainage and to detect SLNs that lie outside the axilla. A prerequisite for the mapping of extra-axillary lymph nodes is deep parenchymal injection of the tracer because only the prepectoral glandular tissue has lymphatic drainage into the nonaxillary regions. When using the cutaneous or periareolar injection technique, SLNs are identified only in exceptional cases outside the axillary cavity. As of today, no data are available to demonstrate that extended staging and improved selection of systemic treatment options may increase the total survival rate. It is also completely unclear whether, and which, local treatment should be performed if a positive mediastinal SLN is identified and what effects this treatment may have on local relapses or on the total survival rate. Because of potential additional morbidity, all international recommendations discourage a systematic search for extra-axillary SLN (Goldhirsch et al, 2003; Kuehn et al, 2005; Lyman et al, 2005; Schwartz et al, 2002).

Open Questions / New Developments

The objective of SLND is to reduce surgery-related morbidity in the shoulder–arm region without reducing the staging accuracy or the safety of local tumor control. In recent years, SLND has become a firmly established clinical procedure. Progress toward further reduction in radical surgical in the lymphatic drainage regions is therefore still in a state of flux. The range of indications for SLND has continuously widened in previous years, and ALND may have become unnecessary in >90% of all women with negative nodal status. The scientific discussion focuses on the following questions:

- What is the value of SLND for the neoadjuvant treatment approach? Should SLND be performed prior to or after chemotherapy? How reliable is SLND in the downstaged axilla? The German SENTINA study is investigating these questions by using a prospective protocol.
- Should axillary dissection always be performed in patients with micrometastases in the SLN? This question is studied by the Breast Cancer International Research Group (BCIRG 23–01 trial).
- Should axillary dissection always be performed in patients with positive SLN? About 60% of women with positive SLNs do not show metastases in subsequent lymph nodes. Can this patient group be identified by predictive factors? Van Zee et al (2003) have developed a nomogram for predicting the individual risk of NSLN involvement by looking at eight risk factors. The value of the nomogram is still being discussed by scientists.
- Also unclear is the question of how to proceed with intramammary relapses after breast-conserving therapy and SLND. Initial data indicate that even in case of a relapse, repeat SLND may be possible and may reliably predict a secondary involvement of residual axillary lymph nodes. Because of insufficient data, secondary ALND is currently still recommended for intramammary relapses.

Quality Assurance

Despite excellent data available from meta-analyses, some breast centers frequently report unacceptable results. It is essential to perform SLND under conditions of quality assurance—using the method in a standardized form according to the recommendations of national and international specialist associations. Sole use of the dye method is therefore unsuitable for bringing about reproducible results regarding detection and FNR. The most important quality assurance measures include: excluding advanced lymph node involvement, careful screening of the axilla and removal of all SLNs according to the recommendations of specialist associations, reexamining scintigraphic findings and intraoperative site for plausibility, and safeguarding adequate histopathologic processing.

11

References

Bauerfeind I, Kuehn T, on behalf of the SENTINA Study Group. Stellenwert der Sentinel-Lymphknotenbiopsie im Rahmen neoadjuvanter Therapiekonzepte beim Mammakarzinom. Überblick und aktuelles Studienkonzept. Geburtshilfe Frauenheilkd 2007;67 : 22–27

Bedrosian I, Reynolds C, Mick R, et al. Accuracy of sentinel lymph node biopsy in patients with large primary breast tumors. Cancer 2000;88(11):2540–2545

Borgstein PJ, Meijer S, Pijpers RJ, van Diest PJ. Functional lymphatic anatomy for sentinel node biopsy in breast cancer: echoes from the past and the periareolar blue method. Ann Surg 2000;232(1):81–89

Chung MH, Ye W, Giuliano AE. Role for sentinel lymph node dissection in the management of large (>or = 5 cm) invasive breast cancer. Ann Surg Oncol 2001;8(9):688–692

Fehr MK, Hornung R, Varga Z, et al. Axillary staging using positron emission tomography in breast cancer patients qualifying for sentinel lymph node biopsy. Breast J 2004;10(2):89–93

Ferrari A, Dionigi P, Rovera F, et al. Multifocality and multicentricity are not contraindications for sentinel lymph node biopsy in breast cancer surgery. World J Surg Oncol 2006;4 : 79

Fleissig A, Fallowfield LJ, Langridge CI, et al. Post-operative arm morbidity and quality of life. Results of the ALMANAC randomised trial comparing sentinel node biopsy with standard axillary treatment in the management of patients with early breast cancer. Breast Cancer Res Treat 2006;95(3):279–293

Goldhirsch A, Wood WC, Gelber RD, Coates AS, Thürlimann B, Senn HJ. Meeting highlights: updated international expert consensus on the primary therapy of early breast cancer. J Clin Oncol 2003;21(17):3357–3365

Kennedy RJ, Kollias J, Gill PG, Bochner M, Coventry BJ, Farshid G. Removal of two sentinel nodes accurately stages the axilla in breast cancer. Br J Surg 2003;90(11):1349–1353

Keramopoulos A, Tsionou C, Minaretzis D, Michalas S, Aravantinos D. Arm morbidity following treatment of breast cancer with total axillary dissection: a multivariated approach. Oncology 1993;50(6):445–449

Kim T, Giuliano AE, Lyman GH. Lymphatic mapping and sentinel lymph node biopsy in early-stage breast carcinoma: a metaanalysis. Cancer 2006;106(1):4–16

Knauer M, Konstantiniuk P, Haid A, et al. Multicentric breast cancer: a new indication for sentinel node biopsy—a multi-institutional validation study. J Clin Oncol 2006;24(21):3374–3380

Kuehn T, Bembenek A, Decker T, et al; Consensus Committee of the German Society of Senology. A concept for the clinical implementation of sentinel lymph node biopsy in patients with breast carcinoma with special regard to quality assurance. Cancer 2005;103(3):451–461

Kuehn T, Klauss W, Darsow M, et al. Long-term morbidity following axillary dissection in breast cancer patients—clinical assessment, significance for life quality and the impact of demographic, oncologic and therapeutic factors. Breast Cancer Res Treat 2000;64(3):275–286

Kuehn T, Santjohanser C, Grab D, Klauss W, Koretz K, Kreienberg R. Endoscopic axillary surgery in breast cancer. Br J Surg 2001;88(5):698–703

Kuehn T, Vogl FD, Helms G, et al; German multi-institutional trial. Sentinel-node biopsy for axillary staging in breast cancer: results from a large prospective German multi-institutional trial. Eur J Surg Oncol 2004;30(3):252–259

Kuehn T, Santjohanser C, Koretz K, et al. Die Sentinel-node-biopsie beim Mammakarzinom nach farbstoffinduzierter Lymphografie. Geburtshilfe Frauenheilkd 1999;59:142–149

Lyman GH, Giuliano AE, Somerfield MR, et al; American Society of Clinical Oncology. American Society of Clinical Oncology guideline recommendations for sentinel lymph node biopsy in early-stage breast cancer. J Clin Oncol 2005;23(30):7703–7720

Nathanson SD, Wachna DL, Gilman D, Karvelis K, Havstad S, Ferrara J. Pathways of lymphatic drainage from the breast. Ann Surg Oncol 2001;8(10):837–843

Palesty JA, Foster JM, Hurd TC, Watroba N, Rezaishiraz H, Edge SB. Axillary recurrence in women with a negative sentinel lymph node and no axillary dissection in breast cancer. J Surg Oncol 2006;93(2):129–132

Rajesh YS, Ellenbogen S, Banerjee B. Preoperative axillary ultrasound scan: its accuracy in assessing the axillary nodal status in carcinoma breast. Breast 2002;11(1):49–52

Rieber A, Schirrmeister H, Gabelmann A, et al. Pre-operative staging of invasive breast cancer with MR mammography and/or PET: boon or bunk? Br J Radiol 2002;75(898):789–798

Romrell LJ, Bland KI. Anatomy of the breast, axilla, chest wall and related metastatic sites. In: Bland KI, ed. The Breast. Philadelphia: Saunders; 1998: 19–37

Roumen RM, Geuskens LM, Valkenburg JG. In search of the true sentinel node by different injection techniques in breast cancer patients. Eur J Surg Oncol 1999;25(4):347–351

Schirrmeister H, Kühn T, Guhlmann A, et al. Fluorine-18 2-deoxy-2-fluoro-D-glucose PET in the preoperative staging of breast cancer: comparison with the standard staging procedures. Eur J Nucl Med 2001;28(3):351–358

Schwartz GF, Giuliano AE, Veronesi U; Consensus Conference Committee. Proceeding of the consensus conference of the role of sentinel lymph node biopsy in carcinoma or the breast. April 19–22, 2001, Philadelphia, PA, USA. Breast J 2002;8(3):124–138

Smidt ML, Janssen CM, Kuster DM, Bruggink ED, Strobbe LJ. Axillary recurrence after a negative sentinel node biopsy for breast cancer: incidence and clinical significance. Ann Surg Oncol 2005;12(1):29–33

Tanis PJ, Nieweg OE, Valdés Olmos RA, Kroon BB. Anatomy and physiology of lymphatic drainage of the breast from the perspective of sentinel node biopsy. J Am Coll Surg 2001;192(3):399–409

Veronesi U, Paganelli G, Viale G, et al. A randomized comparison of sentinel-node biopsy with routine axillary dissection in breast cancer. N Engl J Med 2003;349(6):546–553

Xing Y, Foy M, Cox DD, Kuerer HM, Hunt KK, Cormier JN. Meta-analysis of sentinel lymph node biopsy after preoperative chemotherapy in patients with breast cancer. Br J Surg 2006;93(5):539–546

Yoshimura G, Sakurai T, Oura S, et al. Evaluation of axillary lymph node status in breast cancer with MRI. Breast Cancer 1999;6(3):249–258

Van Zee KJ, Manasseh DM, Bevilacqua JL, et al. A nomogram for predicting the likelihood of additional nodal metastases in breast cancer patients with a positive sentinel node biopsy. Ann Surg Oncol 2003;10(10):1140–1151

11

12 Cytologic Evaluation

T. Decker, W. Boecker

Basics of Cytologic Diagnosis

History

Fine needle aspiration biopsy (FNAB) was introduced by H.E. Martin for the diagnosis of solid tumors almost 80 years ago (Martin and Ellis, 1930). Following the analysis of over 3000 FNAB of palpable mammary lesions by Franzén and Zajicek (1968), this noninvasive method was used to replace diagnostic excision biopsy. Until the early 1990s, this was the only established minimally invasive method available for making a preoperative diagnosis of mammary carcinoma.

Material and Criteria

FNAB essentially yields single cells and cell clusters, and only in rare cases also tiny pieces of tissue. For this reason, one of the most important criteria in pathologic diagnosis—the evaluation of invasive growth—cannot be used here. FNAB is based on the recognition of malignant cells, without the possibility of evaluating their relationship to the surrounding tissue. The method thus requires that the evaluating cytologist has special training and the corresponding experience and expertise in histologic diagnosis.

The cytologic criteria of malignancy (**Table 12.1**) vary in their expression, both qualitatively and quantitatively. This makes it necessary that the evaluating cytologist considers the findings carefully and matches them consistently to the clinical and imaging findings using the triple approach (physical examination, mammography, and FNA cytology). Palpable tumors are the domain of FNAB. The method is less effective for the diagnosis of small, nonpalpable tumors, even under ultrasonic or stereotactic guidance, and even less so in cases of architectural distortion and microcalcification of the tissue.

Table 12.1 Criteria of malignancy in fine needle aspiration biopsy.

Criterion	Expression
Cell count	High
Cell arrangement	Overlapping 3D
Cell types	Uniform
Cells with naked nuclei	Missing
Background	Necrotic material, desmoplastic stroma
Size of nuclei	Variable, mostly increased
Nuclear pleomorphy	Severe
Nuclear demarcation	Irregular
Nucleoli	Mostly prominent, often multiple
Chromatin structure	Irregular, clumpy

C Categories

The aim of the cytologic examination is to differentiate between benign and malignant lesions as accurately as possible. The histologic findings of both types of lesions vary considerably, and the same is true for the cytologic material obtained by FNAB. Difficulties with interpretation not only occur because of insufficient yield of cells. To better understand the results of FNAB, the following C categories for cytologic malignancy have been published and recommended for the screening program (NHSBSP, 1992; Shabot et al, 1982). In addition to the verbal diagnosis, they should help determine—unambiguously and for all persons involved—the various degrees of reliability of the statement.

C1—Inadequate (Insufficient Material)

Inadequate aspirates include:
* samples with very few cells and with less than five cell clusters
* compromised samples (too bloody material, very thick smears, air-drying artifacts, and the like)

The reasons for classification as C1 should always be stated.

C2—Benign

Benign aspirates are moderately rich in cells. They may contain cohesive clusters of uniform epithelial cells with bland cytologic properties, naked bipolar cells (myoepithelial cells), and stromal fragments. Cystic lesions may contain, in addition to the above, apocrine cells with nuclei of various sizes and prominent nucleoli and with a distinctly eosinophilic, granulated cytoplasm, as well as foam cells, cell detritus, and microcalcification.

Category C2 requires a minimum amount of five cell clusters. Some findings, such as fatty tissue necrosis, fibroadenoma, lymph nodes, abscesses, and granuloma may permit a definitive diagnosis based on their cytology.

C3—Equivocal / Atypia Probably Benign

Equivocal aspirates may show all findings listed under C2. In addition, the following changes are observed, either individually or in combination: high cell density, polymorphic nuclei, loss of cohesion, reduction in the number of cells with naked nuclei, and nuclear changes due to proliferation, involution, or lactation.

C4—Suspicious of Malignancy

This category includes atypical findings highly suspicious of malignancy, but do not permit a definite diagnosis of malignant growth. Three principal constellations of findings prompt classification as C4:

12

- highly atypical cells present in low numbers or in a cohesive arrangement
- cell-rich benign aspirate with solitary, but highly atypical cells
- compromised aspirate with recognizable, highly atypical cells

All atypical criteria in this group surpass the ones listed under C3; nuclear criteria are identical to those under C5.

C5—Malignant

This category indicates that the aspirate is derived from a malignant tumor. The atypical cells meet all criteria of malignancy (**Table 12.1**) and are present in high numbers. Incomplete fulfillment of malignancy criteria and low cell numbers exclude classification as C5.

Quality Indicators for Cytologic Diagnosis

The following quality indicators are the sole basis for assessing the method. A prerequisite is the analysis of the definitive histologic findings as well as the follow-ups of those patients who did not undergo surgery.

Absolute sensitivity. This indicates the rate of carcinomas that were properly recognized by FNAB as being malignant.

Complete sensitivity. This expresses the sensitivity of FNAB and corresponds to the percentage of all nonbenign FNAB results (C3, C4, and C5 findings) in the total of all histologically confirmed carcinomas.

Specificity. This corresponds to the percentage of biopsies correctly classified as benign (C2) by cytology and confirmed by histology in the total of benign FNAB results.

False-negative rate (FNR). This indicates the percentage of FNAB falsely classified as benign (C2) in the total of all carcinomas. (It does not include insufficient FNAB samples.)

False-positive rate (FPR). This corresponds to the percentage of FNAB falsely classified as malignant (C5) in the total of all carcinomas.

Rate of inadequate samples. This is the percentage of all inadequate samples (C1) out of the total of FNAB results.

Rate of suspicious findings. This is the percentage of the total of all C3 and C4 findings out of all cytologic findings.

Influencing factors. The results are influenced by the quality of how the biopsy is performed, by the expertise of the evaluating cytologist, and by the characteristics of the lesion (see above). The properties of the lesion during imaging procedures determine the choice of guidance for FNAB and, therefore, the quality of the biopsy (**Table 12.2**).

Possibilities and Limitations of Breast Cytology Diagnosis

FNAB is quick, simple, and minimally invasive, thus leading to a diagnosis with minimal costs. This applies particularly to cysts and well-demarcated palpable masses. However, it no longer applies to all mammary lesions that are discovered under contemporary circumstances. In the older literature, there are numerous reports on the diagnostic equivalence of FNAB and core needle biopsy (CNB; Pedersen et al, 1986; Shabot et al, 1982). These reports refer to historic biopsy conditions using CNBs that produced predominantly just one sample and were neither performed with automated devices nor under image guidance. These lesions were mostly palpable.

Cysts. The uncontested domain of FNAB remains the definitive confirmation (and therapy) of noncomplex cysts. The use of FNAB is not recommended in cases of complex or complicated cysts (with intraluminar vegetations detected by imaging procedures). A definitely malignant result is almost never observed, and any other suspicious finding requires further invasive diagnosis anyway. Finally, even in case of suspicious cytologic findings, there may be problems with regard to locating the lesion again after the cyst has collapsed due to the intervention.

Results with focal lesions. In cases of focal lesions, the FNAB results vary considerably under contemporary circumstances. Although positive FNAB results are largely considered accurate with a FPR of only 1 to 2% (Stanley et al, 2000), the sensitivity and the accuracy of the method vary. In a meta-analysis of 17 108 FNAB in 31 publications, Britton and coworkers calculated a mean sensitivity of 62% for stereotactic and 83.1% for US-guided FNAB as compared with 90.5% for stereotactic and 96.7% for US-guided CNB (Britton, 1999). The specificity was 86.9% and 84.0%, respectively, for stereotactic and US-guided FNAB as compared with 98.3% and 98.7% for stereotactic and US-guided CNB.

Table 12.2 Quality indicators of fine needle aspiration biopsy and core needle biopsy: a comparison of biopsy guidance methods (Britton, 1999).

Parameter	Stereotactic		US	
	FNAB (%)	CNB (%)	FNAB (%)	CNB (%)
Absolute sensitivity	62.4	90.5	83.1	96.7
Complete sensitivity	83.1	94.6	95.1	98.5
Specificity	86.9	98.3	84.0	98.7
Positive predictive value (PPV) (5)	99.3	99.5	98.0	100.0
False-positive rate (FPR)	0.5	0.4	3.0	0.0
Rate of inadequate samples	6.4	1.0	1.4	0.05

Results with nonpalpable tumors. In cases of exclusively non-palpable tumors, Leifland and coworkers found 68% sensitivity and 99.6% specificity for FNAB as compared with 90% and 98.8%, respectively, for CNB (Leifland et al, 2003a). The smaller the diameter of the tumor, the least favorable are the FNAB results. For example, Cariaggi and coworkers demonstrated for a series of 1609 FNAB with a FNR of 2.9% that the FNR for the subgroup of pT1a and pT1b tumors was clearly higher, namely, 4.2% and 7.6%, respectively (Cariaggi et al, 1995). Most of the errors were due to the high degree of carcinoma differentiation and the difficulty with distinguishing them from benign lesions, rather than to poor hit rates.

Screening. The problem with the diagnosis of small, well-differentiated carcinomas becomes particularly clear when screening. The results of the NHS Breast Screening Program in Britain demonstrate the superiority of CNB with regards to sensitivity, specificity, positive predictive value (PPV) of C5 and B5 categories, and FPR (Ellis, 2001) (**Table 12.3**).

Inadequate biopsies. Another problem of FNAB is the high rate of inadequate biopsies, particularly with nonpalpable lesions. In a multicenter study in Italy on 23 063 women involving various fine needle aspiration techniques, this rate was 6.5% for carcinomas and 23.2% for benign lesions. In a multicenter study in the United States (by the radiologic diagnosis oncology group V), involving 377 women and US-guided FNAB, a total of 34% of samples were inadequate (Pisano et al, 2001).

Therapy planning. Distinction between invasive and intraductal carcinomas by FNAB is not possible with the certainty required for clinical decision making (Jacobs et al, 1999; Leifland et al, 2003b; Silverman et al, 1993; Sneige et al., 1989, Wang et al, 1989). Hence, a decision about axillary staging surgery is not possible prior to surgery. Other parameters important for surgery planning, such as the presence of a DCIS component with invasive carcinoma and its association with microcalcification, cannot be determined by FNAB preoperatively either.

Benign results. The biggest problem, however, is the definitive diagnosis of a lesion that looks suspicious on the mammogram, but is actually benign. A small portion of benign results is also specific for certain entities, such as biphasic fibroadenoma formation, lymph nodes, and granuloma. Provided there is no contradiction to clinical findings, the cytologic findings may be regarded as the definitive diagnosis. Benign findings are nonspecific in the majority of cases. Before refraining from further diag-

nosis in case of a benign cytologic result, triple negativity (cytology, imaging, clinical examination) is therefore absolutely essential. Should there be the slightest suspicion based on clinical examination or imaging, on no account will it be invalidated by the FNAB result.

Risk stratification. When the appropriate diagnostic tools are used, proliferative lesions demanding a risk assessment are detected far more often. Hence, the dichotomy of the diagnostic approach of FNAB for palpable lesions classified as benign or malignant are no longer sufficient. The intermediate categories C3 and C4 contain not only difficult-to-classify lesions of these two categories, but also proliferative lesions belonging to neither of them and carrying different risks (e.g., various forms of adenosis, flat epithelial atypia, lobular neoplasia, atypical epithelial proliferation of the ductal type). Accurate classification and the associated risk stratification are not possible here (Maygarden et al, 1994; Page, 1992; Stanley et al, 1993, 2000).

Guidelines

FNAB results are therefore no longer suitable as the sole basis for decision making on the next diagnostic approach. This has also been included in the European Guidelines for Quality Assurance in Breast Cancer Screening and Diagnosis (2006) and in the EUSOMA position paper for quality assurance in diagnosis (Perry, 2001). Mammographic screening, core needle biopsy, and vacuum-assisted biopsy—but not fine needle aspiration biopsy—are intended to be used exclusively as minimally invasive biopsy methods.

Conclusion

The trend in modern breast diagnosis, particularly under screening conditions, is toward the biopsy of smaller, clinically occult lesions while simultaneously increasing the detection of proliferative lesions. Here are the limitations of FNAB. In the diagnosis of nonpalpable lesions, FNAB is clearly inferior to CNB; furthermore, it does not allow for the accurate discrimination between intraductal and invasive carcinoma. In the case of identified proliferative lesions, FNAB cannot distinguish those that require further invasive diagnosis from those that are harmless.

12

Table 12.3 National Health Service Breast Screening Program: results of a comparison between fine needle aspiration biopsy and core needle biopsy (Ellis, 2001).

Parameter	Median FNAB (%)	Median CNB (%)
Absolute sensitivity	57.1	76.4
Complete sensitivity	81.5	84.5
Specificity	58.5	81.2
PPV C5/B5	99.6	100.0
FPR	0.2	0.0

References

Britton PD. Fine needle aspiration or core biopsy. Breast 1999;8 : 1–4

Cariaggi MP, Bulgaresi P, Confortini M, et al. Analysis of the causes of false negative cytology reports on breast cancer fine needle aspirates. Cytopathology 1995;6(3):156–161

Ellis IO. Guidelines for non-operative diagnostic procedures and reporting in breast cancer screening (50). NHS Breast Screening Programme. Sheffield, UK: NHSBSP Publications; 2001

Franzén S, Zajicek J. Aspiration biopsy in diagnosis of palpable lesions of the breast. Critical review of 3479 consecutive biopsies. Acta Radiol Ther Phys Biol 1968;7(4):241–262

Jacobs TW, Silverman JF, Schroeder B, Raza S, Baum JK, Schnitt SJ. Accuracy of touch imprint cytology of image-directed breast core needle biopsies. Acta Cytol 1999;43(2):169–174

Leifland K, Lagerstedt U, Svane G. Comparison of stereotactic fine needle aspiration cytology and core needle biopsy in 522 non-palpable breast lesions. Acta Radiol 2003a;44(4):387–391

Leifland K, Lundquist H, Lagerstedt U, Svane G. Comparison of preoperative simultaneous stereotactic fine needle aspiration biopsy and stereotactic core needle biopsy in ductal carcinoma in situ of the breast. Acta Radiol 2003b;44(2):213–217

Martin HE, Ellis EB. Biopsy by needle puncture and aspiration. Ann Surg 1930;92(2):169–181

Maygarden SJ, Novotny DB, Johnson DE, Frable WJ. Subclassification of benign breast disease by fine needle aspiration cytology. Comparison of cytologic and histologic findings in 265 palpable breast masses. Acta Cytol 1994;38 (2):115–129

NHSBSP. NHS Breast Screening Programme: Guidelines for Cytology Procedures and Reporting in Breast Cancer Screening (No.22). Sheffield, UK: NHSBSP Publications; 1992

Page DL. FNA identification of familial breast disease. Am J Clin Pathol 1992;97 (2):291–293

Pedersen L, Guldhammer B, Kamby C, Aasted M, Rose C. Fine needle aspiration and Tru-Cut biopsy in the diagnosis of soft tissue metastases in breast cancer. Eur J Cancer Clin Oncol 1986;22(9):1045–1052

Perry NM; EUSOMA Working Party. Quality assurance in the diagnosis of breast disease. Eur J Cancer 2001;37(2):159–172

Perry N, Broeders M, de Wolf C, Törnberg S, Holland R, von Karsa L. European Guidelines for Quality Assurance in Breast Cancer Screening and Diagnosis. 4th ed. Ann Oncol 2008;19(4):614–622

Pisano ED, Fajardo LL, Caudry DJ, et al. Fine-needle aspiration biopsy of nonpalpable breast lesions in a multicenter clinical trial: results from the radiologic diagnostic oncology group V. Radiology 2001;219(3):785–792

Shabot MM, Goldberg IM, Schick P, Nieberg R, Pilch YH. Aspiration cytology is superior to Tru-Cut needle biopsy in establishing the diagnosis of clinically suspicious breast masses. Ann Surg 1982;196(2):122–126

Silverman JF, Masood S, Ducatman BS, Wang HH, Sneige N. Can FNA biopsy separate atypical hyperplasia, carcinoma in situ, and invasive carcinoma of the breast?: Cytomorphologic criteria and limitations in diagnosis. Diagn Cytopathol 1993;9(6):713–728

Sneige N, White VA, Katz RL, Troncoso P, Libshitz HI, Hortobagyi GN. Ductal carcinoma-in-situ of the breast: fine-needle aspiration cytology of 12 cases. Diagn Cytopathol 1989;5(4):371–377

Stanley MW, Henry-Stanley MJ, Zera R. Atypia in breast fine-needle aspiration smears correlates poorly with the presence of a prognostically significant proliferative lesion of ductal epithelium. Hum Pathol 1993;24(6):630–635

Stanley MW, Sidawy MK, Sanchez MA, Stahl RE, Goldfischer M. Current issues in breast cytopathology. Am J Clin Pathol 2000; **113**(5, Suppl 1)S49–S75

Wang HH, Ducatman BS, Eick D. Comparative features of ductal carcinoma in situ and infiltrating ductal carcinoma of the breast on fine-needle aspiration biopsy. Am J Clin Pathol 1989;92(6):736–740

12

13 Histologic Evaluation of Core Needle Biopsy Specimens

T. Decker, W. Boecker

Requirements for Pathologic Diagnosis

Core needle biopsy. Sampling cores of tissue through minimally invasive biopsy (MIB) now plays an important role in breast diagnosis. Core needle biopsy (CNB) and vacuum-assisted biopsy (VAB) are two widely used techniques. A core biopsy specimen is well suited for histologic examination: it can provide a definite diagnosis of benign lesions routinely—not just in individual cases —unlike the cytologic specimen obtained by fine needle aspiration biopsy (FNAB). Furthermore, far better information regarding microcalcification and architectural distortion can be obtained from tissue samples than from single cells of cytologic specimens.

Sensitivity and specificity. The sensitivity and specificity of CNB depend on the biopsy target and on the method of guidance selected. Ultrasound (US)-guided CNB of focal lesions is associated with higher absolute specificity and sensitivity than stereotactic core biopsy, which is mostly used to examine microcalcifications and architectural distortion and, far less often, focal lesions. In a meta-analysis of 17 108 biopsies, Britton and coworkers determined a sensitivity of 90.5% and a specificity of 96.7% for stereotactic core biopsy and 98.3% and 98.7%, respectively, for US-guided CNB (Britton, 1999). CNB is therefore superior to FNAB in both these diagnostic situations (for detailed data and a comparison with FNAB, see Chapter 12) and is the preferred method for the diagnosis of nonpalpable lesions (Ibrahim et al, 2001; Shannon et al, 2001; Britton and McCann, 1999; European Guidelines for Quality Assurance in Breast Cancer Screening and Diagnosis, 2006).

Classification systems. Although a diagnosis based on the results garnered from CNBs poses far higher intellectual demands on the pathologist, the basic principles of morphologic breast diagnosis are valid here. In recent years, the Royal College of Pathologists (Guidelines Working Group of the National Coordinating Committee for Breast Pathology, 2005), the College of American Pathologists (Fitzgibbons et al, 1998), the European Working Group for Breast Screening Pathology (Wells et al, 2006a), and the World Health Organization (WHO; Tavassoli and Devilee, 2003) have issued almost identical classification systems for proliferative lesions of the mammary gland. In the present chapter, we use a three-pronged classification system of benign proliferative lesions, precursor lesions, and invasive carcinoma.

Progenitor Cell Concept

Proliferative lesions. The progenitor cell concept of the mammary epithelium has led to a better understanding of proliferative breast lesions. Data obtained by using immunofluorescence microscopy show that the normal mammary epithelium contains progenitor cells that develop into differentiated glandular and/or myoepithelial cells (Boecker et al, 2002; Dontu et al, 2003). These cell types differ in morphology and in their immunohistochemical properties. Progenitor cells contain the cytokeratins CK5 and CK14, whereas differentiated glandular epithelia contain the cytokeratins CK8 and CK18. Myoepithelia express smooth muscle actin (α-SM actin), p63, and CD10 (**Fig. 13.1**). Apart from very rare exceptions (microglandular adenosis and syringomatous adenoma of the mammilla), all benign proliferative lesions mimic the normal glandular epithelium. Side-by-side, these lesions contain CK5/14-positive progenitor cells (CK5/14+), glandular cells (CK8/18+), and/or myoepithelial cells (CD10+, α-SM actin+, etc.), and this can be demonstrated by immunohistochemistry. Another important component of benign lesions is the stroma with its extracellular matrix; it is present not only in fibroadeno-

13

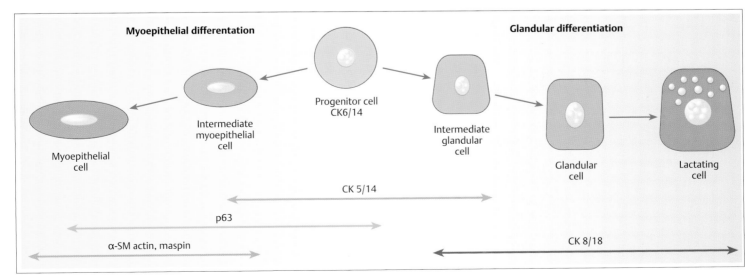

Fig. 13.1 Progenitor cell concept of the mammary epithelium.

mas, but also in papillomas, adenomas, radial scars, sclerosing adenoses, etc. Recently, it was found that the interactions seen between the epithelium and stroma of benign proliferative lesions are similar to those seen during the normal developmental process of the mammary gland (Osin et al, 1998; Boecker et al, 2006). In summary, these findings show that simple epithelial hyperplasia is a benign lesion and is completely unrelated to carcinogenesis.

Carcinogenesis. The traditional view of breast cancer development has assumed a linear development, with the simple epithelial hyperplasia being the initial lesion that develops into atypical ductal hyperplasia, ductal carcinoma in situ (DCIS), and finally, invasive mammary carcinoma (Boecker et al, 2001).

This hypothesis has been challenged by a series of recent findings. Thus, ductal hyperplasia of usual type (HUT) and DCIS/invasive carcinoma show basic genetic differences (e.g., in the comparative genomic hybridization [CGH] analysis) that make a

transformation from ductal hyperplasia to neoplasia unlikely (Buerger et al, 1999, 2001; Farabegoli et al, 2002). This is also demonstrated by basic differences in the immunohistochemical expression of the markers listed above. In contrast to benign proliferative lesions with a mixture of cells from normal tubules, most carcinomas have a strictly glandular phenotype. More than 97 % of in situ lesions and approx. 90 % of invasive carcinomas are CK8/18+ (**Fig. 13.2**).

Most mammary carcinomas develop de novo from the glandular epithelium of the terminal ductal-lobular units (TDLUs). Development of lobular and/or ductal neoplasia in situ within primarily benign epithelial proliferative lesions is relatively rare. The diagram shown in **Fig. 13.3** reflects the current state of knowledge regarding breast cancer development. Thus, the majority of benign proliferative mammary gland lesions may be interpreted as proliferative lesions that represent a developmental "cul-de-sac" and are therefore unrelated to carcinogenesis.

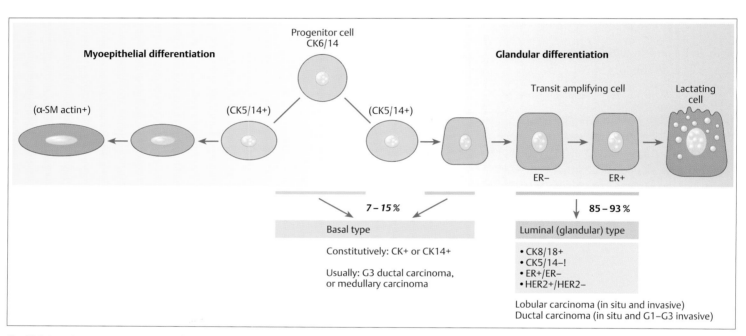

Fig. 13.2 Invasive carcinomas positive for CK8/18.

13

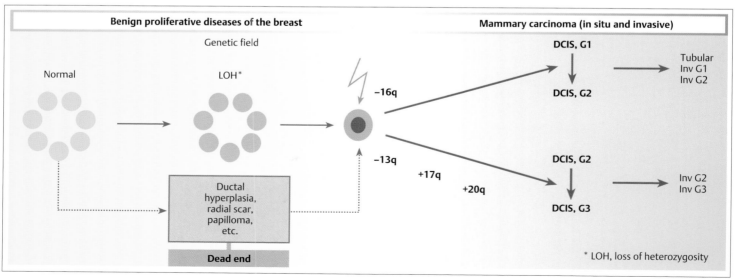

Fig. 13.3 Hypothetical model of breast cancer development.

Diagnostic Implications of the Progenitor Cell Concept

The progenitor cell concept not only contributes to the basic understanding of the pathogenesis of benign and malignant lesions, but it is also becoming a valuable diagnostic aid. The detection of cellular components that correspond to those of a normal tubule allows for the classification of a proliferative lesion as definitely benign. However, when a lesion is comprised exclusively of differentiated glandular cells, this strongly suggests a precancerous lesion or carcinoma.

Immunohistochemistry. In difficult cases, the pathologist may use immunohistochemistry for histologic pattern recognition in addition to conventional histology with routine staining. Based on the progenitor cell concept, immunohistochemistry is used to analyze the cellular constituents of the lesions even when this is not possible with conventional histology. This method thus provides the key for making a correct diagnosis. Breast pathology preferentially uses antibodies directed against basal cytokeratins (CK5, CK14) and luminal cytokeratins (CK8, CK18), as well as smooth muscle (SM) proteins as myothelial markers (e.g., α-SM actin, calponin, maspin, myosin heavy-chain [SMMHC], CD10, and p63). Whereas benign proliferating lesions are characterized by a mixture of different cellular constituents, precancerous lesions and invasive carcinomas are composed of just one cell type. **Table 13.1** lists the lesions in question and cell type-specific marker proteins.

Carcinomas of the luminal type (CK8/18+) represent more than 90% of breast carcinomas found. Basal cell carcinomas, which represent a small percentage of breast carcinomas, were described more than 20 years ago (Nagle et al, 1986; Wetzels et al, 1989). Ever since its description in the journal, *Nature,* by Perou et al (2000), this type of breast cancer has been the center of today's breast research (Abd El-Rehim et al, 2004; Jacquemier et al, 2005; Korsching et al, 2008; Livasy et al, 2006; Sørlie et al, 2001). These basal cell carcinomas express CK5 and CK14, which should be taken into account when interpreting CK5/14 immunohistochemistry. Normally, CK5/14+ cells are characteristic for benign proliferative lesions and are distributed in a mosaic-like fashion. In basal cell carcinomas, these cells occur as homogenous (monotonous) clonal cell populations and exhibit distinct cytologic signs of malignancy.

Requirements for Optimal Pathologic Diagnosis of Biopsy Specimens

Qualification of the pathologist. CNB diagnosis demands far more from the pathologist than the diagnosis of excision (open surgical) biopsy. A decision on patient management is based on the pathologic findings from quantitatively limited material; however, communicating the results in an interdisciplinary context is much more demanding. Although the pathologic result is exclusively based on tissue samples, the pathologist must nevertheless assume that the biopsy may contain only parts of the target lesion. Experience and training for examining CNBs as well as excision biopsies are required for optimal pathologic diagnosis. Furthermore, the pathologic findings are correlated with those of mammography, US, and magnetic resonance imaging (MRI). Hence, the pathologist should also have a basic knowledge of diagnostic imaging. Specialization in the field of breast diagnosis thus seems to be essential.

Nevertheless, the pathologist can only meet the special demands of CNB when the minimum requirements on patient information and handling of biopsy specimens are fulfilled.

Accompanying information. Interpretation of the histopathologic results of a CNB is best achieved when the pathologist has detailed knowledge about the indication and biopsy method

Table 13.1 Role of immunohistochemistry in breast cancer diagnosis using antibodies against various cell-type specific marker proteins.

Question	Marker proteins	Remarks
Hyperplasia of usual type or ductal and lobular neoplasia	CK5/14 and CK8/18	CK5 and/or CK14 or CK8/18 mosaic is typical for HUT, whereas neoplasia in situ* is CK5- and/or CK14-negative
Sclerosing adenosis or classic tubular carcinoma and invasive lobular carcinoma (ILC)	α-SM-actin, CD10, calponin, p63, SMMHC, maspin, CK5/14	Loss of myothelial cell layer in carcinomas Carcinomas are p63-negative and CK5- and/or CK14-negative
Papilloma or papillary carcinoma	α-SM-actin, CD10, calponin, p63, maspin, CK5/14	Myothelial cell layer is present in papillomas, but usually absent in carcinomas For exceptions, see below†
Squamous epithelial differentiation	CK6, 10, 11	Sensitive markers for squamous epithelial differentiation
Adenomyothelial tumors or phyllodes tumors and spindle cell lesions	CK5/14, α-SM-actin, CK8/18	Note that all markers are expressed in adenomyothelial tumors Tumors of mesenchymal origin are usually CK5- and/or CK14-negative The mesenchymal portion of phyllodes tumors is CK5- and/or CK14-negative
Tubular carcinoma and other G1 and G2 carcinomas, as well as most G3 carcinomas	p63, α-SM-actin, CD10, calponin, CK5/14, CK8/18	With few exceptions,* carcinomas are negative for these markers Note that myofibroblasts stain intensely for α-SM-actin

* G1 and G2 carcinomas in situ and invasive carcinomas are generally all CK5- and/or CK14-negative, G3 carcinomas in situ and invasive carcinomas may express CK5 and/or CK14; some special forms (adenoid-cystic carcinoma, adenosquamous carcinoma) express CK5 and/or CK14 constitutively.
† Some papillary carcinomas in situ contain a fully developed myothelial cell layer.

13

Table 13.2 Minimum of accompanying information for the pathologic examination of core needle biopsy.

Patient data	Surname
	First name
	Date of birth
Biopsy localization	Left/right side
	Time, distance from the nipple
	Region (subregion according to the International Classification of Diseases for Oncology [ICDO]: quadrant, central glandular body, axillary process)
Clinical examination	Palpation
	Inspection
	Findings on skin and nipple
	Relevant patient history and family history
Findings of imaging	Mammography (focal lesion, architectural distortion, microcalcification)
	US
	MRI
	BI-RADS category
Size of lesion	Maximum diameter in mm, with indication of method
Differential diagnosis	With indication of method
Overall clinical and image assessment	Suspected grade (for scoring, see text)
Yield of tissue	Number of specimens obtained
Results of specimen radiography	Number of samples containing microcalcification

used, as well as the target lesion characteristics. Detailed information on clinical findings, mammography, US, and other imaging results are absolutely essential. The situation is optimal when the corresponding images are all available. **Table 13.2** lists the minimum information required for the pathologic examination of specimens obtained from a CNB.

Handling of specimens after biopsy. The specimen capsules must be moved with small forceps using great care to prevent fragmentation and artifacts due to squeezing. All specimens obtained during the biopsy of microcalcification lesions must undergo specimen radiography. This is the only way to start a targeted histologic search for microcalcification. For this purpose, the microcalcification-containing specimen capsules are separated from the others and submitted for pathologic examination together with the specimen radiographs. Ideally, the radiologist has already placed the specimens in special tissue-embedding cassettes for histologic processing. Buffered 4% formaldehyde should be used for fixation.

> **Tips and Tricks**
>
> Fixation should be performed as quickly as possible to prevent irreversible artifacts by air-drying. The specimens should be moistened with physiologic saline when they cannot be placed directly into the shipping container after biopsy (e. g., prior to specimen radiography after VAB).

Histotechnical processing. Examination of frozen sections of CNB tissue is risky and unnecessary; it should be avoided (Step 3–Guideline for Early Detection of Breast Cancer in Germany; Leitlinie Brustkrebs-Früherkennung in Deutschland, 2008; Heywang-Köbrunner et al, 2003; Ellis et al, 2004). The emotional stress caused by waiting for the results from regular histologic sections, which is occasionally cited as justification for frozen sections, can certainly be reduced by appropriate patient education and optimal interdisciplinary time management. This is true especially in modern breast diagnostics where suspicious, but usually benign lesions dominate. The minimum time for optimal tissue fixation is 6 hours. Shorter fixation times lead to reduced quality of the conventional histologic diagnosis (e. g., when grading the lesions; Start et al, 1991) and of the immunohistochemical examination (Cattoretti, 1994), particularly when a diagnosis involves the detection of estrogen receptor (ER) and human epithelial growth factor receptor 2 (HER2) (Goldstein et al, 2003). This should also be taken into account when planning rapid embedding programs. After fixation, the tissue samples should be embedded in paraffin in a horizontal position (**Fig. 13.4**) and poured into paraffin blocks. No more than four specimens should be placed into one embedding cassette (Wells et al, 2000). Microtome sections of a maximum 4 μm in thickness are best. The number of sections or sectioning levels depends on the target lesion. Although in

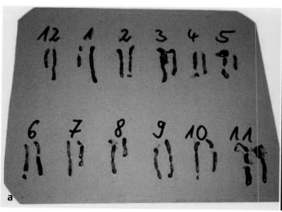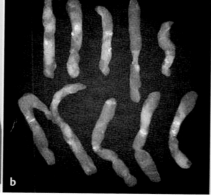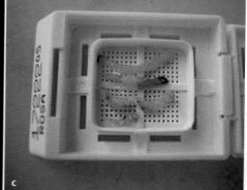

Fig. 13.4a–c Paraffin embedding of tissue samples.
a Samples arranged in the order of 1 to 12.
b Part of a specimen radiograph.
c Samples placed in an embedding cassette.

theory, a single section may suffice for the diagnosis of a focal lesion, most laboratories dealing with early detection diagnosis prepare sections from three sectioning levels for focal lesions and architectural distortion. If microcalcifications are the biopsy target, sectioning levels are obligatory. This approach has found its way into international and national guidelines (Heywang-Köbrunner et al, 2003; Ellis et al, 2004; Wells et al, 2006b; Stufe-3-Leitlinie Brustkrebs-Früherkennung in Deutschland, 2008). The first section should be used for examination to prevent loss of calcification.

B Categories

The simple classification of CNB findings into histologically benign or malignant lesions no longer accommodates the diagnostic and management problems in modern breast cancer diagnosis. Individual lesions differ greatly in their clinical importance, and there is a wide scope of further diagnostic and therapeutic options. The suggestion of expressing the pathologic findings of biopsies in categories stems from mammographic screening programs. In 1997, the B categories for breast CNBs were introduced in the UK for the first time by the National Coordinating Group for Breast Screening Pathology (National Coordinating Group for Breast Screening Pathology, 1997). These categories were then adopted by the European guidelines for mammographic screening (European Guidelines for Quality Assurance in Breast Cancer Screening and Diagnosis, 2001). Their use has now extended outside the screening setting, and they are recognized internationally.

Five categories. The five-category classification system (**Table 13.3**) helps the pathologist to formulate the biopsy assessment to facilitate a decision on further management.

Importance of the B categories. The categories permit a clear statement regarding the diagnosis after CNB. It is not always possible to establish a definitive histologic diagnosis; nevertheless, the histopathologic results as documented are often used in further decisions. In most cases, the results are either benign (B2) or malignant (B5). In the remaining cases, the biopsies are either normal or unsatisfactory (insufficient amounts of tissue) (B1), of uncertain malignant potential (B3), or suspicious of malignancy (B4). The B categories are also used as a basis for standardized

Table 13.3 The five-category classification system for pathologic findings of core needle biopsy (Wells et al, 2006b).

Category	Definition
B1	Normal tissue / unsatisfactory biopsy
B2	Benign lesion
B3	Lesion of uncertain malignant potential
B4	Lesion suspicious of malignancy
B5	Malignant lesion
B5a	DCIS
B5b	Invasive carcinoma
B5c	Invasion not assessable
B5d	Other malignant lesion

quality assurance (see the section, Quality Indicators of the Pathologic Diagnosis, p. 196). This requires that the B categories be derived exclusively based on microscopic findings, without influence from any information derived from imaging and clinical findings. In an interdisciplinary conference between the pathologist and clinician, correlation between the pathologic and image findings is confirmed. The procedural consequences are the result of this analysis. When using the B categories, it is essential that the pathologist strictly applies the definitions as provided in his or her country's accepted guidelines.

B1—Normal Tissue/Unsatisfactory Biopsy

This category includes biopsies with normal tissue as well as biopsies unsatisfactory for evaluation. Biopsies unsatisfactory for pathologic evaluation contain insufficient amounts of tissue and/or are comprised predominantly of blood clots or show severe artificial alterations. The pathologic report should always state the reason for classification as B1.

If the tissue is normal, the report should distinguish biopsies containing glandular tissue from those without parenchyma. Minor pathologic changes at the microscopic level, which are unlikely to show up on the radiograph, should be classified as B1. Lesions with microcalcifications of <80 µm should also be classified as B1.

A B1 result with normal tissue is an indication that the target lesion may not have been hit. But this is by no means the only explanation. The normal glandular tissue may be part of a hamartoma, and normal fatty tissue may be part of a lipoma. Islets of normal parenchyma in a mostly involuted breast may cause small dense areas on the mammogram.

Conclusions. Category B1 largely includes biopsies that do not represent the target lesion, but this does not necessarily apply to all biopsies classified as B1. Some B1 biopsies do correlate with the lesion to be examined and thus permit a diagnosis. Such a connection must then be definitively confirmed or excluded by radiologic–pathologic correlation.

B2—Benign Lesion

This category implies that the biopsy contains a benign lesion that, in principle, may have been responsible for the results in the mammogram, both qualitatively and quantitatively. Whether this holds true for the case in question will have to be clarified by the subsequent radiologic–pathologic correlation. In cases of doubt, minor pathologic changes should be classified as B1 instead.

Typical lesions. Typical B2 lesions include fibroadenomas, sclerosing adenoses, blunt duct adenoses, periductal mastitis, microcysts, macrocysts, abscesses, and fatty tissue necroses. Apart from fibroadenomas and macrocysts, almost all of these lesions may also occur as a minor microscopic lesion of a few hundred micrometers in diameter, thus calling for classification as B1. In some cases, unambiguous diagnosis of a hamartoma in the CNB specimen is nevertheless possible, thus qualifying the lesion for category B2. In some cases, it is even possible for the pathologist to confirm that a papilloma is completely contained in the biopsy specimen. In that case, the lesion is classified as B2, although it would otherwise be assigned to category B3 (**Fig. 13.5**).

13

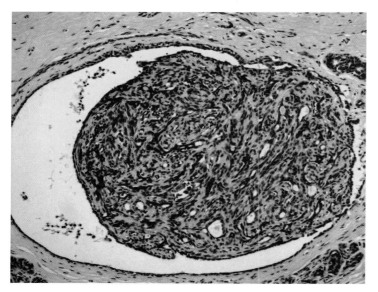

Fig. 13.5 Papilloma, category B2. Microcyst containing a papilloma of 1.5 mm in diameter, completely included within the biopsy specimen.

Conclusions. Category B2 contains only lesions that are definitely benign according to histopathologic criteria, even though this classification is based exclusively on the microscopic findings. However, assignment of the biopsy to category B2 does not complete the diagnosis of a lesion detected by imaging; a definitive diagnosis is only possible after radiologic–pathologic correlation.

B3—Lesion of Uncertain Malignant Potential

This category includes lesions where the biopsy specimen does not meet the criteria for malignancy, but rather indicates a risk of associated malignancy. Although some of the lesions in this group are known markers for an increased risk of bilateral and diffuse breast cancer later in life, a classification of B3 signals a synchronous and local risk at the time of biopsy and in the immediate surrounding of the biopsy site.

Typical lesions. Category B3 consists basically of two groups:
- lesions with a known heterogeneous structure, the clinically relevant portion of which may not have been hit by the biopsy
- lesions that frequently occur together with intraductal or invasive carcinomas

The first group (heterogeneous lesions) includes papillary lesions (**Fig. 13.6**) (unless they are completely contained in the biopsy specimen and classified as B2, see above), radial scars, phyllodes tumors, mucocele-like lesions, cystic hypersecretory lesions, and spindle cell proliferations. In the case of these lesions, it is possible that a malignant portion remains in situ because of the limited amount of tissue removed by CNB.

The second group (high-risk lesions preferentially associated with intraductal or invasive carcinomas) includes lobular neoplasia (LN; except special cases listed under B5a), flat epithelial atypia, and atypical ductal hyperplasia (ADH).

Conclusions. Diagnostic excision is by far not the only conclusion for category B3. As with other B categories, the conclusion depends on the radiologic–pathologic correlation. The various combinations of specific histologic findings and the findings of diagnostic imaging after biopsy will determine the next approach (see the section, Radiologic–Pathologic Correlation, p. 188).

B4—Lesion Suspicious of Malignancy

Due to technical problems during the biopsy procedure, not enough tissue of the target lesion may have been obtained. This may lead to a situation where a definitive histologic diagnosis is not possible; nevertheless, the lesion is clearly abnormal and suspicious of malignancy (**Fig. 13.7**). A similar situation may arise due to artifacts, such as squeezing, air-drying, or insufficient fixation.

Conclusions. Category B4 does not provide a basis for therapeutic decisions. Lesions of this category do not necessarily require clarification by excision biopsy. Any further approach should be

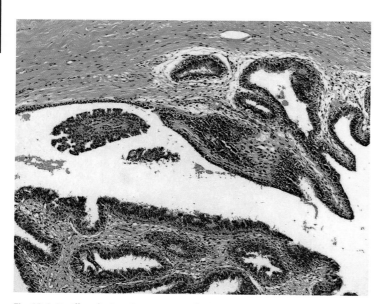

Fig. 13.6 Papillary lesion. Cross-section of a dilated duct with part of a benign papilloma.

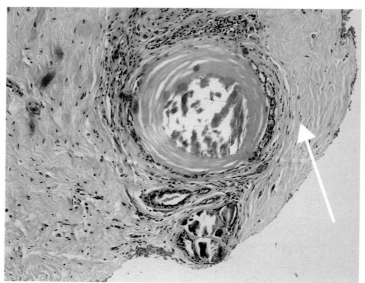

Fig. 13.7 Suspected malignant lesion, category B4. Non-high-grade atypical cell clusters in minute amounts near an intraductal calcification (arrow). Intraductal neoplasia is suspected. However, the findings do not allow a definitive diagnosis.

13

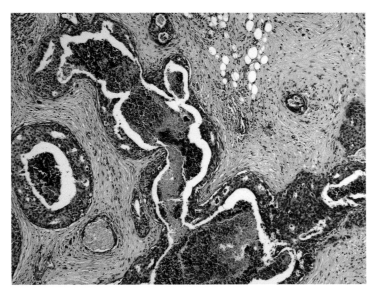

Fig. 13.8 Ductal carcinoma in situ (DCIS) in a CNB specimen. Cross-section of a branching duct showing a DCIS with central comedo necroses (red) and calcifications (blue).

determined by the interdisciplinary team after analyzing what has led to the B4 classification.

B5—Malignant Lesion

This category only includes lesions that are definitively malignant and for which treatment is possible without having to reevaluate its state of malignancy. In the case of carcinomas, it is essential that the invasive growth is subclassified.

B5a (carcinoma in situ). Category B5a includes all lesions classified as DCIS (**Fig. 13.8**), Paget disease of the nipple (the only cancer where B categories may be applied to excision biopsy), and also a small portion of lobular neoplasia (LN of the extended type, LN with comedo necrosis, and pleomorphic LN) (**Fig. 13.9**); according to expert opinion, treatment similar to that of DCIS is indicated. Category B5a applies when a DCIS present in the CNB can be definitely diagnosed without further intervention, independently of the possible detection of an invasive component in the excision biopsy.

B5b (invasive carcinoma). Category B5b includes all types of primarily invasive carcinomas, such as invasive ductal carcinoma (IDC) and invasive lobular carcinoma (ILC), independently of whether and to what extent they contain a DCIS (**Fig. 13.10**).

B5c (invasion not assessable). Category B5c characterizes lesions that definitely contain at least a DCIS without allowing a definitive statement regarding invasion. This uncertainty refers to the findings in the CNB and not to the possibility that an invasive tumor might be found in the excision biopsy.

B5 d (other malignant lesions). Category B5 d includes primary nonepithelial malignancies (sarcoma) and all metastases of extramammary tumors (carcinoma and sarcoma) of the breast.

Conclusion

The B categories not only represent diagnostic groups, but also the histologic findings, which are based exclusively on the microscopic examination of the CNB specimens. They form the basis for the radiologic–pathologic correlation, which, in turn, is the foundation of any decision made by the interdisciplinary team on how to proceed. Hence, the B categories are neither a simplified histologic classification nor instructions for diagnostic or therapeutic action.

Clinical Management after Histologic Diagnosis

Clinical management after the CNB diagnosis requires specialty and interdisciplinary collaboration; this is best served by a designated breast care team. All participants must have at least a basic knowledge of the other disciplines and must be familiar with the current literature on diagnosis and treatment. The team's tasks after CNB include

- radiologic–pathologic correlation
- assessing the status of the diagnosis
- establishing a joint recommendation on how to proceed

All recommendations, particularly any treatment suggestions for the patient, require a consensus.

13

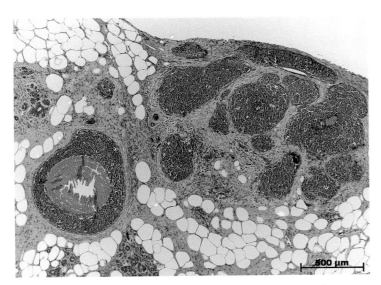

Fig. 13.9 LN of the extended type. Cross-section of an LN with typical duct involvement. The center of the neoplasia (left) shows comedo necrosis (red).

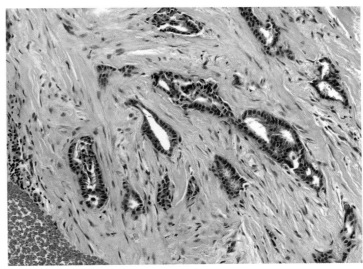

Fig. 13.10 Primary invasive carcinoma, category B5b. Cross-section of a core specimen showing parts of a well-differentiated, G1 invasive ductal carcinoma (IDC).

Radiologic–Pathologic Correlation

When the pathologist has completed the histologic evaluation and specified the B category, a decision is made on how to proceed. Before this is possible, however, the pathologist and radiologist together must confirm that the histologic findings actually represent the biopsy target on the radiograph. Exact radiologic–pathologic correlation is the basis for subsequent management decisions by the interdisciplinary team.

Prior to the actual correlation, the radiologist should confirm that the biopsied lesion is, in fact, the lesion to be examined. In theory, the pathologist is able to identify nearly all breast lesions present in the CNB as accidental microscopic findings, i.e., without reference to the biopsy target. In addition to the qualitative assessment, he or she should therefore critically estimate the quantitative relationships within the biopsy specimens and in relation to the target lesion.

Histologic differential diagnosis. The radiologist and pathologist should be familiar with any important histologic differential diagnoses of the specific findings in the imaging diagnosis. **Table 13.4** lists important mammographic or ultrasound findings for focal lesions and architectural distortion, and their histologic differential diagnoses.

Table 13.4 Radiologic–pathologic correlation: Focal lesions and architectural distortion.

Mammographic or US findings	Degree of suspicion	Histologic differential diagnosis
Sharp boundaries, solid	No suspicion of malignancy	Fibroadenoma (**Fig. 13.11**) Hamartoma Phyllodes tumor Tubular adenoma Adenomyoepithelioma Intraductal papilloma
Partly unsharp boundaries, solid	Low suspicion of malignancy	Nodular adenosis (**Fig. 13.12**) Fibroadenoma
Sharp boundaries, solid, radiographically heterogeneous	No suspicion of malignancy	Hamartoma Fibroadenoma (with fatty tissue) Lymph nodes
Partly unsharp boundaries, solid, radiographically heterogeneous	Low suspicion of malignancy	Hamartoma Pseudoangiomatous hyperplasia
Sharp boundaries, cystic	No suspicion of malignancy	Apocrine cyst Duct ectasia Galactocele Small intracystic papilloma
Partly solid, partly cystic	Low suspicion of malignancy	Fibroadenoma (complex) Hamartoma Intraductal papilloma Intraductal papilloma with atypical epithelial proliferation Intraductal papilloma with DCIS
Spheroid, partly unsharp boundaries, solid	High suspicion of malignancy	G3 IDC (**Fig. 13.13**) Medullary carcinoma Mucinous carcinoma Metaplastic carcinoma Lymph node metastasis Fibroadenoma Sclerosing adenosis
Irregularly solid	Extremely high suspicion of malignancy	IDC/ILC Scar Mastitis obliterans/mammary duct ectasia Fatty tissue necrosis
Spicular architectural distortion	High suspicion of malignancy	Radial scar (**Fig. 13.14**) Tubular carcinoma G1 IDC ILC
Architectural distortion		ILC Radial scar Tubular carcinoma (**Fig. 13.15**)

13

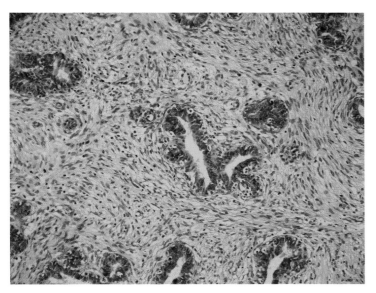

Fig. 13.11 Fibroadenoma. Cross-section of a pericanalicular fibroadenoma.

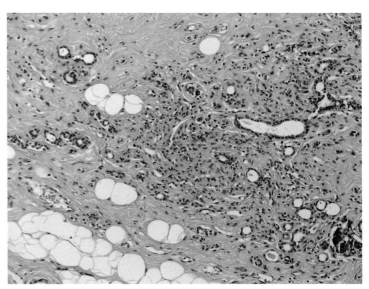

Fig. 13.12 Nodular adenosis. Tumor-producing nodular adenosis with psammomatous calcifications at the lower right.

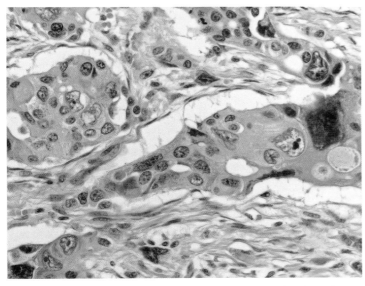

Fig. 13.13 G3 IDC. Section of a solid carcinoma with pronounced nuclear polymorphy, and with numerous mitoses (not shown in this picture).

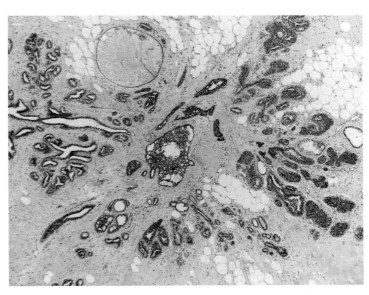

Fig. 13.14 Radial scar. Radial scar showing hyalinosis and elastosis in the center and radial parenchymal extensions.

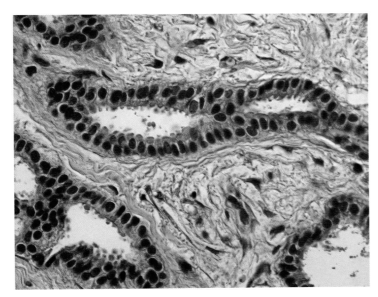

Fig. 13.15 Tubular carcinoma. Tubular carcinoma at high magnification. The neoplastic glands are lined with monomorphic epithelium. These carcinomas are always classified as G1 tumors.

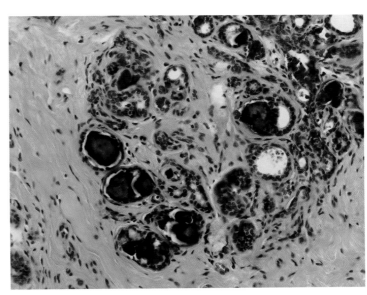

Fig. 13.16 Blunt duct adenosis. Blunt duct adenosis with pronounced psammomatous calcifications.

13

Table 13.5 Radiologic–pathologic correlation: microcalcification types.

Microcalcification type on specimen radiograph	Degree of suspicion	Histologic differential diagnosis
Punctiform/amorphous	Low suspicion of malignancy	Microcysts Sclerosing adenosis Blunt duct adenosis (**Fig. 13.16**) Foreign body granulomas DCIS nuclear grades 1 and 2
Amorphic	Low suspicion of malignancy	Sclerosing adenosis Blunt duct adenosis Non-high-grade DCIS
Pleomorphic	Moderate suspicion of malignancy	Fibroadenoma (**Fig. 13.17**) Blunt duct adenosis DCIS nuclear grades 2 and 3
Linear	High suspicion of malignancy	DCIS nuclear grades 3 and 2 Periductal mastitis/mastitis obliterans (**Fig. 13.18**) Fibroadenoma
Linear branching	Very high suspicion of malignancy	DCIS nuclear grade 3 Fibroadenoma

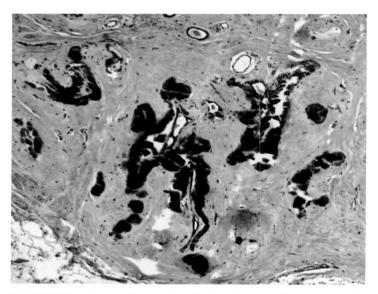

Fig. 13.17 Fibroadenoma. Cross-section of a fibroadenoma with popcorn-shaped polymorphic calcifications.

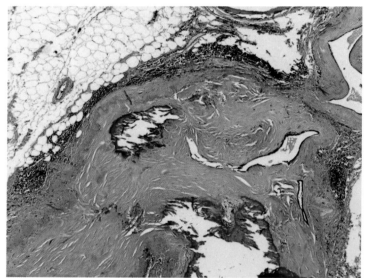

Fig. 13.18 Periductal (interstitial) mastitis. Cross-section of a duct showing severe periductal mastitis, fibrosis, and polymorphic calcifications.

Table 13.5 lists the most important microcalcification types and their histologic differential diagnoses. Here, the findings are strictly limited to comparing specimen radiographs with histologic findings; they do not include the clinically and diagnostically important parameter of microcalcification patterns.

Correlation of findings. In principle, the correlations between the histopathologic result and the imaging diagnosis may lead to the following situations. These correlations apply equally to the findings of mammography, US, and MRI, using the Breast Imaging Reporting and Data System (BI-RADS).

- **Histology B1—imaging BI-RADS 5:**
  Under no circumstances does a lesion classified histologically as B1 correlate to an imaging finding of category BI-RADS 4 or 5. A repeat biopsy is always indicated here.

- **Histology B1—imaging BI-RADS 2, 3, or 4:**
  B1 lesions with normal tissue may originate from a hamartoma, lipoma, or glandular tissue containing microcalcifications associated with involution; imaging procedures may yield a BI-RADS 2 or 3 result, but rarely a BI-RADS 4 result. If the radiologic–pathologic correlation is confirmed, the approach is similar to that in case of a B2 finding with definite correlation.

- **Histology B5—imaging BI-RADS 4 or 5:**
  The suspicious lesion detected by imaging turns out to be malignant based on its histology. Such lesions usually represent highly suspicious, irregularly shaped, and radially demarcated focal lesions that either prove to be invasive carcinomas histologically, or they represent highly suspicious microcalcifications that prove to be DCIS histologically. Here,

Table 13.6 Causes of false-negative CNB results and their quality control.

Cause	Source of error	Quality control
Wrong biopsy target	Biopsy planning	Revision of complete imaging procedure
Heterogeneous biopsy target	Lesion properties	Documentation of biopsy results Correlation with histology
Hit error	Biopsy method	Movement by patient? Function of biopsy device Quality of image guidance
Sample too small	Biopsy method Interruption of biopsy	Function of biopsy device Protocol
Artifacts	Handling after biopsy Histologic processing	Analysis of type of artifacts
Lesion not present in the histologic section	Histologic processing	Specimen radiography in cases of microcalcification Number of sectioning levels
Misinterpretation	Pathologist	Internal/external quality management

the correlation is easy, and the team may start planning the treatment.

- **Histology B5—imaging BI-RADS 2 or 3:**
  This situation is rare and, as a rule, occurs when clinical symptoms (a suspicious palpable mass, skin dimples, or unilateral secretion) had been the indication for CNB. With such a discrepancy in the assessment, the pathologist should check once again the histologic result. Furthermore, any possibility of a mix-up should be ruled out prior to making further decisions. The approach toward the patient is similar to that for concurring malignant findings. Nevertheless, the reasons for underassessment of the imaging result should be analyzed in detail, and they should be subjected to internal quality management.

- **Histology B2—imaging BI-RADS 2 or 3:**
  Even concurring benign findings require radiologic–pathologic correlation because, in theory, both results could be false-negative. When the correlation is certain, no further diagnostic or therapeutic measures are necessary thanks to the benign nature of the findings. Disturbing findings upon palpation, specific symptoms, or cosmetic impairment may, of course, be indications for surgical removal. Different guidelines prescribe imaging follow-ups at different intervals (evidence level 3B of the German S3 guideline; Stufe-3-Leitlinie, Brustkrebs-Früherkennung in Deutschland, 2008). Within mammographic screening programs, check-ups are performed at the next screening round (European Guidelines for Quality Assurance in Breast Cancer Screening and Diagnosis, 2001, 2006).

- **Histology B2—imaging BI-RADS 4 or 5:**
  It is possible, in principle, that a benign lesion causes a suspicious imaging result. In this situation, the radiologic–pathologic correlation is especially important because, if confirmed, no further diagnostic action will be taken. All possible causes of a false-negative biopsy result must therefore be excluded, and comments from both the radiologist and the pathologist are required (**Table 13.6**). In this situation, the German S3 guideline recommends a check-up after 6 months.
  The probability of a benign histopathologic lesion being the correlate to a lesion classified as suspicious of malignancy

increases, first, with the number of biopsy specimens containing the lesion and, second, with the portions occupied by the lesion in the respective biopsy specimens. This applies to focal lesions and architectural distortions, as well as microcalcifications. In case of focal lesions, the detection of a clear border between lesion and normal breast tissue indicates a correlation between pathology and the image findings. If such a border is confirmed, its histologic characteristics (smooth convex, radial, or very irregular) may also be used for correlation with the imaging result. Generally, false-negative results of CNBs are rare, with a reported rate of < 1 %–2 % (Bassett et al, 1997; Dahlstrom et al, 1998).

- **Histology B3—imaging BI-RADS 4 or 5:**
  Here, too, the radiologic–pathologic correlation is decisive. If the correlation is certain, the next approach depends on the respective histologic lesion and the imaging result after biopsy (see section, Interdisciplinary Management, p. 192). If the correlation is uncertain or nonexistent, the assessment is incomplete. The B3 result increases the suspicion of malignancy of the target lesion, and a repeat biopsy should be performed without delay. This does not always have to be excision biopsy. For example, if the target was missed, CNB is the method of choice.

- **Histology B3—imaging BI-RADS 2 or 3:**
  This rare constellation presupposes that a lesion that does not justify biopsy according to the imaging results did undergo biopsy based on clinical symptoms. If the radiologic–pathologic correlation is certain, the histologic findings decide the approach to be taken (see section, Interdisciplinary Management, p. 192). If there is no certain correlation, the assessment is incomplete. Therefore, the histologic B3 result should prompt a thorough revision of the imaging results before and after CNB, with the aim of arriving at a definitive diagnosis.

Documenting the radiologic–pathologic correlation. The correlation should finally be assessed in a joint written statement by the radiologist and pathologist involved, and the result should include comments on the pathologic and radiologic reports. The

13

Table 13.7 Categories of radiologic–pathologic correlation (adapted and modified from Decker et al, 2006).

Category	Statement
CO1	Radiologic–pathologic correlation confirmed
CO2	Radiologic–pathologic correlation excluded
CO3	Radiologic–pathologic correlation uncertain
• CO3a	• Uncertain, but likely
• CO3b	• Unlikely, but not excluded

Table 13.9 Overall clinical and imaging categories (Decker et al, 2006).

Category	Statement
OCI 1	Normal findings
OCI 2	Benign lesion
OCI 3	Uncertain status
OCI 4	Malignant lesion suspected
OCI 5	Malignant lesion, clinical and/or imaging findings

final document should be as clear as possible. In principle, there are only three possibilities: the correlation is certain, the correlation definitely does not exist, or the correlation is uncertain. To simplify the documentation, our interdisciplinary team uses three correlation (CO) categories (Decker et al, 2006) (**Table 13.7**).

Interdisciplinary Management

After documenting the radiologic–pathologic correlation, the interdisciplinary team must decide on the approach to be followed. This is best done by following a fixed protocol.

Action categories. In principle, five approaches are available for deciding on five diagnostic results; our team uses five action (A) categories (**Table 13.8**).

Before the final diagnostic result can be assessed, all clinical and imaging findings, the B category, and the radiologic–pathologic correlation have to be discussed.

Overall clinical and imaging assessment. To begin, the clinical symptoms should be recapitulated together with the overall BI-RADS assessment category resulting from imaging (mammography, US, and/or MRI), and an overall clinical and imaging assessment should be made. The degree of suspected malignancy may be increased based on clinical symptoms in some cases, but not in others. Neither the absence of clinical symptoms nor unsuspicious palpation results have an effect on the overall assessment. Unilateral secretion requires that all BI-RADS 1 and 2 results be classified as uncertain; however, it does not affect the assessment of higher BI-RADS categories. Suspicious palpation results and/or skin symptoms require that all BI-RADS 1 to 3 results be classified as suspicious.

Our interdisciplinary team uses five overall clinical and imaging (OCI) categories for clarification (**Table 13.9**) (Decker et al, 2006).

Inclusion of the radiologic–pathologic correlation. The next step is to include the results of the radiologic–pathologic correlation.

- **CO1—correlation confirmed:**
  If the radiologic–pathologic correlation is confirmed, the team may proceed with combining the overall clinical and imaging score with the B category as outlined below.
- **CO2—correlation excluded:**
  In this case, a decision as outlined below may only be made for lesions of categories B4 and B5. For all lesions of categories B1 to B3, however, the diagnosis is incomplete without correlation; these lesions require that the biopsy is repeated without delay, either as CNB or as excision biopsy (action category A1).
- **CO3—correlation unclear:**
  Here, too, a decision as outlined below may be made for biopsy results of categories B4 and B5. Category B2 results with uncertain correlation are only acceptable with a score of OCI 1 (normal findings) or OCI 2 (benign lesion), but this situation is rare because there is no indication for biopsy. The subcategories CO3a and CO3b are helpful when there is a category B2 lesion with a score of OCI 3 (uncertain status of lesion). If a correlation is uncertain but likely (CO3a), short-term follow-up is a responsible decision. If a correlation is unlikely but not excluded (CO3b), the decision should be to repeat the biopsy (action category A1). The same criteria apply to all lesions of categories B1 and B2 where a correlation with the imaging results is not quite certain.

Final decisions. After clarifying the immediate conclusions drawn from absent or uncertain radiologic–pathologic correlations, the final conclusions for the remaining cases may now be made from the histologic findings (B categories) and the overall clinical and imaging assessment (OCI scores) (**Fig. 13.19**).

- **B1—normal tissue:**
  This biopsy result is only acceptable for lesions classified as benign according to clinical and imaging findings (OCI 2). The

Table 13.8 Action categories according to the decision made by the interdisciplinary team (Decker et al, 2006).

Category	Statement	Final decision
A1	Lesion not evaluated	Repeat biopsy (core needle biopsy or excision)
A2	Confirmed benign lesion	Regular follow-up care
A3	Benign lesion with residual uncertainty	Early check-up
A4	Lesion with risk of malignancy	Repeat biopsy (excision or core needle biopsy)
A5	Confirmed malignant lesion	Start with treatment planning

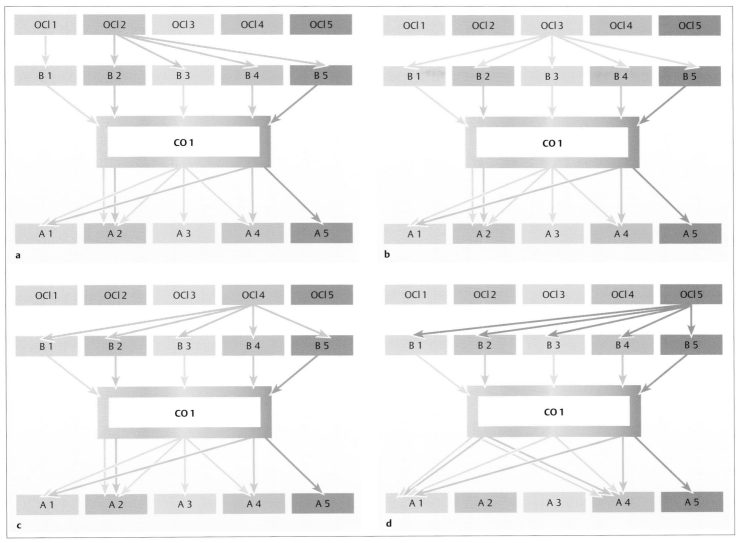

Fig. 13.19a–d Management decisions for confirmed radiologic–pathologic correlation. When a correlation has been verified (CO1), the various combinations of overall clinical and image scores (OCI1–OCI5) and B categories (B1–B5) make it possible to decide between the five categories of action (A1–A5) (see text).
a–c With scores of OCI2 to OCI4 as starting points and with verified correlations, the histologic result alone determines how to proceed further. B2 lesions require no further diagnosis; the correlation should therefore be checked once again, par-

ticularly with OCI3 and OCI4 scores. In the case of B3 lesions, the approach depends on the specific lesion and/or residual findings after the biopsy. B4 lesions always require repeat biopsy, either core needle biopsy (A1) or excision biopsy (A4). In the case of B5 lesions, a treatment plan is indicated (A5).
d In cases with an OCI5 score, a similar approach is only indicated for B5 lesions (A5 treatment plan). All other category B lesions require CNB or excision (A1 or A4), even in the case of (supposed) radiologic–pathologic correlation.

final decision calls for regular follow-up care without further diagnostic intervention (action category A2). For all lesions with scores of OCI3 to OCI5, a B1 result is not acceptable. Here, the diagnosis is incomplete, and a repeat biopsy is indicated (action category A1).

- **B2—benign lesion:**
This result is typical for OCI2 situations in which a biopsy is rarely performed. When the benign status according to clinical and imaging findings is uncertain (OCI3), or when the overall rating is suspicious (OCI4), the notion of positive correlation between imaging and histologic findings should be re-examined. Only if the correlation is confirmed can a B2 result eliminate any uncertainty or suspicion. Regular follow-up without further diagnostic intervention (action category A2) is then justified. A malignant lesion according to the clinical and imaging assessment (OCI5), however, is not invalidated by a B2 result and requires further clarification. This is usually obvious by the lack of correlation. However, even if there is a presumed correlation, the diagnosis should be considered incomplete, and a repeat biopsy should be performed (action category A1).

- **B3—lesion of uncertain malignant potential:**
The high rate of repeat biopsies following histologic B3 results stems less from the lesions themselves than from the fact that many histologic results do not correlate with the imaging results and thus call for reexamination. When dealing with the correlation results, B3 results are not always an indication for repeat biopsy (CNB or excision biopsy).

Indications for regular follow-up care without further diagnostic intervention (action category A2) include

1. Findings of LN or flat epithelial atypia, associated with a benign histologic lesion that correlates with the biopsy target (e.g., fibroadenoma, macrocysts, adenosis with microcalcification—provided the microcalcifications are completely removed).
2. Portions of a papillary lesion not associated with atypical findings—if after the diagnostic intervention no residual findings (focal lesion or residual microcalcification) are detected at the site by imaging.
3. Portions of a radial scar when they are detected as microscopical findings in addition to the benign lesion that called for the

13

biopsy (e.g., fibroadenoma or adenosis with microcalcification —provided the microcalcifications are completely removed) and when no additional architectural distortion is present.

4. Portions of a radial scar, which are only detected because of the microcalcifications associated with it and which have caused neither architectural distortion nor a focal lesion. Here, too, the complete removal of microcalcifications is a precondition for refraining from further invasive examination.

In another group of situations, detection of a B3 lesion with imaging correlate constitutes an indication for further invasive diagnostic intervention because of the increased risk involved (action category A4). Examples include

1. Rare atypical intraductal epithelial proliferations (AIEP) containing microcalcification. This is highly suspicious of non-high-grade DCIS. This is an indication for repeat biopsy of residual microcalcification (either CNB or excision biopsy) or for diagnostic excision of the biopsy area for the complete removal of microcalcification.

2. Atypical intraductal epithelial proliferations associated with another lesion (fibroadenoma, papilloma, adenosis). The risk of synchronous DCIS is lower, yet substantial (see below) and requires complete removal of the lesion containing the atypical epithelial proliferation.

3. LN not belonging to the special group in category B5a (see p. 187), but being confluent or containing microcalcification. This requires complete diagnostic excision of the lesions detected by diagnostic imaging.

4. Flat epithelial atypia associated with microcalcification, and with residual microcalcification detected after the diagnostic intervention. Residual microcalcification should be completely removed by CNB or excision biopsy, and the underlying lesion should be histologically examined.

5. Portions of a papillary lesion or portions of a radial scar with residues of the target lesion (focal lesion or microcalcification) detected by imaging. The residual lesion should be completely removed by excision biopsy and examined histologically.

6. Portions of a phyllodes tumor and biopsies suspicious of phyllodes tumors require complete excision of the focal lesion together with a layer of healthy tissue.

7. Less common lesions representing an indication for excision and definitive identification. Examples include spindle cell proliferations, mucocele-like lesions, and cystic hypersecretory lesions.

Examples 1 to 3 probably carry higher risks than examples 4 to 7. We completely agree with Ibrahim et al (2001) that category B3 may contain subgroups carrying unequal risks. However, these may not play a reproducible role in the decision-making process because of considerable variability in the overall situations. Possible subgroups B3a and B3b, when assigned by the pathologist without any team discussion, are therefore problematic. They may lead to a wrong decision and are therefore not included in the European Guidelines for Quality Assurance in Breast Cancer Screening and Diagnosis (Wells et al, 2006b).

- **B4—suspicious of malignancy:**
  All lesions with this classification are subject to repeat biopsy (action category A4). The interdisciplinary team has only to decide on the safest method to arrive at a definitive diagnosis.

- **B5—malignant lesion:**
  Malignant lesions require a treatment plan adjusted to the respective lesion (action category A5). It is important to obtain as much information as possible from the CNB to help planning the surgery. The situation may also require repeat CNB for detailed planning (e.g., for examining associated microcalcifications in an invasive carcinoma).

Suggested Solution for Borderline Lesion: Atypical Ductal Type Epithelial Proliferation

Definition. The term atypical ductal type epithelial proliferation (AEPDT) is a technical term exclusively used in CNB diagnosis (Wells et al, 2006b). The criteria include

- Proliferation of an atypical cell population (largely monomorphic) of non-high-grade nuclear malignancy (usually low grade; nuclear diameter < that of three to two erythrocytes)
- The neoplastic cells form secondary histologic structures.

These features apply to both atypical ductal hyperplasia (ADH) and non-high-grade DCIS.

ADH and DCIS differ by the following quantitative criterion: ADH is restricted to one glandular lobe, whereas DCIS characteristically involves large extralobular ductal portions (**Fig. 13.20**). When ductal involvement is confirmed, a definitive diagnosis of DCIS by CNB is possible. When extralobular involvement cannot be confirmed within the specimen, this does not mean the lesion is restricted to a lobule. A duct affected by DCIS may be in the immediate area, but did not get included in the biopsy specimen. The conclusion is that a diagnosis of ADH by CNB is never certain. The European Guidelines (European Guidelines for Quality Assurance in Breast Cancer Screening and Diagnosis, 2006) recommend that the diagnostic term ADH should not be applied to CNB results. Instead, the term AEPDT is to be used here for lesions identical to ADH. The term thus carries the information that a decision between ADH and non-high-grade DCIS is not possible (**Fig. 13.21**). Hence, the lesion is assigned to category B3.

Frequency. Under the conditions of population-based mammographic screening, AIEP was with 35.3% the second most common B3 lesion among 5000 consecutive CNB results (unpublished data of the pathology databank of the German mammogram reference center, Pathologie-Datenbank des Referenzzentrums Mammografie, Münster, 2008). In the largest CNB series published so far, with follow-up data from 4035 patients without reference to screening, 46.2% of the B3 lesions were identified as AEPDT (Houssami et al, 2007).

Risk. If the CNB diagnosis is AEPDT, the risk of having a synchronous malignant lesion (DCIS or invasive carcinoma) in the same breast that underwent biopsy is at least 40% (Harvey et al, 2002; Houssami et al, 2007; Jackman et al, 1999; Lee et al, 2003).

Approach. Because of this synchronous risk, the diagnosis of AEPDT requires immediate histologic examination. However, the modus of the repeat biopsy should be selected depending on the overall situation. Although a definitive diagnosis is in many cases only achieved by open (excision) biopsy, this is not unavoidable in every case. The repeat biopsy method should rely on the correlation between the first biopsy and the target lesion because

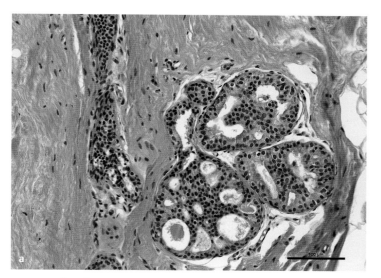
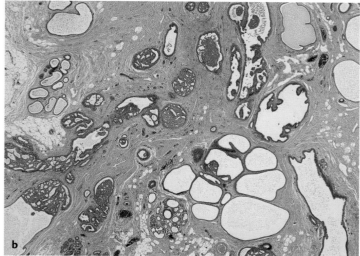

Fig. 13.20a,b Differentiation between ADH and DCIS.
a Cross-section of atypical ductal hyperplasia with involvement of a lobule. The duct on the left is not involved.
b Cross-section of a DCIS, showing the involvement of numerous ducts and cystic dilation of lobules.

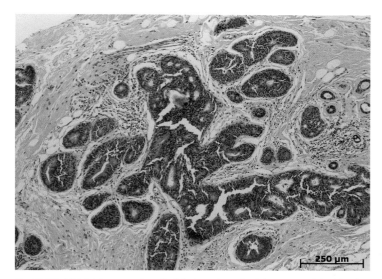
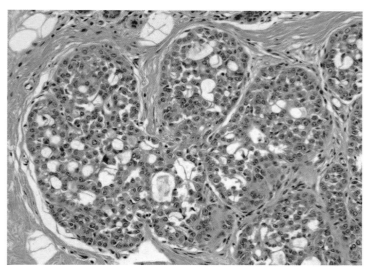

Fig. 13.21 AEPDT. Cross-section of a lobule with marked distension of the glands by atypical cells.

Fig. 13.22 LCIS. Cross-section of an enlarged lobule with dilated acini containing monomorphically atypical tumor cells.

13

AEPDT almost never produces an imaging result on its own. Excision of the area of the previous biopsy is the method of choice when the histologic correlate to the imaging findings is definitely benign and AEPDT is an additional finding. When no such correlate is found in the biopsy, one should consider whether the suspicious target lesion detected by imaging may be reached by repeat CNB.

Suggested Solution for Borderline Lesion: Lobular Neoplasia

Definition. Traditionally, noninvasive LN is classified according to quantitative criteria as atypical lobular hyperplasia (ALH) and lobular carcinoma in situ (LCIS) (Foote and Steward, 1941) (**Fig. 13.22**). Because of the moderate reproducibility particularly with CNB, the term lobular neoplasia (LN) introduced by Haagensen et al (1978) includes both groups; it is often preferred and has also been adopted into the WHO classification (Tavassoli and Devilee, 2003). Further attempts at quantifying LN using the lob-

ular intraepithelial neoplasia (LIN) classification system (Bratthauer and Tavassoli, 2002) has not proven successful internationally (Hanby and Hughes, 2008).

Frequency. It is very difficult to estimate the incidence of LN. Because LN on its own almost never produces a focal lesion and rarely microcalcifications, it is mostly detected accidentally (Simpson et al, 2003; Sonnenfeld et al, 1991; Sapino et al, 2000). The frequency of LN in otherwise benign CNB specimens has been reported at 0.5% to 3.8% (Haagensen et al, 1978; Page et al, 1991). More recent population-based data of over 8 million women from the Surveillance, Epidemiology, and End Results (SEER) program in the United States showed an incidence of 5 in 100000 for 1997–2001, which amounts to an increase by a factor of 2.6 when compared with the period of 1980–1996 (Li et al, 2005). According to the older literature, LN occurs preferentially in women between 40 and 55 years of age and in premenopausal women, with an incidence of >90% (Haagensen et al, 1978; Simpson et al, 2003). In the SEER data, however, the increased incidence during the late 1990s was largely caused by the increased number of women between 50 and 60 years of age.

Risk. The literature on excision biopsy findings after diagnosis of LN in a CNB specimen is confusing and contradictory for the following reasons: the studies were almost exclusively retrospective on small groups of patients, additional risk lesions were present, and the indication for surgical intervention was rarely reported. The largest, partly prospective study by Elsheikh and Silverman (2005) yielded a rate of 28 % for synchronous carcinomas (DCIS or invasive carcinomas); however, it included only a total of 33 patients with LN. The pleomorphic variant of LN is still biologically and clinically insufficiently characterized. First described in 1992 (Eusebi et al, 1992), data on isolated pleomorphic LN (without concurrent invasive carcinoma) were published only in 2002 (Sneige et al, 2002), without clearly demonstrating an increased risk.

Approach. The answer to the question whether a histologic correlate to the radiologic target lesion exists provides a basis for the decision on how to proceed after detecting LN. Only in the rare cases of directly associated microcalcification does LN represent this correlate. LN is usually discovered accidentally when symptomatic findings or imaging results caused by other lesions are examined. Nevertheless, LN may only be considered clinically irrelevant when another histologic finding in the biopsy specimen clearly represents the correlate to the radiologic target lesion, and when no uncertainties remain. The decision on how to proceed is therefore always made by the interdisciplinary team. If the correlation is uncertain, the indication for histologic diagnosis still remains. Repeat biopsy (CNB or diagnostic excision) is indicated without delay. If microcalcification is detected in the LN, LN of the extended type is usually present and the microcalcifications are present in the comedo necroses. This subtype, like pleomorphic LN with which it shares part of the definition, is treated by agreement in the same way as a DCIS without much evidence. When the CNB target is a focal lesion and when a clear correlate to this focal lesion exists (e. g., fibroadenoma), LN may be considered an accidental finding that does not require further diagnosis. A prerequisite is the exclusion of any concurrent malignant lesion. No data on prospective studies exist for the radiologic follow-up after diagnosis of LN and for its relevance to the survival of women who develop metachronous invasive carcinoma. Nevertheless, there is agreement to check up on these women at least according to the medium risk criteria (annual mammograms at two levels on both sides) (Lakhani et al, 2006). Clinical studies on the role of MRI are currently incomplete.

Quality Indicators of the Pathologic Diagnosis

Sensitivity and specificity. CNB requires continuous quality assurance by the interdisciplinary team. Quality assurance in pathology is an integral component. The main indicators are sensitivity and specificity, which are established using the results of surgical interventions and patient follow-up. The interdisciplinary data must therefore be documented and communicated to establish these parameters. This is facilitated by auxiliary means that are easy to handle during the daily routine. These include protocols for histopathologic processing, checklists for clinical data and pathologic findings, the use of diagnostic categories (BI-

RADS categories, B categories), and the use of internationally uniform nomenclature. The nonobligatory categories used by our team for the overall clinical and image score (OCI), the radiologic–pathologic correlation (CO), and the resulting action categories (A) enable us to determine specific sensitivities and specificities for individual components of the interdisciplinary diagnostic process. Furthermore, we can measure the impact of the individual correlation- and decision-making steps by the effect on sensitivity and specificity.

Random-corrected concordance statistics. For the pathologic results within a group of team pathologists as well as among pathologists of large screening programs random-corrected concordance statistics are far more informative than percentage concordance analyses. Using kappa statistics for this purpose also makes it possible to analyze the homogeneity of the diagnostics and is psychologically motivating because individual participants compare their own assessment with that of other participants.

References

Abd El-Rehim DM, Pinder SE, Paish CE, et al. Expression of luminal and basal cytokeratins in human breast carcinoma. J Pathol 2004;203(2):661–671

Bassett L, Winchester DP, Caplan RB, et al. Stereotactic core-needle biopsy of the breast: a report of the Joint Task Force of the American College of Radiology, American College of Surgeons, and College of American Pathologists. CA Cancer J Clin 1997;47(3):171–190

Boecker W, Buerger H, Herbst H. Basic principles of benign proliferative breast disease. In: Boecker W, ed. Preneoplasia of the Breast. Munich: Elsevier; 2006:129–144

Boecker W, Buerger H, Schmitz K, et al. Ductal epithelial proliferations of the breast: a biological continuum? Comparative genomic hybridization and high-molecular-weight cytokeratin expression patterns. J Pathol 2001;195 (4):415–421

Boecker W, Moll R, Dervan P, et al. Usual ductal hyperplasia of the breast is a committed stem (progenitor) cell lesion distinct from atypical ductal hyperplasia and ductal carcinoma in situ. J Pathol 2002;198(4):458–467

Bratthauer GL, Tavassoli FA. Lobular intraepithelial neoplasia: previously unexplored aspects assessed in 775 cases and their clinical implications. Virchows Arch 2002;440(2):134–138

Britton PD, McCann J. Needle biopsy in the NHS breast screening programme 1996/97: how much and how accurate? Breast 1999;8:5–11

Britton PD. Fine needle aspiration or core biopsy. Breast 1999;8:1–4

Buerger H, Otterbach F, Simon R, et al. Comparative genomic hybridization of ductal carcinoma in situ of the breast-evidence of multiple genetic pathways. J Pathol 1999;187(4):396–402

Buerger H, Schmidt H, Beckmann A, Zänker KS, Boecker W, Brandt B. Genetic characterisation of invasive breast cancer: a comparison of CGH and PCR based multiplex microsatellite analysis. J Clin Pathol 2001;54(11):836–840

Bundesmantelvertrag – Ärzte/Ersatzkassen über besondere Versorgungsaufträge im Rahmen des Programms zur Früherkennung von Brustkrebs durch Mammografie-Screening. Anlage 9.2 Versorgung im Rahmen des Programms zur Früherkennung von Brustkrebs durch Mammografie-Screening. Dtsch Arztebl 2004;4:16–44

Cattoretti G. Standardization and reproducibility in diagnostic immunohistochemistry. Hum Pathol 1994;25(10):1107–1109

Dahlstrom JE, Sutton S, Jain S. Histologic–radiologic correlation of mammographically detected microcalcification in stereotactic core biopsies. Am J Surg Pathol 1998;22(2):256–259

Decker T, Boecker W, Kettritz U, et al. Pathological diagnosis in minimal invasive biopsy. In: Boecker W, ed. Preneoplasia of the Breast. Munich: Elsevier; 2006:81–106

Dontu G, Al-Hajj M, Abdallah WM, Clarke MF, Wicha MS. Stem cells in normal breast development and breast cancer. Cell Prolif 2003;36(Suppl 1):59–72

Ellis IO, Humphreys S, Michell M, Pinder SE, Wells CA, Zakhour HD; UK National Coordinating Commmittee for Breast Screening Pathology; European Commission Working Group on Breast Screening Pathology. Best Practice No 179. Guidelines for breast needle core biopsy handling and reporting in breast screening assessment. J Clin Pathol 2004;57(9):897–902

Elsheikh TM, Silverman JF. Follow-up surgical excision is indicated when breast core needle biopsies show atypical lobular hyperplasia or lobular carcinoma in situ: a correlative study of 33 patients with review of the literature. Am J Surg Pathol 2005;29(4):534–543

European Guidelines for Quality Assurance in Breast Cancer Screening and Diagnosis. 4th ed. Luxembourg: Office for Official Publications of the European Communities; 2006

European Guidelines for Quality Assurance in Breast Cancer Screening and Diagnosis. 3rd ed. Luxembourg: European Communities; 2001

Eusebi V, Magalhaes F, Azzopardi JG. Pleomorphic lobular carcinoma of the breast: an aggressive tumor showing apocrine differentiation. Hum Pathol 1992;23(6):655–662

Farabegoli F, Champeme MH, Bieche I, et al. Genetic pathways in the evolution of breast ductal carcinoma in situ. J Pathol 2002;196(3):280–286

Fitzgibbons PL, Henson DE, Hutter RV; Cancer Committee of the College of American Pathologists. Benign breast changes and the risk for subsequent breast cancer: an update of the 1985 consensus statement. Arch Pathol Lab Med 1998;122(12):1053–1055

Foote FW, Steward FW. Lobular carcinoma in situ. Am J Pathol 1941;17 (4):491–496

Goldstein NS, Ferkowicz M, Odish E, Mani A, Hastah F. Minimum formalin fixation time for consistent estrogen receptor immunohistochemical staining of invasive breast carcinoma. Am J Clin Pathol 2003;120(1):86–92

Guidelines Working Group of the National Coordinating Committee for Breast Pathology. The Royal College of Pathologists. Pathology Reporting of Breast Disease. Minimum Dataset for Breast Cancer Histopathology. 2nd ed. Sheffield, UK: NHS Cancer Screening Programmes and The Royal College of Pathologists; 2005

Haagensen CD, Lane N, Lattes R, Bodian C. Lobular neoplasia (so-called lobular carcinoma in situ) of the breast. Cancer 1978;42(2):737–769

Hanby AM, Hughes TA. In situ and invasive lobular neoplasia of the breast. Histopathology 2008;52(1):58–66

Harvey JM, Sterrett GF, Frost FA. Atypical ductal hyperplasia and atypia of uncertain significance in core biopsies from mammographically detected lesions: correlation with excision diagnosis. Pathology 2002;34(5):410–416

Heywang-Köbrunner SH, Schreer I, Decker T, Böcker W. Interdisciplinary consensus on the use and technique of vacuum-assisted stereotactic breast biopsy. Eur J Radiol 2003;47(3):232–236

Houssami N, Ciatto S, Bilous M, Vezzosi V, Bianchi S. Borderline breast core needle histology: predictive values for malignancy in lesions of uncertain malignant potential (B3). Br J Cancer 2007;96(8):1253–1257

Ibrahim AEK, Bateman AC, Theaker JM, et al. The role and histological classification of needle core biopsy in comparison with fine needle aspiration cytology in the preoperative assessment of impalpable breast lesions. J Clin Pathol 2001;54(2):121–125

Jackman RJ, Nowels KW, Rodriguez-Soto J, Marzoni FA Jr, Finkelstein SI, Shepard MJ. Stereotactic, automated, large-core needle biopsy of nonpalpable breast lesions: false-negative and histologic underestimation rates after long-term follow-up. Radiology 1999;210(3):799–805

Jacquemier J, Padovani L, Rabayrol L, et al; European Working Group for Breast Screening Pathology; Breast Cancer Linkage Consortium. Typical medullary breast carcinomas have a basal/myoepithelial phenotype. J Pathol 2005;207 (3):260–268

Korsching E, Jeffrey SS, Meinerz W, Decker T, Boecker W, Buerger H. Basal carcinoma of the breast revisited: an old entity with new interpretations. J Clin Pathol 2008;61(5):553–560

Lakhani SR, Audretsch W, Cleton-Jensen AM, et al; EUSOMA. The management of lobular carcinoma in situ (LCIS). Is LCIS the same as ductal carcinoma in situ (DCIS)? Eur J Cancer 2006;42(14):2205–2211

Lee AHS, Denley HE, Pinder SE, et al; Nottingham Breast Team. Excision biopsy findings of patients with breast needle core biopsies reported as suspicious of malignancy (B4) or lesion of uncertain malignant potential (B3). Histopathology 2003;42(4):331–336

Li CI, Daling JR, Malone KE. Age-specific incidence rates of in situ breast carcinomas by histologic type, 1980 to 2001. Cancer Epidemiol Biomarkers Prev 2005;14(4):1008–1011

Livasy CA, Karaca G, Nanda R, et al. Phenotypic evaluation of the basal-like subtype of invasive breast carcinoma. Mod Pathol 2006;19(2):264–271

Nagle RB, Böcker W, Davis JR, et al. Characterization of breast carcinomas by two monoclonal antibodies distinguishing myoepithelial from luminal epithelial cells. J Histochem Cytochem 1986;34(7):869–881

National Coordinating Group for Breast Screening Pathology. Guidelines for breast pathology. NHSBSP Publication No. 2. Sheffield, UK: NHS Breast Screening Programme; 1997

Osin P, Shipley J, Lu YJ, Crook T, Gusterson BA. Experimental pathology and breast cancer genetics: new technologies. Recent Results Cancer Res 1998;152 : 35–48

Page DL, Kidd TE Jr, Dupont WD, Simpson JF, Rogers LW. Lobular neoplasia of the breast: higher risk for subsequent invasive cancer predicted by more extensive disease. Hum Pathol 1991;22(12):1232–1239

Perou CM, Sørlie T, Eisen MB, et al. Molecular portraits of human breast tumours. Nature 2000;406(6797):747–752

Sapino A, Frigerio A, Peterse JL, Arisio R, Coluccia C, Bussolati G. Mammographically detected in situ lobular carcinomas of the breast. Virchows Arch 2000;436(5):421–430

Shannon J, Douglas-Jones AG, Dallimore NS. Conversion to core biopsy in preoperative diagnosis of breast lesions: is it justified by results? J Clin Pathol 2001;54(10):762–765

Simpson PT, Gale T, Fulford LG, Reis-Filho JS, Lakhani SR. The diagnosis and management of pre-invasive breast disease: pathology of atypical lobular hyperplasia and lobular carcinoma in situ. Breast Cancer Res 2003;5 (5):258–262

Sneige N, Wang J, Baker BA, Krishnamurthy S, Middleton LP. Clinical, histopathologic, and biologic features of pleomorphic lobular (ductal-lobular) carcinoma in situ of the breast: a report of 24 cases. Mod Pathol 2002;15 (10):1044–1050

Sonnenfeld MR, Frenna TH, Weidner N, Meyer JE. Lobular carcinoma in situ: mammographic-pathologic correlation of results of needle-directed biopsy. Radiology 1991;181(2):363–367

Sørlie T, Perou CM, Tibshirani R, et al. Gene expression patterns of breast carcinomas distinguish tumor subclasses with clinical implications. Proc Natl Acad Sci U S A 2001;98(19):10869–10874

Start RD, Flynn MS, Cross SS, Rogers K, Smith JH. Is the grading of breast carcinomas affected by a delay in fixation? Virchows Arch A Pathol Anat Histopathol 1991;419(6):475–477

Stufe-3-Leitlinie, Brustkrebs-Früherkennung in Deutschland. 2nd ed. Munich: Zuckschwerdt; 2008

Tavassoli FA, Devilee P. Pathology and genetics of tumours of the breast and female genital organs. In: World Health Organisation, Classification of Tumours. Lyon: IARC-Press; 2003

Wells CA, Amendoeira I, Apostolikas N, et al. Quality assurance guidelines for pathology. In: Perry NM, Broeders M, de Wolf C, et al. European guidelines for quality assurance in breast cancer screening and diagnosis. 4th ed. Luxembourg: Office for Official Publications of the European Communities; 2006a: 219–311

Wells CA, Amendoeira I, Apostolikas N, et al. Quality assurance guidelines for pathology – Cytological and histological non-operative procedures. In: Perry NM, Broeders M, de Wolf C, et al. European guidelines for quality assurance in breast cancer screening and diagnosis. 4th ed. Luxembourg: Office for Official Publications of the European Communities; 2006b: 219–256

Wells WA, Carney PA, Eliassen MS, Grove MR, Tosteson AN. Pathologists' agreement with experts and reproducibility of breast ductal carcinoma-in-situ classification schemes. Am J Surg Pathol 2000;24(5):651–659

Wetzels RH, Holland R, van Haelst UJ, Lane EB, Leigh IM, Ramaekers FC. Detection of basement membrane components and basal cell keratin 14 in noninvasive and invasive carcinomas of the breast. Am J Pathol 1989;134(3):571–579

13

14 Tumor Cell Displacement

U. Fischer

Of great importance is the serious concern about malignant tumor cell displacement and the possible promotion of tumor recurrence due to iatrogenic seeding during the performance of percutaneous interventions.

Tumor cell displacement. Several studies have reported a tumor cell displacement rate in histologic specimens of 2% to 54%. The most reliable histopathologic study of the actual needle tract in 325 cases reported a rate of approx. 30%. This convincing study also demonstrated that the incidence and amount of tumor cell displacement was inversely related to the time interval between core needle biopsy (CNB) and excision, and suggests that tumor cells do not survive displacement. Tumor cell displacement was seen in 42% of patients with an interval between biopsy and excision of ≤2 weeks, and in only 15% when the tumors were excised >4 weeks after CNB. This study also provides evidence that tumor cell displacement is influenced by the tumor histology. It was found that invasive ductal carcinoma (IDC) has a higher rate of tumor cell displacement than ductal carcinoma in situ (DCIS) or invasive lobular carcinoma (ILC). Comparison of the rate of tumor displacement for CNB and vacuum-assisted biopsy (VAB) showed a lower rate for the VAB technique.

Recurrence. A limited number of studies investigate the relationship between percutaneous biopsy and local recurrence. The grade of evidence of these analyses, however, is level 4 because the number of cases studied were too small and/or no correlation of the recurrence location to the needle tract was made.

Conclusion. In summary, there is no current high-grade evidence for the recommendation to excise the needle tract after percutaneous needle biopsy or tumor localization. It cannot, however, be completely discounted that a local recurrence may develop in the needle tract if it has not been excised, as this has been reported in individual case histories. The cases of such local recurrences reported in the literature, however, developed without exception in patients who did not receive adjuvant radiotherapy.

Further Reading

Diaz LK, Wiley EL, Venta LA. Are malignant cells displaced by large-gauge needle core biopsy of the breast? AJR Am J Roentgenol 1999;173(5):1303–1313

Liberman L, Dershaw DD, Rosen PP, Morris EA, Abramson AF, Borgen PI. Percutaneous removal of malignant mammographic lesions at stereotactic vacuum-assisted biopsy. Radiology 1998;206(3):711–715

Stolier A, Skinner J, Levine EA. A prospective study of seeding of the skin after core biopsy of the breast. Am J Surg 2000;180(2):104–107

Thurfjell MG, Jansson T, Nordgren H, Bergh J, Lindgren A, Thurfjell E. Local breast cancer recurrence caused by mammographically guided punctures. Acta Radiol 2000;41(5):435–440

Youngson BJ, Cranor M, Rosen PP. Epithelial displacement in surgical breast specimens following needling procedures. Am J Surg Pathol 1994;18(9):896–903

15 Guidelines for the Early Detection of Breast Cancer: Interventions and Excision Biopsy

U. Fischer

Condensed Version: Intervention

Percutaneous core biopsy, vacuum-assisted biopsy (VAB), or open biopsy should be performed to obtain tissue samples for histologic assessment of ambiguous breast findings. Percutaneous interventions should be performed according to quality assurance recommendations.

Fine needle aspiration biopsy (FNAB) cannot be recommended as a standard diagnostic method.

Image-guided interventions are performed to obtain tissue samples for histologic verification and therapy planning from mammographic findings in the BI-RADS categories 4 and 5, and/or ultrasonographic findings in the BI-RADS categories 4 and 5, and/or magnetic resonance imaging (MRI) findings in the BI-RADS categories 4 and 5.

Percutaneous large core needle biopsies (CNBs) should be ultrasound (US)-guided. At least four tissue samples using a ≤14-gauge needle should be harvested.

When biopsying microcalcifications, stereotactic VAB technique should be employed.

The VAB technique should also be employed for MRI-guided interventions.

The stereotactic VAB procedure should be standardized. The needle access path and stroke margin must be documented. To document the correct needle position, the following are required: a scout image, the stereo pair images, and the prefire pair and postbiopsy pair images. At least 12 tissue samples should be harvested when using an 11-gauge needle. If using needles with a different caliber (8 to 11 gauge), the number of specimens harvested should yield an equivalent tissue volume.

A specimen radiograph is required to verify correct tissue sampling and should be obtained using a magnification view. Successful sampling is confirmed when representative microcalcifications are detected in the tissue samples. Separating the samples with microcalcifications from those without often facilitates the detection of these for the pathologist.

After VAB, a final mammographic documentation of the biopsied breast in two orthogonal planes should be performed.

After each minimally invasive, image-guided intervention, correlation of imaging with histology should be performed to verify a representative biopsy.

If the biopsy results are benign, a short-term follow-up in the respective imaging modality should be recommended in 6 months.

categories 4 and 5, and/or MR-mammographic findings in the BI-RADS categories 4 and 5 that are histologically verified by an appropriate image-guided biopsy: ≥70%

- The proportion of nonpalpable findings that are histologically verified preoperatively by mammographic-, sonographic-, or MRI-guided CNB or VAB: ≥70%
- The proportion of palpable and nonpalpable findings that are histologically verified preoperatively by mammographic-, sonographic-, or MRI-guided CNB or VAB: ≥90%
- The proportion of interventions for mammographic findings with microcalcifications in the BI-RADS categories 4 and 5 that have representative microcalcifications detected in the specimen radiograph: ≥95%
- The proportion of cases in which surgical excision reveals a malignant finding after image-guided biopsy has yielded a benign finding (B classification 1 or 2) (false-negative): <10%

Condensed Version: Excision Biopsy

The preoperative localization of nonpalpable mammographic lesions should aim to place the localization wire so that it penetrates the target lesion and does not project more than 1 cm past the distal border. If it does not penetrate the lesion, it should be placed ≤ 1 cm from the target lesion. When localizing a nonmass lesion, however, two or more markers/wires can be placed at the surgically relevant borders without adhering to the 1-cm limit.

The preoperative localization of nonpalpable breast lesions and the imaging confirmation of correct excision is indispensable.

The surgical excision of lesions detected only by US should be verified by intraoperative specimen US.

The excision specimen should be clearly marked by the surgeon to ensure proper orientation. It should be sent to the pathologist without further incisions after removal from the breast.

A frozen section to attain an intraoperative statement about a lesion's histology should only be performed in exceptional cases. Prerequisites for a frozen section on a breast specimen are:

- The lesion is palpable intraoperatively and in the specimen.
- The lesion is large enough (generally >10 mm).

Quality indicators with tentative reference values.

- The proportion of mammographic findings in the BI-RADS categories 4 and 5 with a correlating sonographic finding, which undergo a US-guided core biopsy that satisfies the quality standard specifications: ≥70%
- The proportion of mammographic findings that contain microcalcifications, are in the BI-RADS categories 4 and 5, and are without a correlating sonographic finding, which undergo a stereotactic VAB that satisfies the quality standard specifications: ≥70%
- The proportion of MR-mammographic findings in the BI-RADS categories 4 and 5 that are solely seen on MR mammography, which undergo an MRI-guided VAB that satisfies the quality standard specifications: ≥95%
- The proportion of mammographic findings in the BI-RADS categories 4 and 5, and/or sonographic findings in the BI-RADS

Quality indicators with tentative reference values.

- The proportion of breast operations after preoperative wire localization in which the wire is placed ≤1 cm from the lesion border: ≥95%
- The proportion of breast operations after preoperative mammographic localization with intraoperative specimen radiography: ≥95%
- The proportion of breast operations after preoperative US-guided localization with intraoperative specimen US: ≥95%
- The proportion of excision specimens that are clearly topographically marked by the surgeon: ≥95%

15

Evidence-Based Medicine: Interventional Techniques

Basic Principles

Needle biopsy techniques can be performed:
- to verify the presence of a suspected malignancy (before neoadjuvant chemotherapy and for surgical planning)
- for minimally invasive histologic work-up of ambiguous and nonpalpable breast findings

The quality assurance of these procedures encompasses the following aspects:
- the technique used (targeting the lesion, harvesting specimens)
- the processing and assessment of the pathologic/cytologic specimen
- the appraisal of pathologic results and the resultant therapy planning

Choice of Method

Guidance. Palpable findings can be percutaneously biopsied with or without sonographic guidance. For the biopsy of nonpalpable imaging findings, the imaging method used for needle guidance should be chosen according to which method visualizes the lesion best and is the most reliable. This can be mammography (stereotactic), US, or MRI.

Puncture method. The current standard biopsy methods are the large CNB and the VAB. FNAB is reserved for a very few specific indications. Which puncture method to choose is dependent upon the clinical constellation and the attainable accuracy of each method.

In this regard, the puncture methods have significant differences:
- The FNAB cannot be recommended as a standard biopsy method (level of evidence [LOE] 3b–3a). Its application should be limited to special cases (complicated cysts, lymph nodes) where specific cytology results can be expected.
- Using a standardized technique (see below), the large CNB reaches a sensitivity of 85 to 98% (LOE 3b–3a).
- VAB reaches a sensitivity of over 98% using a standardized technique (LOE 3b–3a).

Quality assurance. The practice guidelines of the American College of Radiology (ACR) first included quality assurance measures for breast interventions in 1997. They currently apply to the equipment specifications and technical standards for diagnostic physics performance monitoring of imaging equipment, indications and contraindications for the performance of image-guided breast interventional procedures, and documentation (including image documentation) of the needle position, pathologic results, problems encountered, and follow-up recommendations. In addition, the ACR practice guidelines also include the minimum qualification requirements of the examiner, and the—albeit relatively small—number of interventions the examiner must perform per year to maintain his or her expertise.

To promote the quality of core biopsy and VAB performance, studies pertaining to the optimal needle diameter and the number of specimens to be harvested have been performed and recommendations based on these studies exist in voluntary practice guidelines. In addition, a quality-assured procedural protocol has been developed specifically for the performance of MRI-guided interventions (VAB, preoperative localization; Breast Diagnostics Working Committee of the German Radiology Association).

Independent of the biopsy method performed, it is always essential that histology be correlated with the diagnostic imaging (EU and ACR guidelines) to recognize biopsies that are not representative. Results that are discordant with the imaging assessment must be discussed in an interdisciplinary conference. A therapeutic recommendation can only be made after a representative biopsy has been ensured. If this is not the case, a repeat intervention or open biopsy must be performed.

Summary

Thorough quality assurance on different levels is necessary for the performance of high-standard percutaneous interventions. High accuracy has been reported for CNB and VAB, but not, however, for FNAB. Quality standards for CNB and VAB have been developed.

> **Guidelines**
>
> Each ambiguous finding must be histologically verified using the most effective image-guidance method.

Structural Quality: Interventional Techniques

Percutaneous Biopsy

Personnel requirements
Physician:
1. Extensive knowledge and experience in breast diagnostic imaging, including the diagnostic image work-up of ambiguous findings, is a prerequisite for the reliable identification and localization of the significant lesion(s) on mammography in two orthogonal planes.
2. For the performance of stereotactic interventions: Performance of at least 30 stereotactic breast biopsy procedures under the supervision of a qualified physician, *or* performance of at least 10 stereotactic breast biopsy procedures under the supervision of a qualified company representative and at least 20 stereotactic breast biopsy procedures under the supervision of a qualified physician. Extensive knowledge of how to verify calibration (10 independently performed verification procedures) is also necessary.
3. For the performance of US-guided interventions: Extensive knowledge and experience in diagnostic breast US examination and performance of at least 30 US-guided breast biopsy procedures under the supervision of a qualified physician.
4. For the performance of MRI-guided interventions: Extensive knowledge and experience in diagnostic MR mammography and performance of at least 30 MRI-guided breast biopsy procedures under the supervision of a qualified physician.
5. For the maintenance of competence, the performance of at least 50 stereotactic-guided percutaneous biopsies per year, at least 50 US-guided percutaneous biopsies per year, and/or at least 50 MRI-guided VABs per year are recommended.

Certified radiologist's assistant:

1. Certification after having successfully completed an advanced academic program encompassing specialized training in breast diagnostics
2. For the performance of stereotactic-guided interventions:
   - extensive knowledge pertaining to the mammographic imaging technique, including image quality, breast positioning, radiation protection
   - vocational training in how to verify calibration (at least 10 verifications) and performance of at least 10 stereotactic breast biopsy procedures under the supervision of a an experienced radiologist's assistant, a medical physicist/technologist, or engineer

Technical quality control

Certified radiologist's assistant:

- verification of the stereotactic unit calibration on each day an intervention is performed, at least once a week
- test of localization accuracy once a month for each needle used

Medical physicist:

- quality assurance measures for the mammographic unit according to the manufacturer's specifications

Documentation. The diagnostician must be a member of an interdisciplinary team in which members from the specialties of diagnostic imaging, interventional diagnostics, and pathology cooperate according to a protocol, *or* be a member of a certified breast center. Regular interdisciplinary case conferences should be instituted.

Requirements:

- acquisition of the results data from all percutaneous biopsies for statistical analysis
- follow-up examination of all patients 6 months after percutaneous biopsy with benign histology
- interdisciplinary consultation to confer on histopathologic results that are unclear or discordant with diagnostic imaging

Localization of Nonpalpable Findings

Personnel requirements

Physician:

1. Extensive knowledge and experience in breast diagnostic imaging, including the diagnostic image work-up of ambiguous findings, is a prerequisite for the reliable identification and localization of the significant lesion(s) on mammography in 2 orthogonal planes.
2. For performance using the free-hand technique (fenestrated compression device): Performance of at least 20 localization procedures under the supervision of a qualified physician
3. For the performance using the stereotactic technique: Performance of at least 20 localization procedures under the supervision of a qualified physician, *or* performance of at least 10 stereotactic localization procedures under the supervision of a qualified company representative and at least 10 stereotactic localization procedures under the supervision of a qualified physician. Extensive knowledge of how to verify calibration (10 independent verifications) is also necessary.

4. For the performance of US-guided localization procedures: Extensive knowledge and experience in diagnostic breast US examination and performance of at least 30 US-guided localization procedures under the supervision of a qualified physician (see DEGUM requirements for breast US, level II)
5. For performance of MRI-guided localization procedures: Extensive knowledge and experience in diagnostic MR mammography and performance of at least 30 MRI-guided localization procedures under the supervision of a qualified physician.
6. For the maintenance of competence, the performance of at least 25 stereotactic-guided percutaneous biopsies per year, at least 25 US-guided percutaneous biopsies per year, and/or at least 25 MRI-guided VABs per year are recommended.

Certified radiologist's assistant:

1. Certification after having successfully completed an advanced academic program encompassing specialized training in breast diagnostics
2. For the performance of stereotactic-guided interventions:
   - extensive knowledge pertaining to the mammographic technique, including image quality, breast positioning, radiation protection
   - vocational training in how to verify calibration (at least 10 verifications) and performance of at least 10 stereotactic breast biopsy procedures under the supervision of an experienced radiologist's assistant, a medical physicist/technologist, or engineer

Technical quality control

Certified radiologist's assistant:

- verification of the stereotactic unit calibration on each day a localization is performed, at least once a week
- quality control measures regarding film processing, if film is used (on each day a localization is performed, or at least once a week)
- test of localization accuracy once a month for each needle used
- quality assurance measures for the mammographic unit according to the manufacturer's specifications

Documentation. The diagnostician must be a member of an interdisciplinary team in which members from the specialties of diagnostic imaging, interventional diagnostics, and pathology cooperate according to a protocol, *or* be a member of a certified breast center. Regular interdisciplinary case conferences should be instituted.

Process Quality: Interventional Techniques

The methods available for excluding malignancy or verifying a diagnosis before planning further therapy of breast lesions in the BI-RADS categories 4 and 5 are large CNB, VAB, and open biopsy with or without preoperative localization. The method used depends upon the clinical situation and the required accuracy, and is influenced by the diagnostician's attainable accuracy.

Algorithm. See **Fig. 15.1**.

15

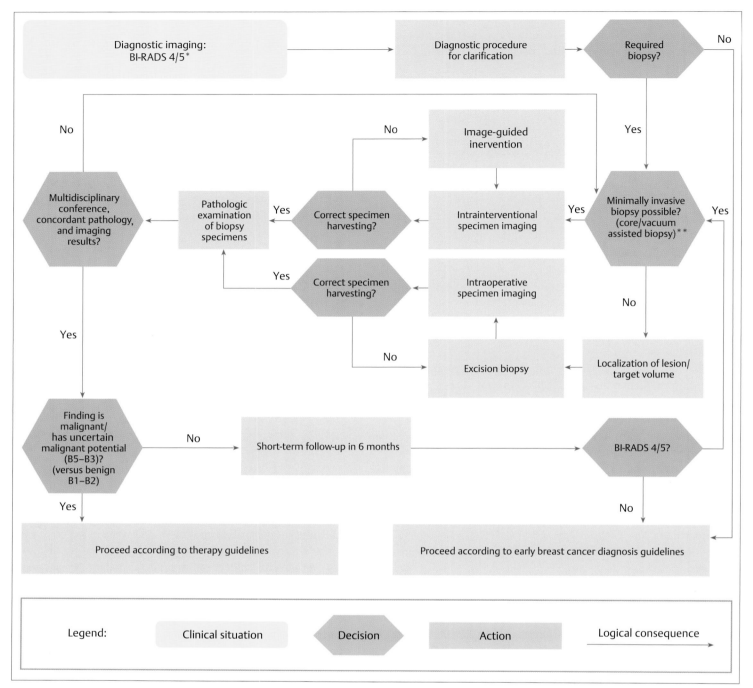

Fig. 15.1 Course of action algorithm for breast findings requiring biopsy in accordance with current guidelines.
 * Basic diagnostic examinations completed (clinical examination, mammography, US).
 ** Accepted reasons for not performing a minimally invasive biopsy (MIB): patient wishes, primary open biopsy preferred (e. g., coagulopathy, medically required anticoagulant therapy, elderly patient, unfavorable lesion position for CNB, suspected intracystic proliferation).

15

Percutaneous Biopsy

Definition. A percutaneous biopsy involves the removal and examination of tissue samples from breast lesions in the BI-RADS categories 4 and 5 to exclude or verify malignancy before planning definitive therapy. The explicit objective of attaining a preoperative, i.e., pretherapeutic histopathologic diagnosis is to reduce the number of open biopsies performed, especially for benign findings, and to optimize the therapeutic course of action. The wishes of an informed patient to undergo primary open surgery, or surgery despite benign histology, however, should be respected. It is the responsibility of the diagnostician to attain a conclusive final diagnosis in cooperation with the pathologist (and, if applicable, the surgeon), taking the diagnostic imaging and pathohistologic results into account.

Choice of biopsy and guidance method. The decision of whether to perform a CNB or VAB is based on the clinical objective and required accuracy. The preoperative verification of malignancy for a highly suspicious breast lesion (BI-RADS 5) does not necessarily require the highest sensitivity, for example, because if the histologic results of percutaneous biopsy are benign, a rebiopsy or open biopsy would result. The choice of biopsy method is also influenced by the physician's personal accuracy, which can be derived from the performance assessment based on his or her collected biopsy and follow-up data.

Guidance:
- stereotactic-mammographic (digital)
- US
- MRI

Criteria influencing the choice of guidance method:
- The lesion to be biopsied must be clearly visible with the chosen imaging method.
- When possible, the most cost-efficient method should be chosen.
- CNBs should preferably be performed when interventions are US-guided.
- VABs should preferably be performed when interventions are stereotactic or MRI-guided.
- The objective with overriding importance is the reliable acquisition of representative tissue specimens.

Indications and contraindications

Indication:
- To exclude or verify malignancy of breast findings in the BI-RADS categories 4 and 5 before planning definitive therapy

Contraindications:
- Existing contraindications for the administration of normally used medication (e.g., local anesthetic)
- Severe coagulopathy (relative contraindication: risk must be compared with surgical risk and the risk of postponing diagnosis).

Specimen acquisition under stereotactic, US, or MRI guidance

Core biopsy of mass lesions:
Acquisition of ≥ four tissue samples ≤ 14 gauge

VAB of microcalcifications:
Acquisition of ≥ 12 tissue samples with 11-gauge biopsy needle, or volume equivalent number of tissue samples with 8- to 11-gauge biopsy needles

Our phantom study using VAB needles of different sizes yielded the following number of tissue samples to be the volume equivalent of 12 tissue samples obtained with an 11-gauge needle:
- 11-gauge: 12 tissue samples
- 10-gauge: eight tissue samples
- 9-gauge: six tissue samples
- 8-gauge: four tissue samples

Specific aspects pertaining to microcalcifications:
- Diagnostic biopsy should be performed in VAB technique.
- Specimen radiography with magnification. If representative microcalcifications are visualized, the biopsy is considered adequate. Separate tissue samples with and without microcalcifications for the pathologist.
- A final mammography should be performed in two orthogonal planes after biopsy

Stereotactic VAB:
The following should be observed when performing a VAB:
1. Before performing a VAB, a strict lateral mammographic projection (mediolateral [ML] or lateromedial [LM]) should be available for exact spatial orientation.

2. Documentation of biopsy approach (e.g., craniocaudal [CC], ML, LM, 30°-, 45°- 60°-oblique view) and stroke margin (if not already documented on laser film).
3. Taking the orthogonal mammographic view into account, the expected target depth and the stereotactically calculated target depth should be compared to avoid error. The recorded depth values may also be of assistance if a stereotactic localization is performed prior to later open surgery.
4. VABs are typically performed using 11- to 8-gauge biopsy needles.
5. The number of harvested tissue samples should be ≥ 12 using an 11-gauge biopsy needle, or volume equivalent number of tissue samples when using a biopsy needle of a different caliber.
6. The objective of percutaneous biopsy is the acquisition of representative tissue samples from ambiguous breast findings. The diagnostic VAB is not a therapeutic procedure when the histologic results reveal an invasive or noninvasive carcinoma, or findings with uncertain malignant potential (e.g., ADH). In these cases, open surgical excision with therapeutic objective is always required.
7. The following images are considered essential for documentation:
   - scout image and stereo pair (0°, +15°, -15°)
   - stereo prefire images (+15°, -15°)
   - stereo postfire images (+15°, -15°)
8. After completion of the VAB (on the following workday at the latest), a final mammographic documentation is performed in two orthogonal planes to again verify the correct biopsy depth, and in case a preoperative localization of a verified malignancy is necessary.

MRI-guided vacuum-assisted biopsy[1]

Indications:
To acquire a definitive histologic diagnosis of MRI breast findings in the MRI-BI-RADS categories 4 and 5 (in exceptional cases MRI-BI-RADS category 3, e.g., patient wishes), which are not clinically palpable or clearly visible with another imaging technique (mammography, US).

Equipment:
- MRI unit with at least 1.0 T
- open breast biopsy coil allowing access to the breast
- MRI-compatible targeting and biopsy equipment

MRI-compatible biopsy equipment:
- VAB system (preferred)
- large CNB (only used in exceptional cases)

Procedure:
- A contrast-enhanced MR mammography is performed with targeting equipment in place to reproduce the lesion to be percutaneously biopsied.
- If the target finding is not or only questionably reproduced, the intervention should be terminated and a short-term follow-up MR mammography performed within 6 months.

---

[1] Recommendations made by the Breast Diagnostics Working Group of the German Radiology Association.

15

- If the target finding is clearly identified, then the puncture coordinates (x-, y-, and z-axes) are calculated. The skin puncture site is marked (e.g., with an oil-containing marker) and a MRI T1-weighted series (without additional contrast administration) is performed to check the correct positioning.
- If the marker position is found to be incorrect, coordinates are calculated anew and the marker position corrected. If the marker position is correct, the skin is disinfected, local anesthesia administered to the puncture site, and a nick-incision performed (if required). The coaxial introduction needle is then introduced (e.g., with a metal puncture stylet) to the appropriate depth (z-axis). The appropriate depth position is dependent upon the VAB system being used.
- The metal puncture stylet is then replaced by a MRI-compatible mandrin and the position of the coaxial introduction needle checked by performing an MRI T1-weighted series (without contrast). If the position is incorrect, then a new calculation is performed and the needle is repositioned and rechecked. If the position is correct, then the MRI-compatible mandrin is removed and replaced with a VAB needle.
- Tissue samples are then harvested in a contiguous manner with the VAB needle by rotating the biopsy notch. It is recommended to obtain ≥12 tissue samples, which is the equivalent of one complete rotation around the clock time positions (1 to 12 o'clock). When appropriate, a MRI-check can be performed during the intervention to confirm the representative position of the biopsy cavity or to redirect further sampling.
- A postinterventional MRI-check (when indicated with contrast administration, e.g., mass lesions) is carried out as a final documentation of representative tissue sampling (target size is reduced, target is no longer detected, the biopsy cavity position is representative). If necessary, further sampling should be performed.
- Placement of a marker coil/clip in the biopsy cavity through the coaxial introduction cannula is optional; MRI documentation (without contrast) of intramammary coil position.
- The coaxial introduction needle is removed; the puncture channel compressed and cooled; a compression bandage is applied.
- A final mammography is performed (optional) in the CC and ML (or LM) projections for topographic orientation with respect to the biopsy cavity position and/or documentation of the marker coil position in case surgery is required at a later date.

Intervention report:
- target is reproduced (yes/no)
- target position (quadrant, clock-time position, distance from the skin)
- VAB needle size (e.g., 11 gauge, 9 gauge)
- number of specimens primarily (if applicable, secondarily) acquired
- occurrence of relevant complications (description)

Image documentation:
- MRI documentation of target lesion (subtraction image)
- MRI documentation of coaxial introduction needle in place
- MRI documentation of biopsy cavity or VAB needle position after tissue acquisition
- contrast-enhanced MR mammography after biopsy (optional)

- X-ray mammography in CC and ML (or LM) projections after biopsy (optional)

Quality criterion:
- complete or partial removal of the targeted MRI finding

Consequences for histologic results in the following pathologic categories:
- B1 or B2: Short-term follow-up MR mammography in 6 months (sometimes earlier)
- B3 or B4: Interdisciplinary conference concerning further proceedings (e.g., MR mammography follow-up, rebiopsy, open biopsy)
- B5a or B5b: Initiation of appropriate definitive therapy

Documentation of stereotactic, ultrasound-, or MRI-guidance
Written report and documentation (for all methods):
- procedural description (sketch): includes compression axis/angle, biopsy approach (medial, lateral, cranial, caudal), stroke margin, and compression thickness
- description of relevant complications (if applicable)
- statement about whether biopsy is representative
- therapeutic recommendations based upon histologic results (after interdisciplinary conference or case discussion with the pathologist, and considering the biopsying physician's personal accuracy)

Image documentation for stereotactic interventions:
- scout image (0°) and stereo pair (from two opposite angles)
- stereo prefire images (from two opposite angles)
- stereo postfire images (from two opposite angles)
- mammography in two orthogonal projections after biopsy

Documentation and evaluation (for all methods):
- data collection for statistical analysis of all percutaneous biopsy results
- follow-up examinations in 6 months of all patients with benign histologic results after percutaneous biopsy (preferably at the same facility that performed the biopsy)
- mandatory interdisciplinary conference to evaluate histologic results that are ambiguous or discordant with primary imaging results

Localization of Nonpalpable Breast Findings

Definition. Localization of nonpalpable breast findings involves the preoperative placement of a localization wire to mark a nonpalpable breast finding. A dye solution or simple needle should only be used in special, justified cases for such localizations.

Guidance:
- free-hand after mammography in two orthogonal planes
- stereotactic
- US
- MRI

Indication and contraindications
Indication:
- to localize and mark nonpalpable breast findings preoperatively

Contraindications:
- no absolute contraindications

Choice of guidance method
- The lesion to be biopsied must be clearly visible with the chosen imaging method.
- If a mammographic lesion has a correlating ultrasonographic finding, the preoperative localization should be performed under US guidance and final mammographic documentation performed (reason: the number of mammographic images required is substantially reduced resulting in lower costs and lower radiation exposure). MRI-guided localizations are performed when a suspicious MRI-finding has no correlating lesion on mammography or US.

Objectives
- The localization wire should penetrate the target lesion and project less than 1 cm past the distal border.
- If the wire does not penetrate the target lesion, then it should lie within 1 cm of the lesion border.
- When localizing a nonmass lesion, several markers/wires can be placed at the surgically relevant borders without adhering to the 1-cm limit.

Documentation
1. A final mammographic documentation in two orthogonal planes should be performed after the localization of all non-palpable mammographic findings (if applicable, sonographic documentation).
2. Exact elucidation of wire localization with respect to the target lesion (possibly with sketch).
3. Description of relevant complications (if applicable).
4. Documentation 1 and 2 must be made available to the operating surgeon.

Specimen radiography (and specimen ultrasound, if applicable)
- A specimen radiograph should be taken whenever nonpalpable, mammographically visible masses or lesions with microcalcifications are surgically excised.

- The specimen radiograph should be performed with compression applied. If the excised lesion contains microcalcifications, the specimen radiograph should be performed with magnification.
- A radiograph of the specimen blocks can be taken when necessary.
- A specimen US scan can be additionally performed after US-guided localization (this allows for an especially rapid intraoperative communication to the surgeon).

Specimen radiography (ultrasound) report
- statement with findings and assessment:
  - The target finding is definitely contained:
    - and completely contained within the specimen
    - but questionably complete within the specimen
    - and incompletely contained within the specimen
  - The target finding is definitely not contained within the specimen.
  - The target finding is questionably contained within the specimen.

The findings must be reported to the surgeon intraoperatively in a verbal communication. A written report must be sent to the pathologist along with the specimen, and to the surgeon postoperatively.

Audit of localization results
- documentation of histologic results
- statement as to whether excisional biopsy is representative
- if biopsy is not representative, then initiation of further diagnostic work-up postoperatively within 14 days: 2-view mammography/stereotactic relocalization and renewed open biopsy
- Interdisciplinary conference

15

16 Case Studies

S. Luftner-Nagel, F. Baum, U. Fischer

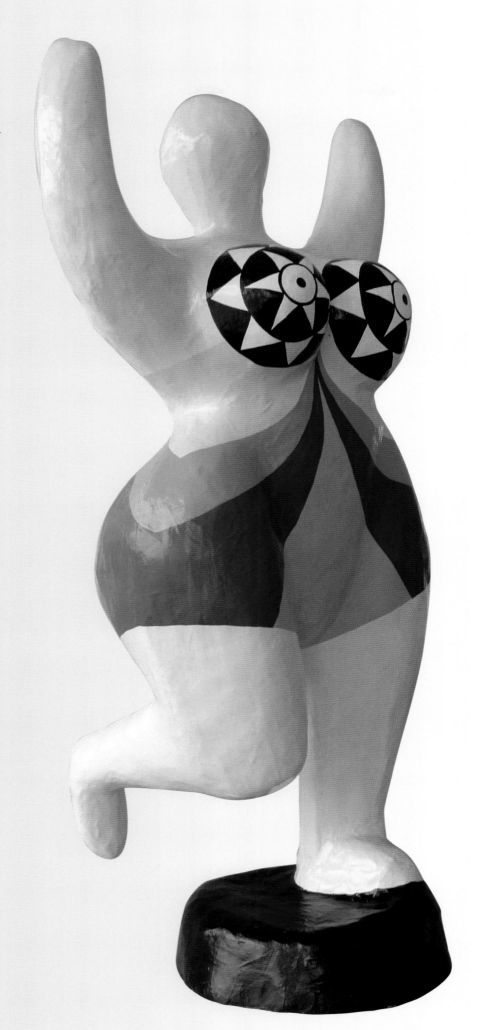

Case Studies Sonography: Cases 1 to 16

Case 1

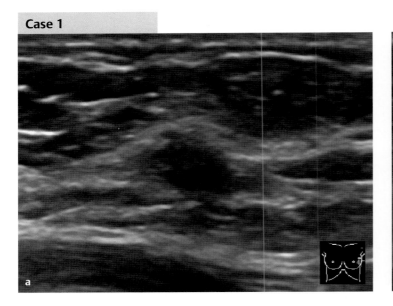
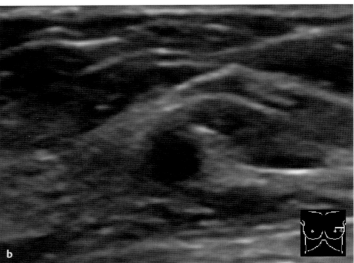

Case 2

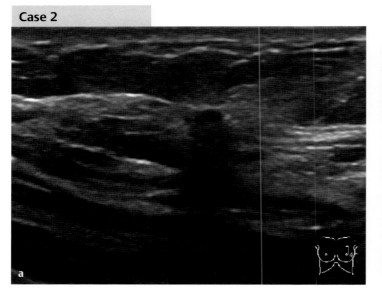
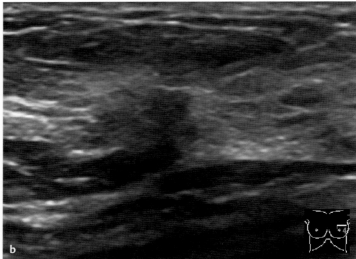

Case 1 solution

Finding:	Mass
Shape:	Round
Margin:	Indistinct
Lesion boundary:	Echogenic halo
Echogenicity:	Hypoechoic
Internal structure:	Inhomogeneous
Surrounding tissue alterations:	Architectural distortion
Posterior acoustic features:	None
US BI-RADS:	**4**
Histology:	Tubular breast cancer
Pathologic category:	**B5b**
Resulting procedure:	Breast conserving therapy
Final histology:	Tubular breast cancer, pT1b

Case 2 solution

Finding:	Mass
Shape:	Irregular
Margin:	Indistinct
Lesion boundary:	Echogenic halo
Echogenicity:	Hypoechoic
Internal structure:	Inhomogeneous
Surrounding tissue alterations:	Architectural distortion
Posterior acoustic features:	Shadowing
US BI-RADS:	**5**
Histology:	Invasive ductal carcinoma (IDC)
Pathologic category:	**B5b**
Resulting procedure:	Breast conserving therapy
Final histology:	IDC, pT1c

16

Case 3

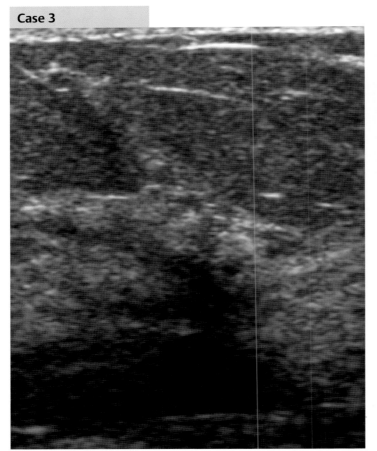

Case 4

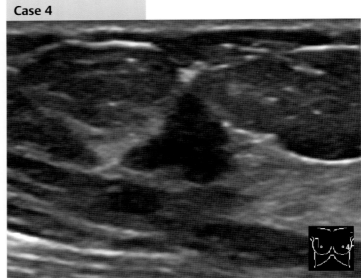

Case 5

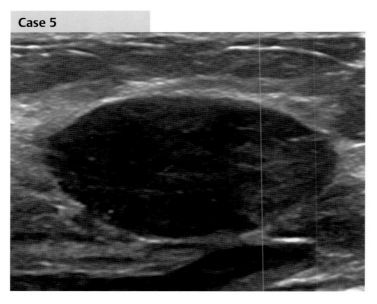

Case 6

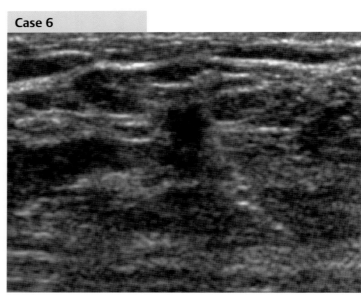

Case 3 solution

Finding:	Architectural distortion
Shape:	Irregular
Margin:	Indistinct
Lesion boundary:	No sharp demarcation
Echogenicity:	Hypoechoic
Internal structure:	Inhomogeneous
Surrounding tissue alterations:	Architectural distortion
Posterior acoustic features:	Shadowing
US BI-RADS:	**4**
Histology:	Invasive lobular carcinoma (ILC)
Pathologic category:	**B5b**
Resulting procedure:	Breast conserving therapy
Final histology:	ILC, pT1b

Case 4 solution

Finding:	Mass
Shape:	Macrolobulated
Orientation:	Perpendicular to the skin
Margin:	Circumscribed
Lesion boundary:	Abrupt interface
Echogenicity:	Hypoechoic
Internal structure:	Homogeneous
Surrounding tissue alterations:	Architectural distortion
Posterior acoustic features:	None
US BI-RADS:	**4**
Histology:	Fibroadenoma
Pathologic category:	**B2**
Resulting procedure:	Short-term US in 6 months

Case 5 solution

Finding:	Mass
Shape:	Oval
Orientation:	Horizontal to the skin
Margin:	Circumscribed
Lesion boundary:	Abrupt interface
Echogenicity:	Hypoechoic
Internal structure:	Homogeneous
Surrounding tissue alterations:	Compression due to displacement
Posterior acoustic features:	None
US BI-RADS:	**3**
Histology:	Fibroadenoma
Pathologic category:	**B2**
Resulting procedure:	Short-term US in 6 months

Case 6 solution

Finding:	Mass
Shape:	Round
Margin:	Spiculated
Lesion boundary:	Echogenic halo
Echogenicity:	Hypoechoic
Internal structure:	Inhomogeneous
Surrounding tissue alterations:	Architectural distortion
Posterior acoustic features:	Shadowing
US BI-RADS:	**5**
Histology:	IDC
Pathologic category:	**B5b**
Resulting procedure:	Breast conserving therapy
Final histology:	IDC, pT1a

16

Case 7

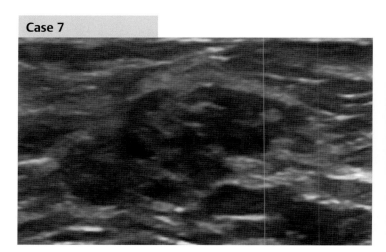

Case 8

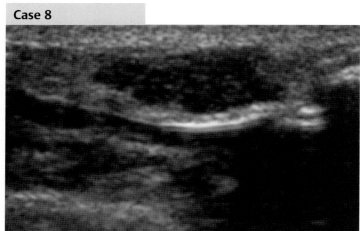

Case 9

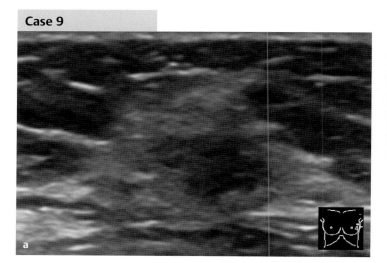

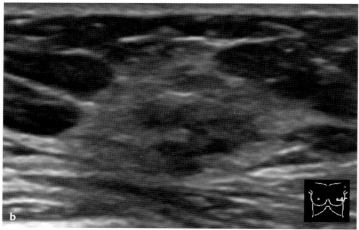

Case 7 solution

Finding:	Mass
Shape:	Irregular
Orientation:	Horizontal to the skin
Margin:	Indistinct
Lesion boundary:	Compression due to displacement
Echogenicity:	Hypoechoic
Internal structure:	Inhomogeneous
Surrounding tissue alterations:	Architectural distortion
Posterior acoustic features:	None
US BI-RADS:	**4**
Histology:	Nodular sclerosing adenosis
Pathologic category:	**B2**
Resulting procedure:	Short-term US in 6 months

Case 8 solution

Finding:	Mass
Shape:	Macrolobulated
Orientation:	Horizontal to the skin
Margin:	Partially indistinct
Lesion boundary:	Abrupt interface
Echogenicity:	Hypoechoic
Internal structure:	Inhomogeneous
Posterior acoustic features:	Indifferent
US BI-RADS:	**4**
Histology:	IDC
Pathologic category:	**B5b**
Resulting procedure:	Breast conserving therapy
Final histology:	Medullary carcinoma

Case 9 solution

Finding:	Mass
Shape:	Irregular
Margin:	Indistinct
Lesion boundary:	Echogenic halo
Echogenicity:	Hypoechoic
Internal structure:	Inhomogeneous
Surrounding tissue alterations:	Architectural distortion
Posterior acoustic features:	Shadowing
US BI-RADS:	**5**
Histology:	ILC
Pathologic category:	**B5b**
Resulting procedure:	Breast conserving therapy
Final histology:	ILC, pT1c

16

Case 10

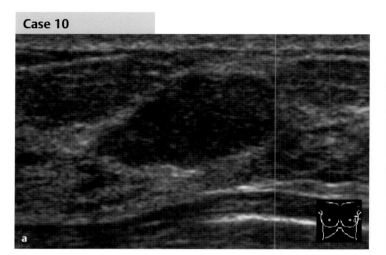

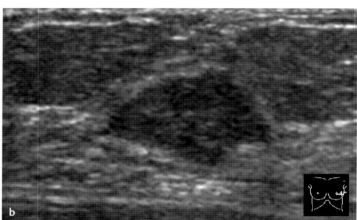

Case 11

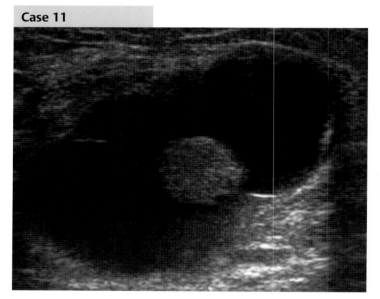

Case 12

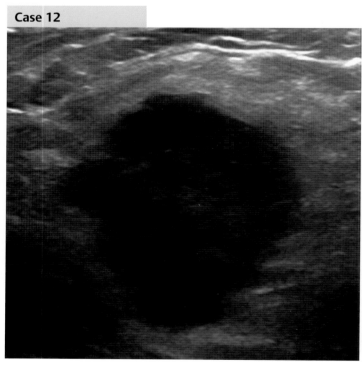

Case 10 solution

Finding:	Mass
Shape:	Macrolobulated
Orientation:	Horizontal to the skin
Margin:	Circumscribed
Lesion boundary:	Abrupt interface
Echogenicity:	Hypoechoic
Internal structure:	Homogeneous
Surrounding tissue alterations:	Compression due to displacement
Posterior acoustic features:	None
US BI-RADS:	**4**
Histology:	Fibroadenoma
Pathologic category:	**B2**
Resulting procedure:	Short-term US in 6 months

Case 11 solution

Finding:	Intracystic proliferation
Shape:	Round
Margin:	Indistinct
Echogenicity:	Hyperechoic
Internal structure:	Homogeneous
Posterior acoustic features:	Indifferent
US BI-RADS:	**4**
Histology:	Papilloma
Pathologic category:	**B3**
Resulting procedure:	Surgical excision
Final histology:	Intracystic papilloma with apocrine metaplasia

Case 12 solution

Finding:	Mass
Shape:	Irregular
Orientation:	Perpendicular to the skin
Margin:	Indistinct
Lesion boundary:	Echogenic halo
Echogenicity:	Hypoechoic
Internal structure:	Inhomogeneous
Surrounding tissue alterations:	Architectural distortion
Posterior acoustic features:	None
US BI-RADS:	**5**
Histology:	IDC with necrosis
Pathologic category:	**B5b**
Resulting procedure:	Neoadjuvant chemotherapy
Final histology:	IDC, ypT1c

16

Case 13

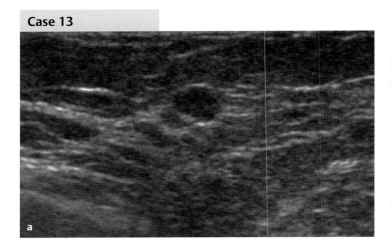

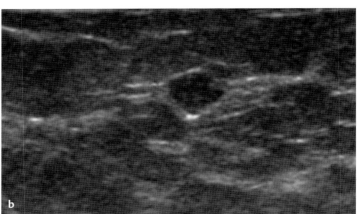

Case 14

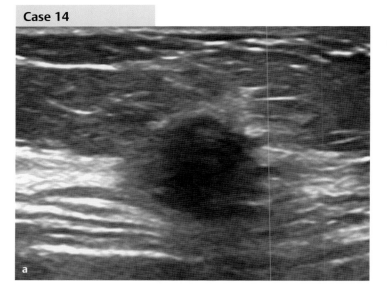

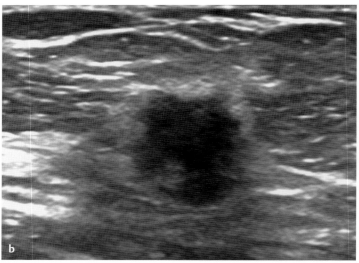

Case 13 solution

Finding:	Mass
Shape:	Round
Margin:	Circumscribed
Lesion boundary:	Abrupt interface
Echogenicity:	Hypoechoic
Internal structure:	Homogeneous
Surrounding tissue alterations:	Compression due to displacement
Posterior acoustic features:	None
US BI-RADS:	**4**
Histology:	Papilloma
Pathologic category:	**B3**
Resulting procedure:	Surgical excision
Final histology:	Intraductal papilloma

Case 14 solution

Finding:	Mass
Shape:	Round
Margin:	Indistinct
Lesion boundary:	Echogenic halo
Echogenicity:	Hypoechoic
Internal structure:	Inhomogeneous
Surrounding tissue alterations:	Architectural distortion
Posterior acoustic features:	Shadowing
US BI-RADS:	**5**
Histology:	ILC
Pathologic category:	**B5b**
Resulting procedure:	Breast conserving therapy
Final histology:	ILC, pT2

16

Case 15

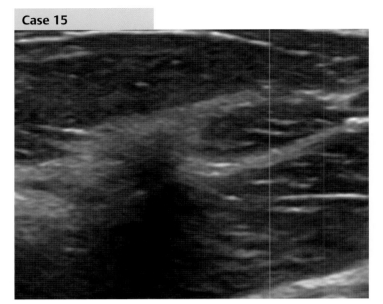

Case 16

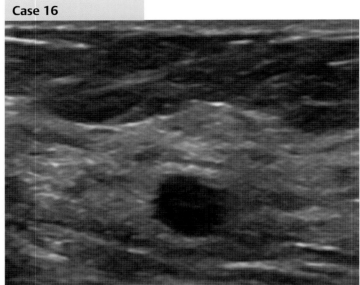

Case 15 solution

Finding:	Mass
Shape:	Irregular
Margin:	Spiculated
Lesion boundary:	Echogenic halo
Echogenicity:	Hypoechoic
Internal structure:	Inhomogeneous
Surrounding tissue alterations:	Architectural distortion
Posterior acoustic features:	Shadowing
US BI-RADS:	**5**
Histology:	IDC
Pathologic category:	**B5b**
Resulting procedure:	Breast conserving therapy
Final histology:	IDC, pT1a

Case 16 solution

Finding:	Mass
Shape:	Round
Margin:	Indistinct
Lesion boundary:	Abrupt interface
Echogenicity:	Hypoechoic
Internal structure:	Homogeneous
Surrounding tissue alterations:	None
Posterior acoustic features:	None
US BI-RADS:	**4**
Histology:	Benign phyllodes tumor
Pathologic category:	**B3**
Resulting procedure:	Surgical excision
Final histology:	Benign phyllodes tumor

16

Case Studies Mammography: Cases 17 to 34

Case 17: Screening Mammography

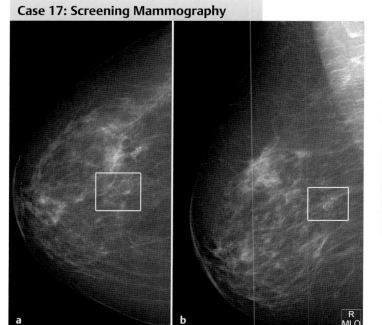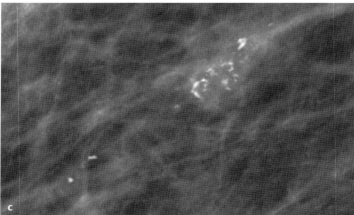

Fig. 16.17a–c Mammography: right breast in craniocaudal (CC) and mediolateral oblique (MLO) projection (a, b). Enlarged partial image in MLO projection (c).

Case 18: Follow-up Mammography after Lumpectomy

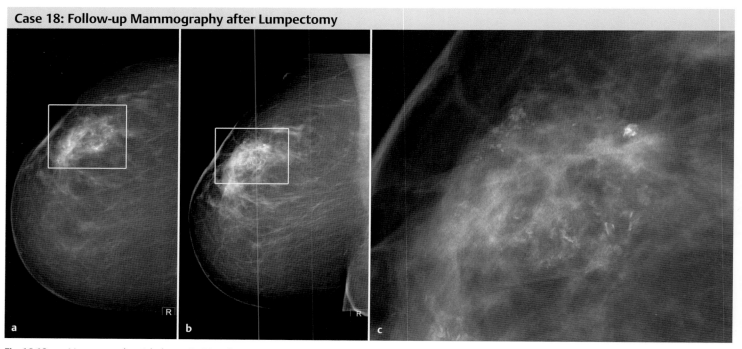

Fig. 16.18a–c Mammography: right breast in CC and MLO projection (a, b). Enlarged partial image in MLO projection (c).

Case 17 solution

Finding:	Microcalcifications
Morphology:	Coarse heterogeneous
Distribution:	Linear
Position:	Central aspect of the right breast, 11 o'clock, 6 cm from the nipple
BI-RADS:	**4**
Histology:	Papillomatosis
Pathologic category:	**B3**
Resulting procedure:	Segmental resection
Final histology:	Papillomatosis

Case 18 solution

Personal history:	Lumpectomy of the right breast 3 years ago
Finding:	Microcalcifications, architectural distortion
Morphology:	Coarse heterogeneous
Distribution:	Regional
Position:	Upper outer quadrant of the right breast, 11 o'clock, 3 cm from the nipple
BI-RADS:	**4**
Histology:	Scar tissue
Pathologic category:	**B2**
Resulting procedure:	Follow-up mammography in 6 months

Case 19: Screening Mammography

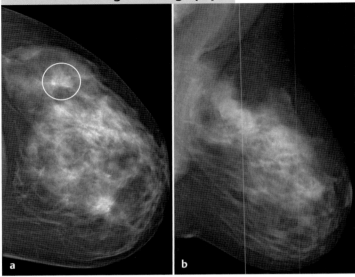

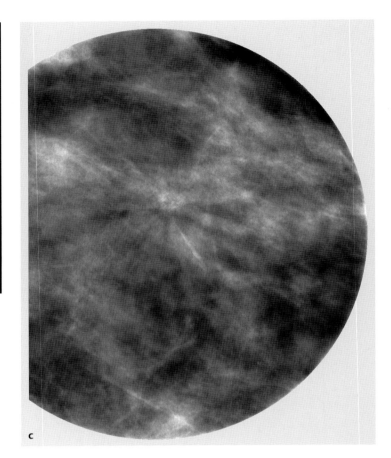

Fig. 16.19a–c Mammography: left breast in CC and MLO projection (**a, b**). Spot compression image in CC projection (**c**).

Case 20: Screening Mammography

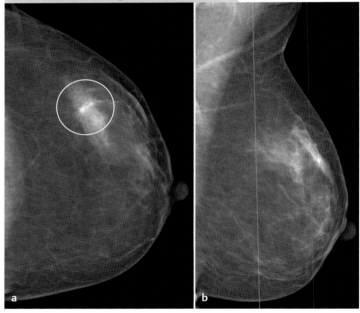

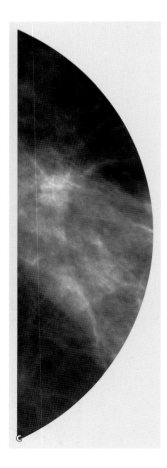

Fig. 16.20a–c Mammography: left breast in CC and MLO (**a, b**). Spot compression image in CC projection (**c**).

Case 19 solution

Finding:	Architectural distortion
Position:	Upper outer quadrant of the left breast, 2 o'clock, 6 cm from the nipple
BI-RADS:	**4**
Histology:	Radial scar
Pathologic category:	**B3**
Resulting procedure:	Surgical excision
Final histology:	Tubular carcinoma pT1a within a radial scar

Case 20 solution

Finding:	Mass lesion (7-mm diameter)
Shape:	Irregular
Margins:	Spiculated
Density:	Hyperdense
Position:	Upper outer quadrant of the left breast, 2 o'clock, 5 cm from the nipple
BI-RADS:	**4**
Histology:	Tubular carcinoma
Pathologic category:	**B5b**
Resulting procedure:	Lumpectomy
Final histology:	Tubular carcinoma pT1b

16

Case 21: Screening Mammography

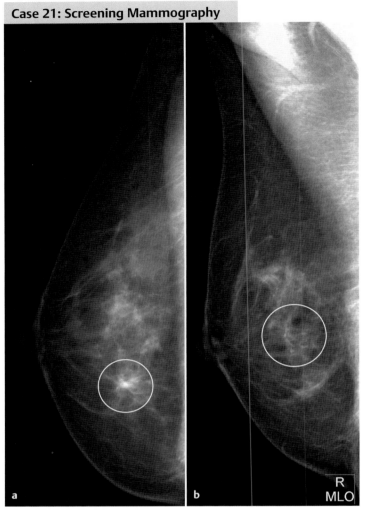

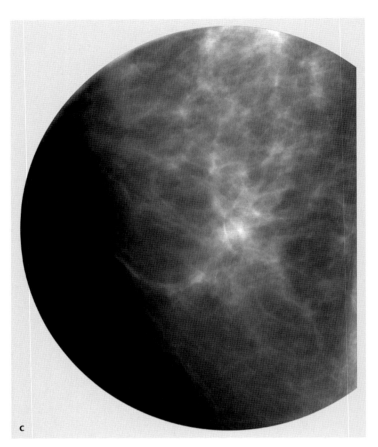

Fig. 16.21a–c Mammography: right breast in CC and MLO projection (a, b). Spot compression image in CC projection (c).

Case 22: Screening Mammography

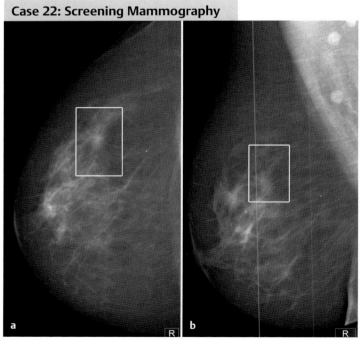

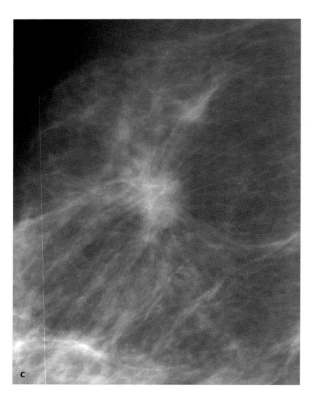

Fig. 16.22a–c Mammography: right breast in CC and MLO projection (a, b). Spot compression image in CC projection (c).

Case 21 solution

Finding:	Mass lesion (5-mm diameter) with architectural distortion
Shape:	Irregular
Margins:	Indistinct
Density:	Isodense
Position:	Inner aspect of the left breast, 2 o'clock, 5 cm from the nipple
BI-RADS:	**4**
Histology:	ILC
Pathologic category:	**B5b**
Resulting procedure:	Lumpectomy
Final histology:	ILC pT1b

Case 22 solution

Finding:	Mass lesion (10-mm diameter)
Shape:	Oval
Margins:	Spiculated
Density:	Isodense
Position:	Upper outer quadrant of the right breast, 10 o'clock, 6 cm from the nipple
BI-RADS:	**4, after spot compression 5**
Histology:	IDC
Pathologic category:	**B5b**
Resulting procedure:	Lumpectomy
Final histology:	IDC pT1c

16

Case 23: Screening Mammography

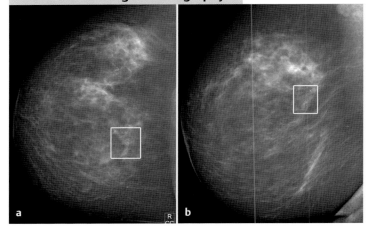

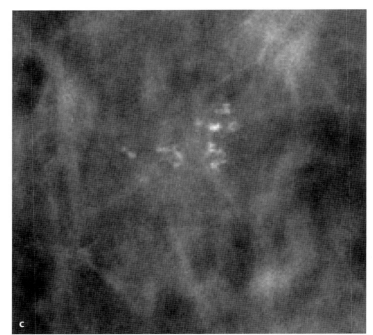

Fig. 16.23a–c Mammography: right breast in CC and lateromedial (LM) projection (**a, b**). Magnification image in CC projection (**c**).

Case 24: Screening Mammography

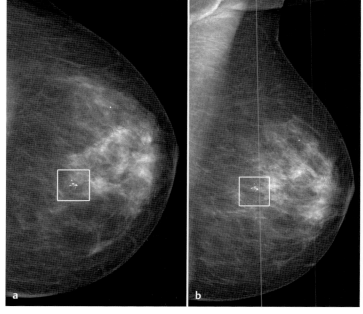

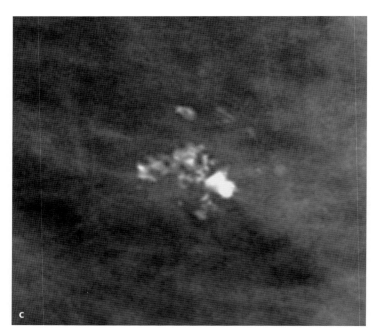

Fig. 16.24a–c Mammography: left breast in CC and MLO projection (**a, b**). Enlarged partial view in CC projection (**c**).

Case 23 solution

Finding:	Microcalcifications
Morphology:	Fine-pleomorphic
Distribution:	Clustered
Position:	Central aspect of the right breast, 1 o'clock, 7 cm from the nipple
BI-RADS:	**4**
Histology:	Fibroadenoma with degenerative calcifications
Pathologic category:	**B2**
Resulting procedure:	Follow-up mammography in 6 months

Case 24 solution

Finding:	Micro- and macrocalcifications
Morphology:	Coarse heterogeneous
Distribution:	Clustered
Position:	Central aspect of the left breast, 7 cm from the nipple
BI-RADS:	**4**
Histology:	Fibroadenoma with degenerative calcifications
Pathologic category:	**B2**
Resulting procedure:	Follow-up mammography in 6 months

16

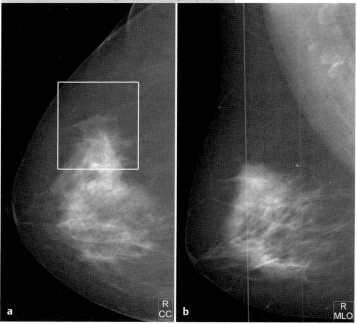

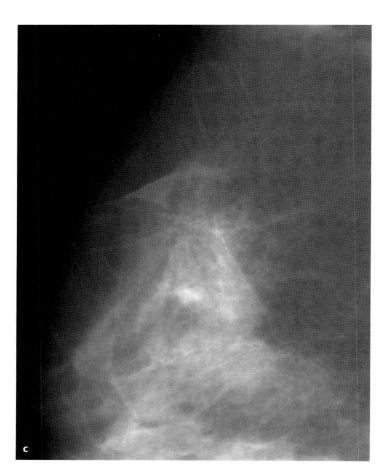

Fig. 16.25a–c Mammography: right breast in CC and MLO projection (**a, b**). Spot compression image in CC projection (**c**).

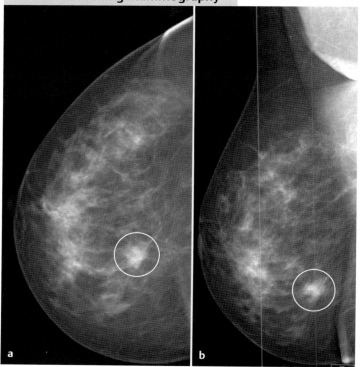

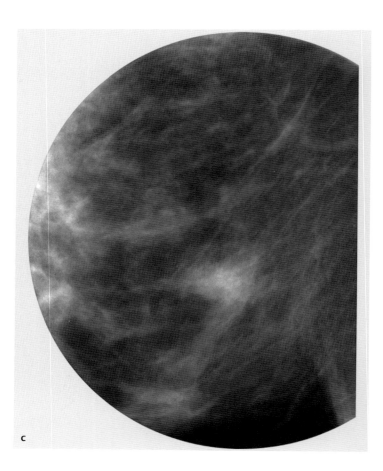

Fig. 16.26a–c Mammography: right breast in CC and MLO projection (**a, b**). Spot compression image in MLO projection (**c**).

Case 25 solution

Finding:	Architectural distortion visible in one plane
Position:	Lateral aspect of the right breast, 5 cm from the nipple
BI-RADS:	**4**
Histology:	Radial scar
Pathologic category:	**B3**
Resulting procedure:	Surgical excision
Final histology:	Radial scar

Case 26 solution

Finding:	Mass lesion (12-mm diameter)
Shape:	Lobulated
Margins:	Indistinct
Density:	Isodense
Position:	Lower inner quadrant of the right breast, 4 o'clock, 5 cm from the nipple
BI-RADS:	**4**
Histology:	Invasive lobular carcinoma (ILC)
Pathologic category:	**B5b**
Resulting procedure:	Lumpectomy
Final histology:	ILC pT1c

16

Case 27: Screening Mammography

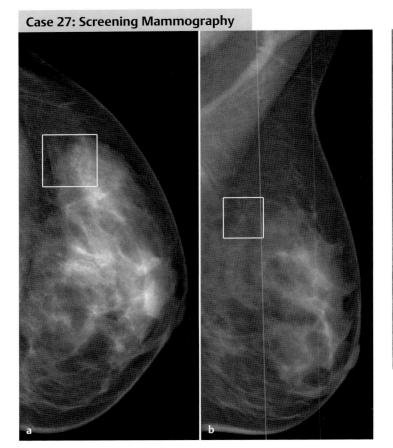
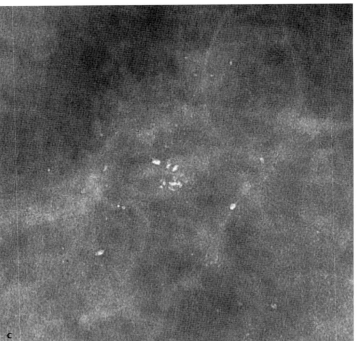

Fig. 16.27a–c Mammography: left breast in CC and LM projection (a, b). Magnification image in MLO projection (c).

Case 28: Follow-up Mammography after Left Side Lumpectomy

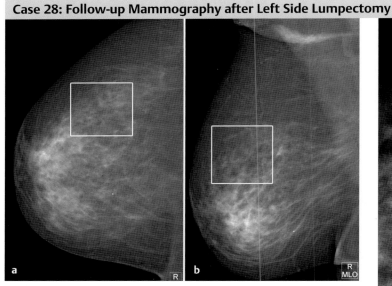
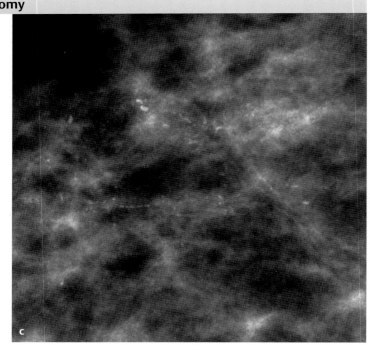
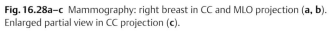

Fig. 16.28a–c Mammography: right breast in CC and MLO projection (a, b). Enlarged partial view in CC projection (c).

Case 27 solution

Finding:	Microcalcifications
Morphology:	Punctate
Distribution:	Clustered
Position:	Upper outer quadrant of the left breast, 2 o'clock, 7 cm from the nipple
BI-RADS:	**4**
Histology:	Sclerosing adenosis
Pathologic category:	**B2**
Resulting procedure:	Follow-up mammography in 6 months

Case 28 solution

Finding:	Microcalcifications
Morphology:	Fine-pleomorphic and fine-linear
Distribution:	Segmental
Position:	Upper outer quadrant of the right breast, 10 o'clock, 7 cm from the nipple
BI-RADS:	**5**
Histology:	High-grade DCIS
Pathologic category:	**B5a**
Resulting procedure:	Mastectomy (DCIS >4 cm)
Final histology:	High-grade ductal carcinoma in situ (DCIS)

16

Case 29: Screening Mammography

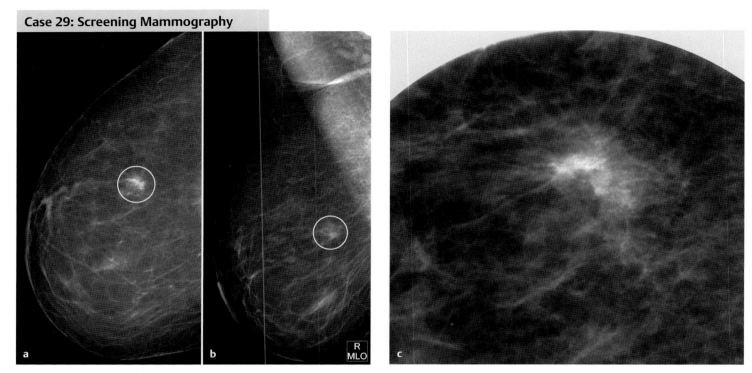

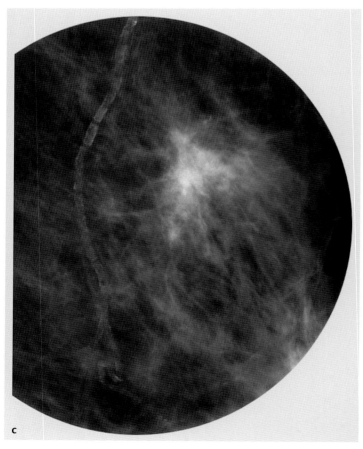

Fig. 16.29a–c Mammography: right breast in CC and MLO projection (**a, b**). Spot compression image in CC projection (**c**).

Case 30: Screening Mammography

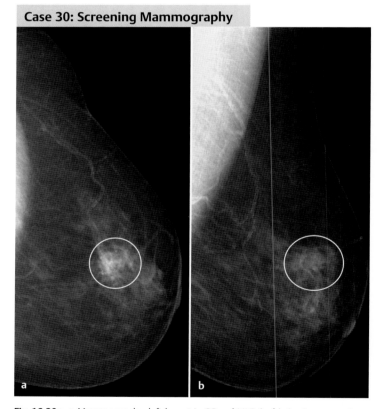

Fig. 16.30a–c Mammography: left breast in CC and MLO (**a, b**). Spot compression image in CC projection (**c**).

Case 29 solution

Finding:	Mass lesion (13-mm diameter)
Shape:	Irregular
Margins:	Indistinct
Density:	Hyperdense
Position:	Lateral aspect of the right breast, 9 o'clock, 5 cm from the nipple
BI-RADS:	**4**
Histology:	IDC
Pathological category:	**B5b**
Resulting procedure:	Lumpectomy
Final histology:	IDC pT1c

Case 30 solution

Finding:	Mass lesion (11-mm diameter)
Shape:	Irregular
Margins:	Indistinct
Density:	Isodense
Position:	Upper aspect of the left breast, 1 o'clock, 3 cm from the nipple
BI-RADS:	**4**
Histology:	ILC
Pathologic category:	**B5b**
Resulting procedure:	Lumpectomy
Final histology:	ILC pT1c

16

Case 31: Screening Mammography

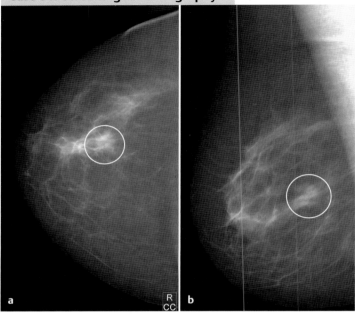

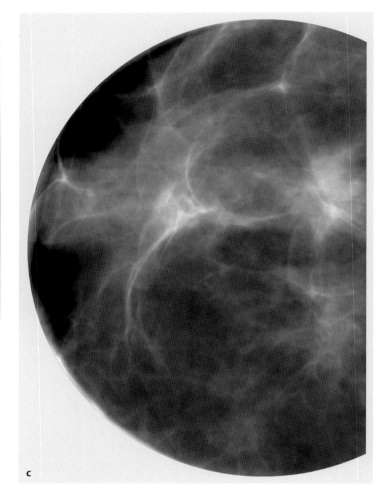

Fig. 16.31a–c Mammography: right breast in CC and MLO (**a, b**). Spot compression image in CC projection (**c**).

Case 32: Screening Mammography

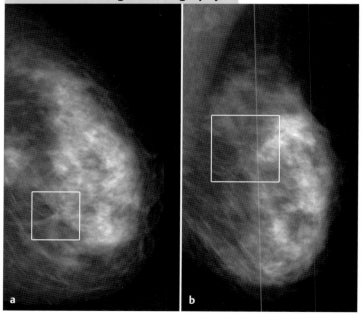

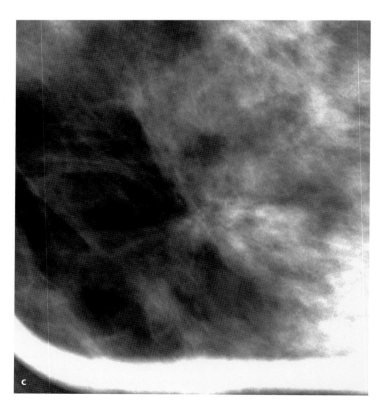

Fig. 16.32a–c Mammography: left breast in CC and MLO (**a, b**). Spot compression image in CC projection (**c**).

Case 31 solution

Finding:	Mass lesions (9-mm and 7-mm diameter)
Shape:	Round
Margins:	Spiculated
Density:	Isodense
Position:	Central aspect of the right breast, 4 cm from the nipple
BI-RADS:	**5**
Histology:	IDC
Pathologic category:	**B5b**
Resulting procedure:	Lumpectomy
Final histology:	Bifocal, IDC pT1b

Case 32 solution

Finding:	Architectural distortion
Position:	Central aspect of the left breast, 6 cm from the nipple
BI-RADS:	**4**
Histology:	Radial scar
Pathologic category:	**B3**
Resulting procedure:	Surgical excision
Final histology:	Radial scar

16

Case 33: Screening Mammography

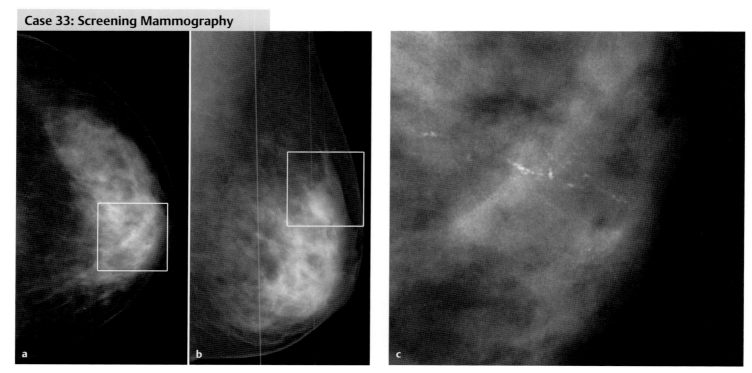

Fig. 16.33a–c Mammography: left breast in CC and LM projection (**a, b**). Magnification image in CC projection (**c**).

Case 34: Screening Mammography

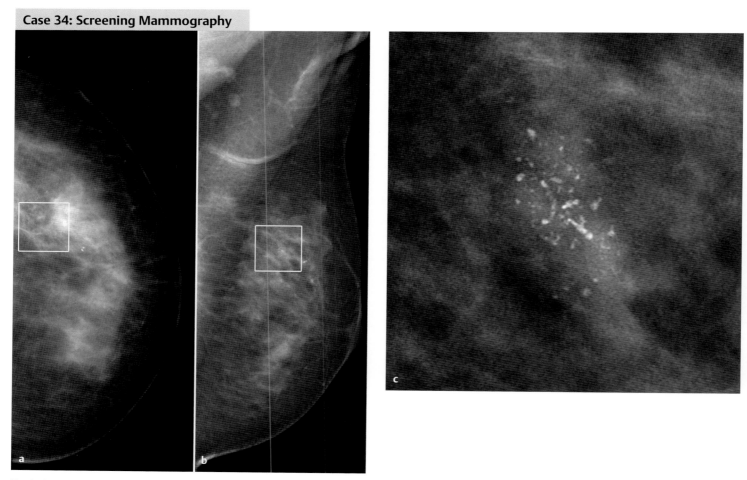

Fig. 16.34a–c Mammography: left breast in CC and MLO projection (**a, b**). Enlarged partial image in MLO projection (**c**).

Case 33 solution

Finding:	Microcalcifications
Morphology:	Fine linear
Distribution:	Segmental
Position:	Upper inner quadrant of the left breast, 11 o'clock
BI-RADS:	5
Histology:	DCIS
Pathologic category:	B5a
Resulting procedure:	Primary lumpectomy, secondary mastectomy due to size >4 cm
Final histology:	Low-grade DCIS

Case 34 solution

Finding:	Microcalcifications
Morphology:	Fine-pleomorphic
Distribution:	Clustered
Position:	Upper aspect of the left breast, 12 o'clock, 7 cm from the nipple
BI-RADS:	5
Histology:	DCIS
Pathologic category:	B5a
Resulting procedure:	Lumpectomy
Final histology:	High-grade DCIS

16

Case Studies MR Mammography: Cases 35 to 42

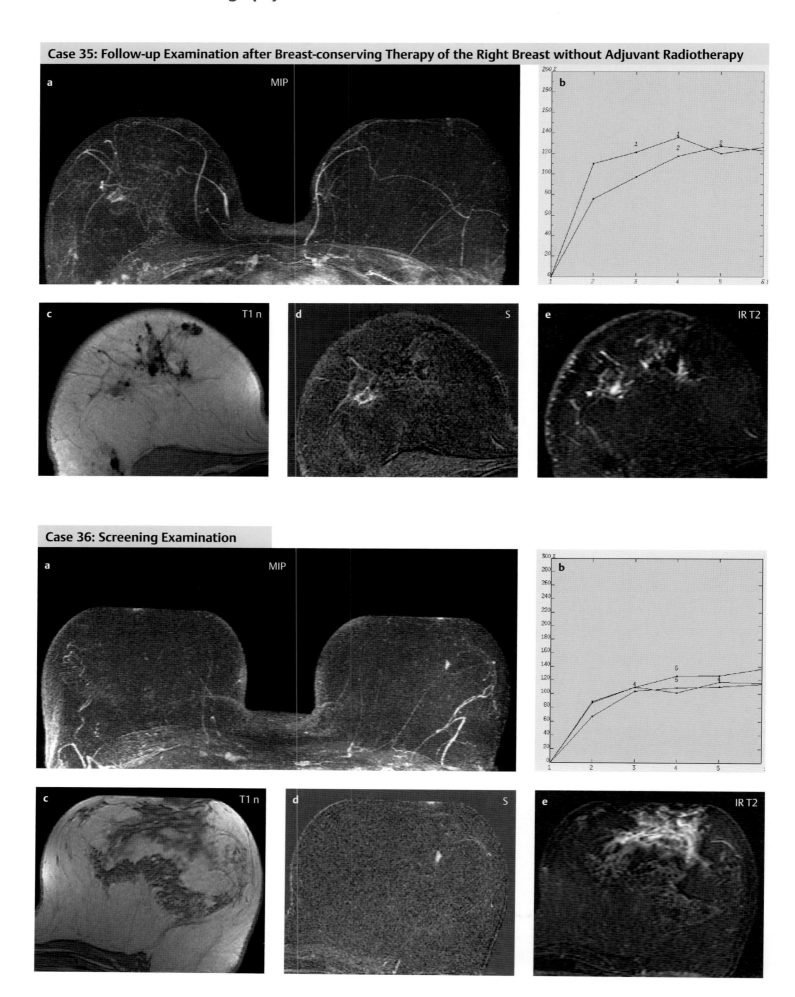

Case 35: Follow-up Examination after Breast-conserving Therapy of the Right Breast without Adjuvant Radiotherapy

a   MIP

b

c   T1 n   d   S   e   IR T2

Case 36: Screening Examination

a   MIP

b

c   T1 n   d   S   e   IR T2

Case 35 solution

Finding:	Nonmass lesion	
Position:	Central aspect of the right breast	
Shape:	Irregular	1 point
Margins:	Indistinct	1 point
T1-weighted postcontrast:	Ring enhancement	2 points
Initial signal increase:	>100%	2 points
Postinitial signal behavior:	Plateau	1 point
Total points:		**7 points**

MRM-BI-RADS 5

T2-weightedw:	Isointense (compared with parenchyma)
Other aspects:	Significant susceptibility artifacts (due to electrocautering during prior surgery)
MRI-guided VAB histology:	IDC recurrence
Pathological category:	**B5b**
Resulting procedure:	Lumpectomy
Final histology:	IDC pT1c

Case 36 solution

Finding:	Focus	
Position:	Central aspect of the left breast	
Shape:	Irregular	1 point
Margins:	Well-circumscribed	0 points
T1-weighted postcontrast:	Homogeneous	0 points
Initial signal increase:	>100%	2 points
Postinitial signal behavior:	Plateau	1 point
Total points:		**4 points**

MRM-BI-RADS 4

T2-weighted:	Isointense (compared with parenchyma)
Other aspects:	None
MRI-guided VAB histology:	Papilloma of 3-mm diameter, completely excised
Pathological category:	**B3**
Resulting procedure:	MRI follow-up in 6 months

16

Case 37: Screening Examination

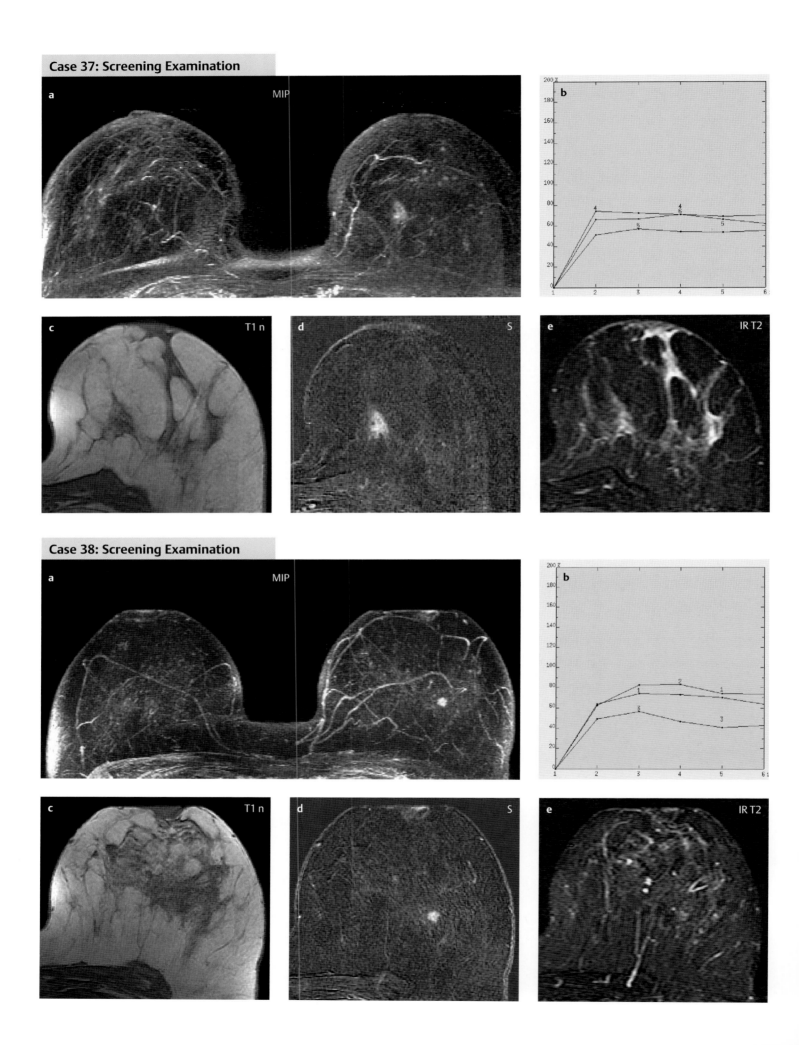

Case 38: Screening Examination

Case 37 solution

Finding:	Nonmass lesion	
Position:	Lower inner quadrant of the left breast	
Shape:	Irregular	1 point
Margins:	Indistinct	1 point
T1-weighted postcontrast:	Inhomogeneous	1 point
Initial signal increase:	80%	1 point
Postinitial signal behavior:	Plateau	1 point
Total points:		**5 points**
MR mammography BI-RADS 4		
T2-weighted:	Hyperintense (compared with parenchyma)	
Other aspects:	None	
MRI-guided vacuum-assisted biopsy (VAB) histology:	Radial scar	
Pathologic category:	**B3**	
Resulting procedure:	Surgical excision	
Final histology:	Radial scar	

Case 38 solution

Finding:	Mass lesion	
Position:	Central aspect of the left breast	
Shape:	Round	0 points
Margins:	Indistinct	1 point
T1-weighted postcontrast:	Inhomogeneous	1 point
Initial signal increase:	50–100%	1 point
Postinitial signal behavior:	Plateau	1 point
Total points:		**4 points**
MR mammography BI-RADS 4		
T2-weighted:	Isointense (compared with parenchyma)	
Other aspects:	None	
MRI-guided VAB histology:	IDC	
Pathologic category:	**B5b**	
Resulting procedure:	Lumpectomy	
Final histology:	IDC pT1b	

16

Case 39: Follow-up Examination after Mastectomy of the Right Breast and Implant Reconstruction

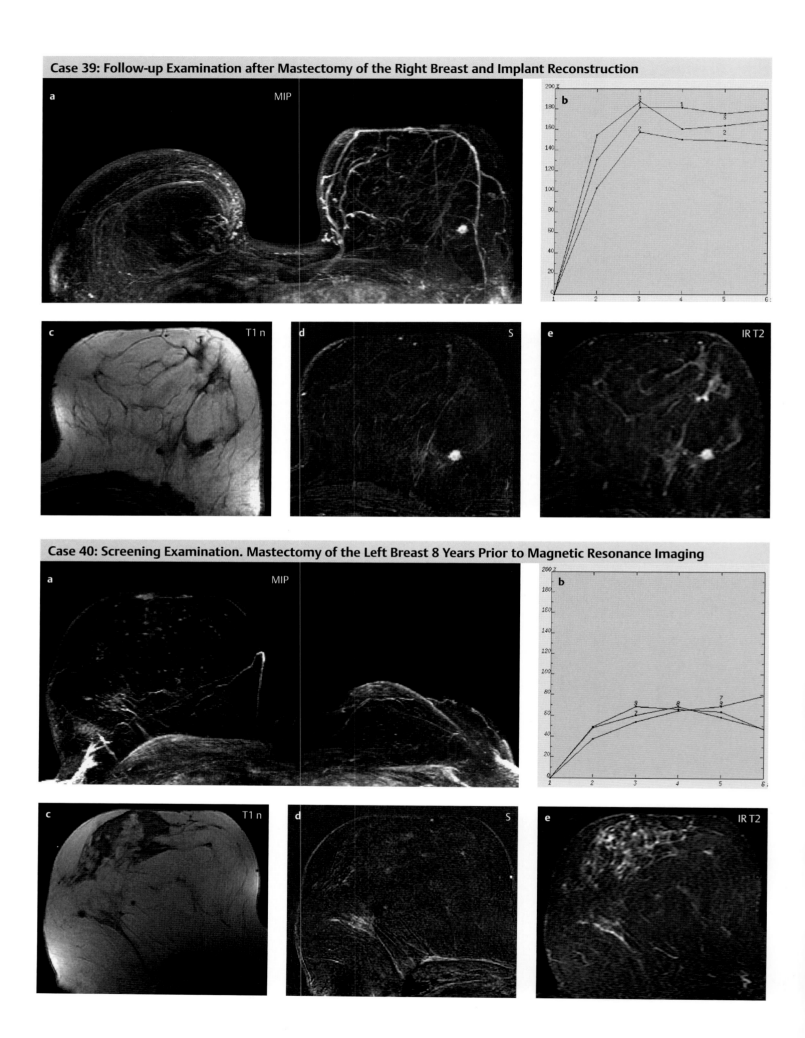

Case 39 solution

Finding:	Mass lesion	
Position:	Lower outer aspect of the left breast	
Shape:	Round	0 points
Margins:	Indistinct	1 point
T1-weighted: postcontrast:	Ring enhancement	2 points
Initial signal increase:	>100%	2 points
Postinitial signal behavior:	Plateau	1 point
Total points:		**5 points**

MR mammography BI-RADS 4

T2-weighted:	Hyperintense (compared with parenchyma)
Other aspects:	Significant susceptibility artifacts (due to electrocautering during prior surgery for benign finding)
MRI-guided VAB histology:	Fibroadenoma
Pathologic category:	**B2**
Resulting procedure:	MRI follow-up in 6 months

Case 40 solution

Finding:	Nonmass lesion	
Position:	Upper outer quadrant of the right breast	
Shape:	Irregular	1 point
Margins:	Indistinct	1 point
T1-weighted: postcontrast:	Inhomogeneous	1 point
Initial signal increase:	50–100%	1 point
Postinitial signal behavior:	Plateau	1 point
Total points:		**5 points**

MR mammography BI-RADS 4

T2-weighted:	Hyperintense (compared with parenchyma)
Other aspects:	Significant susceptibility artifacts (due to electrocautering during prior surgery), prior left mastectomy and reconstruction
MRI-guided VAB histology:	Invasive lobular carcinoma
Pathological category:	**B5b**
Resulting procedure:	Primary mastectomy according to patient wishes
Final histology:	ILC pT1c

16

Case 41: Local Preoperative Magnetic Resonance Mammography Staging. Proven Breast Cancer in the Inner Aspect of the Right Breast (Circle, Correlating Mammographic Lesion in American College of Radiology Density Type 2)

Case 42: Screening examination

Case 41 solution

Finding:	Nonmass lesion	
Position:	Lower inner quadrant of the right breast	
Shape:	Ductal	1 point
Margins:	Indistinct	1 point
T1-weighted: postcontrast:	Homogeneous	0 points
Initial signal increase:	>50–100%	1 point
Postinitial signal behavior:	Plateau	1 point
Total points:		**4 points**

MR mammography BI-RADS 4

T2-weighted:	Hyperintense (compared with parenchyma)
Other aspects:	3-cm distance from the index tumor

No preoperative VAB of this secondary lesion. Instead: preoperative MRI-guided localization

Procedure:	Extended segmental resection with excision of both MRI lesions
Final histology:	*Index tumor*: IDC pT1b. *Secondary lesion*: High-grade DCIS

Case 42 solution

Finding:	Architectural distortion (see T1-weighted image) with central enhancement (focus, see subtraction image)	
Position:	Central aspect of the left breast	
Shape:	Irregular	1 point
Margins:	Partially indistinct	1 point
T1-weighted postcontrast:	Inhomogeneous	1 point
Initial signal increase:	>100%	2 points
Postinitial signal behavior:	Wash-out	2 points
Total points:		**7 points**

MRM BI-RADS 5

T2-weighted:	Hyperintense (compared with parenchyma)
Other aspects:	Insignificant enhancement asymmetry of parenchymal structures
MRI-guided VAB histology:	Radial scar (pathologic category B3)
Final pathology report:	Tubular carcinoma within a radial scar
Pathologic category:	**B5b**
Resulting procedure:	Lumpectomy
Final histology:	Tubular carcinoma pT1a

16

Index

I

I

I